LIVING IN SHITVILLE

What an Invisible Brain Injury Feels Like

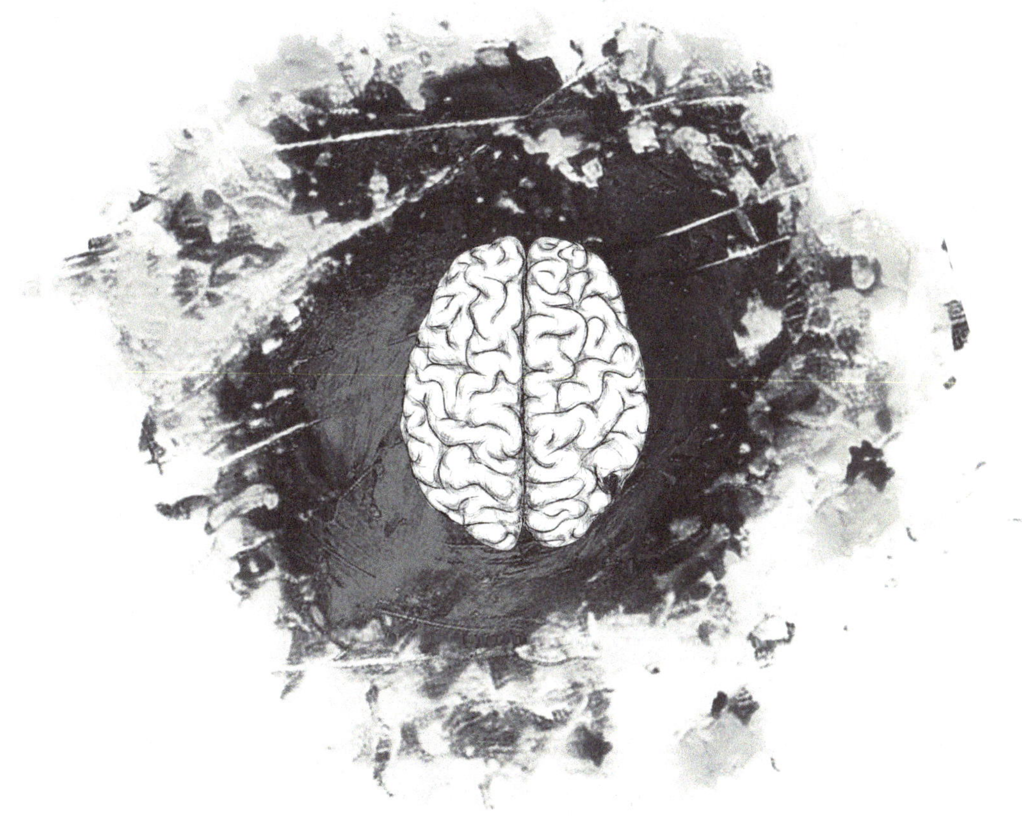

René Ready

Occupational Therapist

To John

Enjoy ♡

René

PICTURES AND WORDS
PUBLISHING

COPYRIGHT

Photography and art by René Ready
Brain image provided by iStock
Maps provided by Google Maps
Cover design by Daniel Fairweather
Book design by René Ready and Erik Jacobson
Edited by Anne Remaley

Paperback ISBN: 978-0-9995345-7-1
Ebook ISBN: 978-0-9995345-8-8

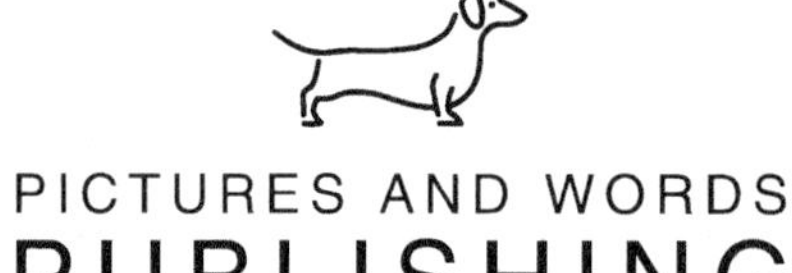

PICTURES AND WORDS
PUBLISHING
949 6th St. #431
Clarkston, WA 99403

www.ReneReady.com
Rene@ReneReady.com

Publisher's Cataloging-in-Publication data

Names: Ready, René, author.
Title: Living in Shitville - what an invisible brain injury feels like /
René Ready, Occupational Therapist.
Description: Clarkston, WA: Pictures and Words Publishing, 2024.
Identifiers: LCCN: 2024901802 | ISBN: 978-0-9995345-7-1 | 978-0-9995345-8-8
Subjects: LCSH Ready, René--Health. | Brain damage--Patients--United States--Biography. |
BISAC BIOGRAPHY & AUTOBIOGRAPHY / Memoirs
Classification: LCC RC387.5 .R43 2024 | DDC 362.1/97481--dc23

DEDICATIONS

My husband Mark Ready
for keeping the shit show together,
no matter what.

The Invisibles.

"Could someone please fix my brain?"
In memory of
Alexis Jordan Bening
01/26/1996 – 11/11/2022

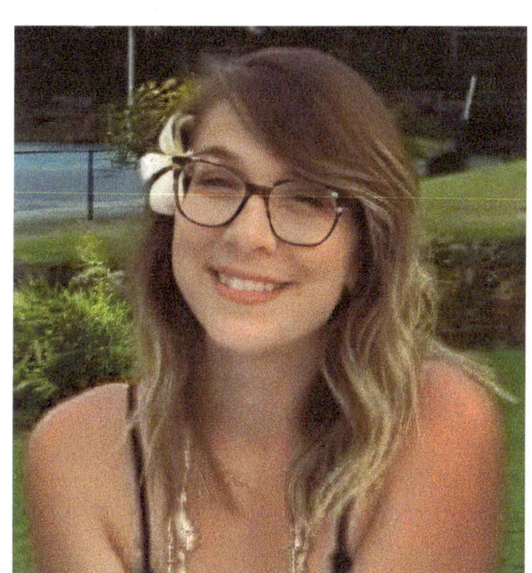

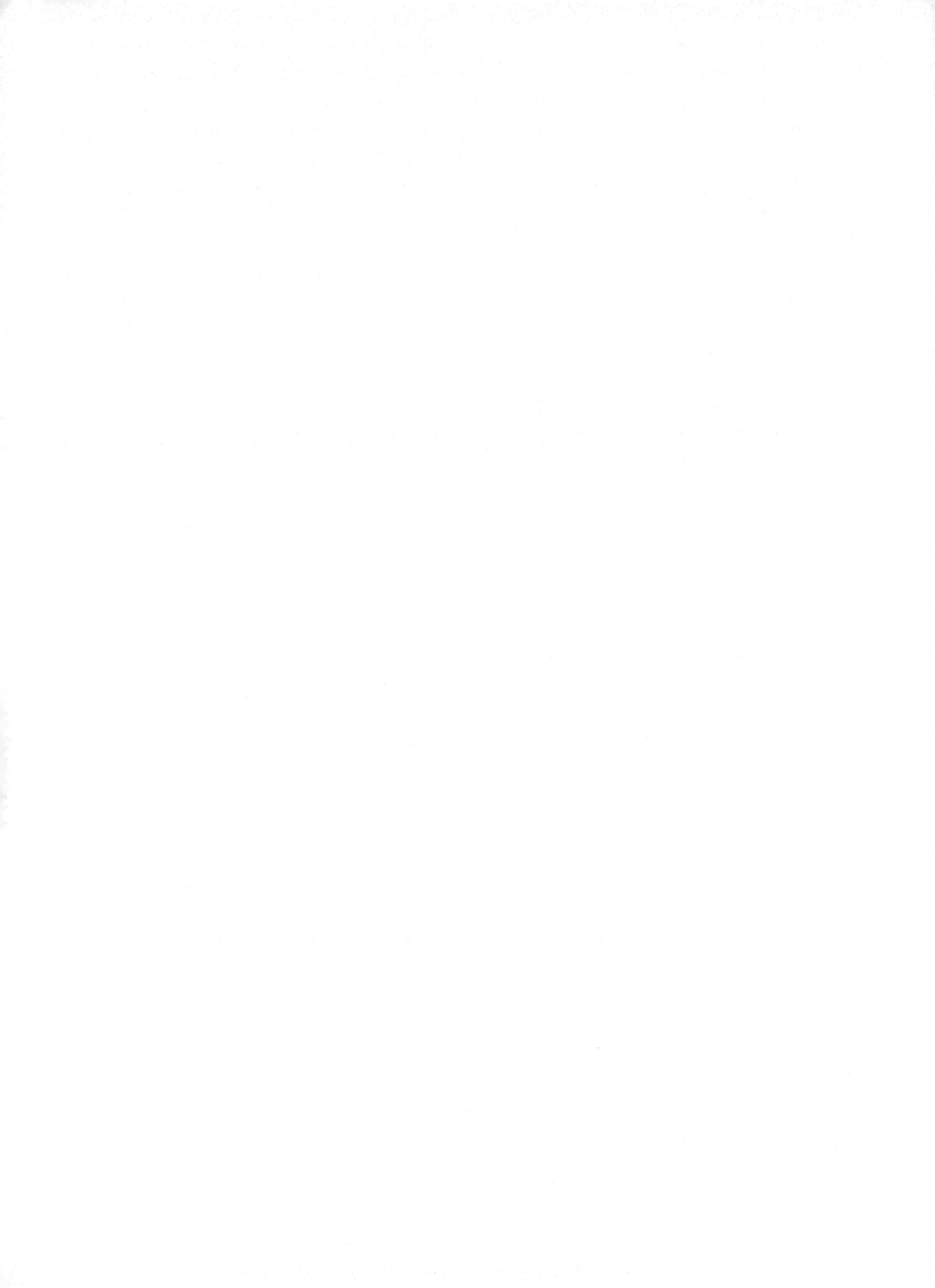

FOREWORD

This story is one of hope and resilience
derived from unexpected hurdles in life.
René uses prose and imagery
that takes the reader on her journey
from brain injury to living in a van
as she travels across the country
to find her new identity.

René demonstrates the characteristics of resilience
I have found over the years as I have dealt with
the impact of brain injury both personally and professionally.
The fact that she was willing to take on the daunting task
of driving across the country alone
is an experience many people would be afraid of
(without the added visual-perceptual
and language challenges René faced).

I met René at one of the stops on her road trip.
She visited the occupational therapy program
at which I am a faculty member
to speak to students and faculty
about her experiences traveling with a brain injury.

She also showed us her van turned into a camper.
The van alone was a testament to her Independence,
ingenuity and drive to accomplish her goal.

René's story resonated with me.
I too am an occupational therapist
and had a mild brain injury when I was in a car wreck at age 18.
During my first semesters of college,
I experienced feelings of isolation, anxiety and depression,
and difficulty attending to tasks.
Since then, I have experienced vestibular and vision issues
related to perception and motion sickness.

In my more than 20 years as an occupational therapist,
I have worked with many individuals
with brain injury who have similar stories that needed to be told.

This led to my dissertation topic related to factors
that contribute to or negatively impact resilience
of young individuals and their caregivers
who did not have visible symptoms after their brain injury.

The individuals in my study were very much like René,
high achieving with no visible symptoms of their injury.
But all experienced vision and vestibular issues
in addition to depression and anxiety related to their brain injury.

René's story is told in a way
that allows the reader to gain a firsthand account
of experiences many face after brain injury.

It serves as an inspiration
to those individuals and their caregivers
who may not be able to express
how their lives have been impacted.

Lauren Woods, PhD, OTR/L
Assistant Professor
University of Tennessee Health Science Center
College of Health Professions

Living in Shitville

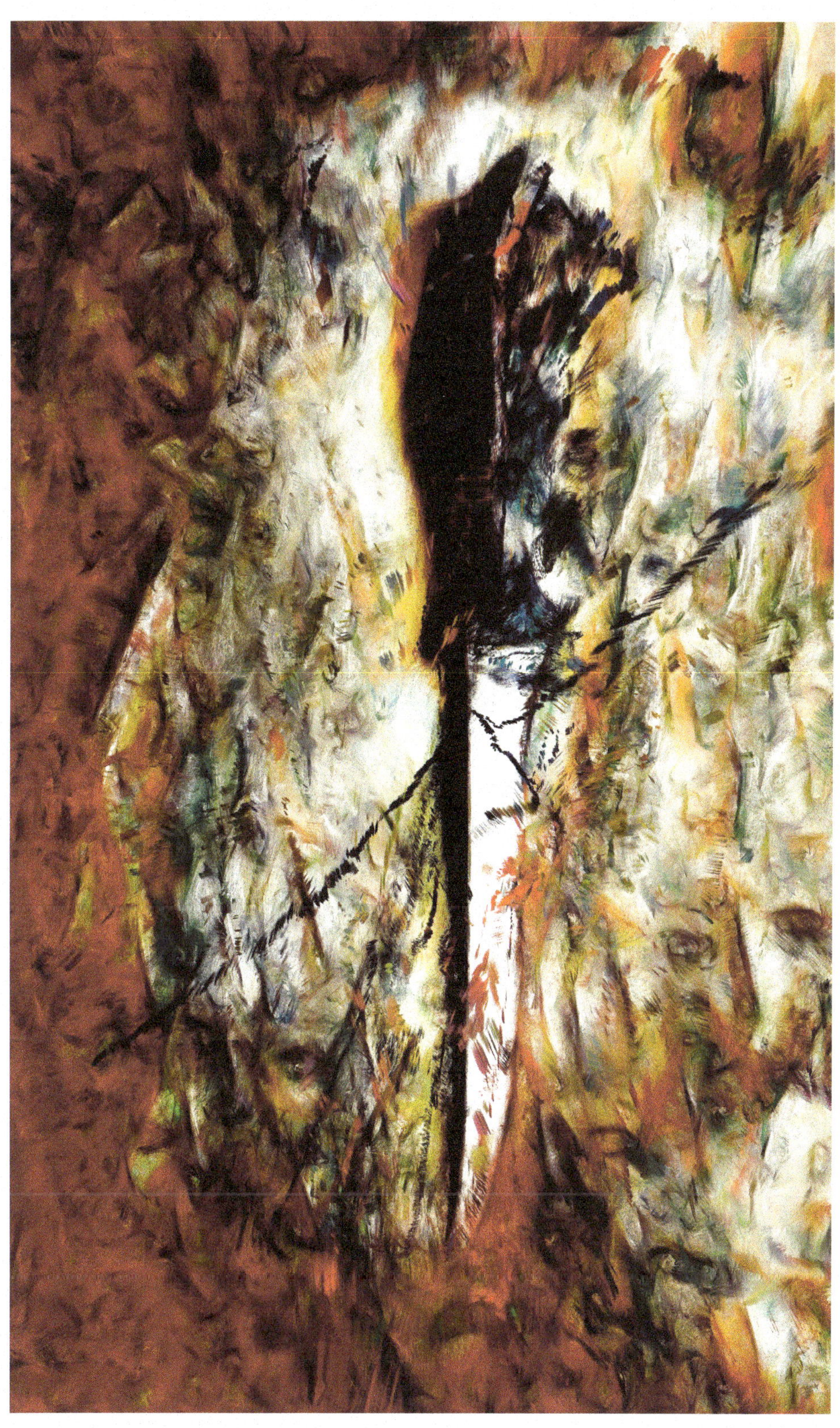

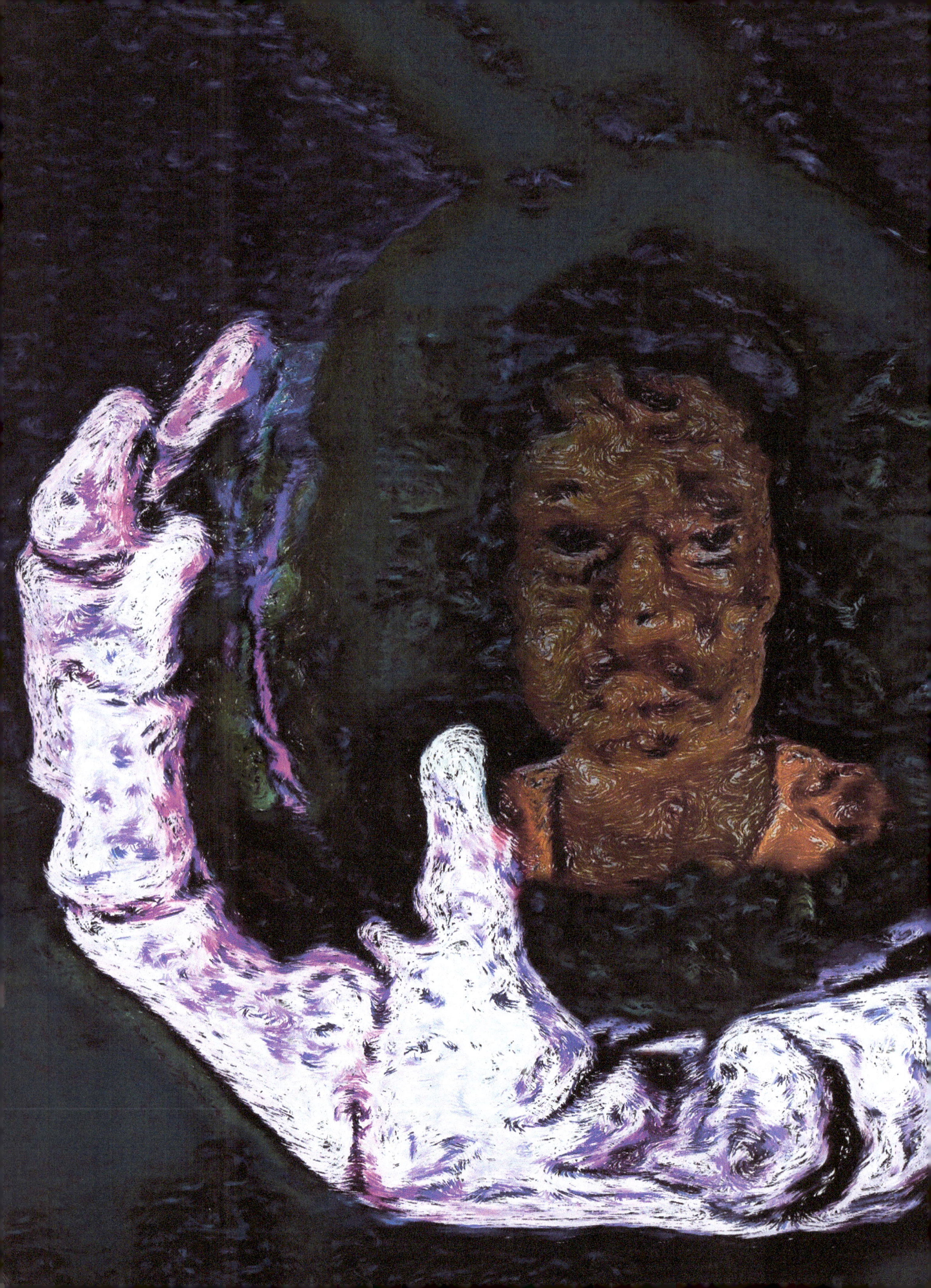

PREFACE

I bought a book about living with brain injury
written by a doctor.
Got as far as the third page before giving up.
It was Times New Roman font,
overwhelming to look at.
Tracking the lines from left to right
and moving on to a new line was torturous.
I hated reading.
It used to be my favorite pastime.

The book is purposely written in a sans-serif font,
wide spacing,
short phrases
with narrow columns
on the left side of the page.

The punctuation in the book is inconsistent.
It depends on how my brain worked that day.
Not enough commas or periods (full stops).
Too many of them are exhausting to look at.

Enjoy the book.

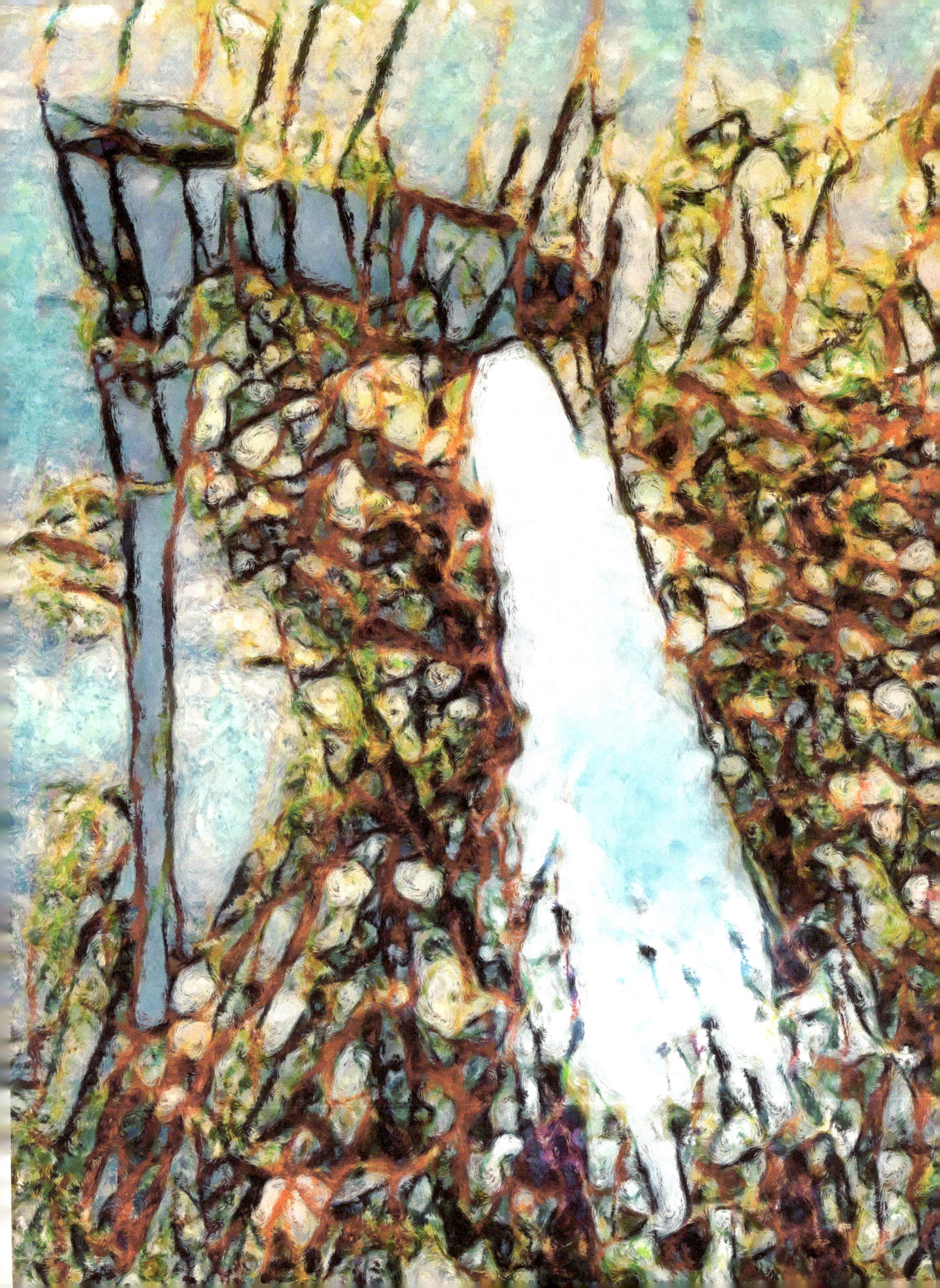

Prologue

I fell out of the sky one day
and landed in Shitville.
Didn't know what hit me.
A town of a lot of trouble.
No roads leading out of Shitville.
I'm stuck here.
Alone.

Brain Injury Boulevard

Visual Dysfunction Avenue
Dizziness Street
Cardiac Dysfunction Drive
Difficulty Swallowing Lane

Nasty street names.

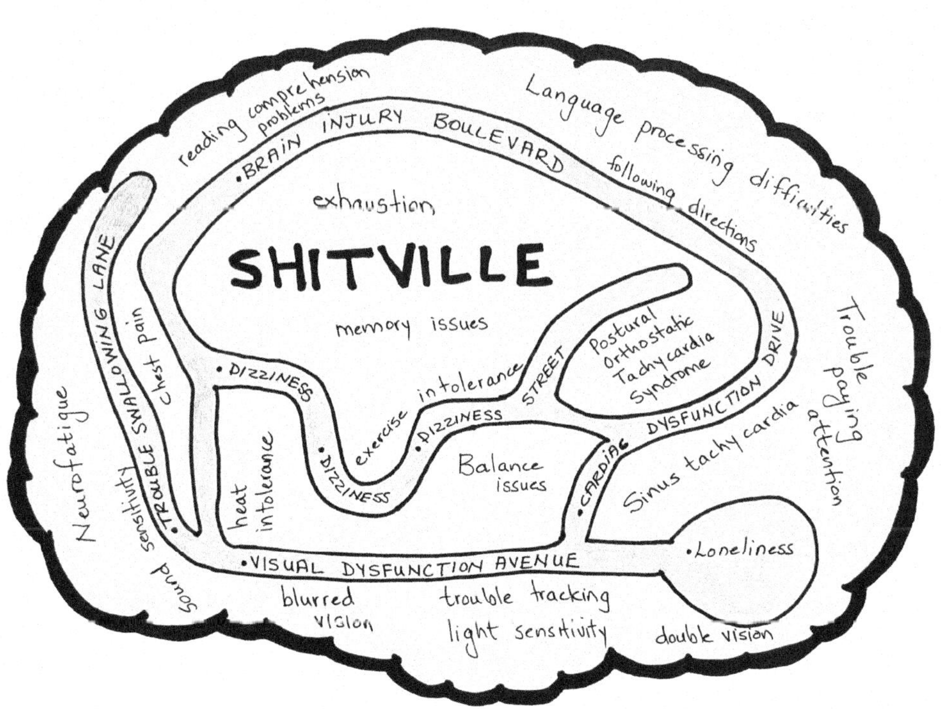

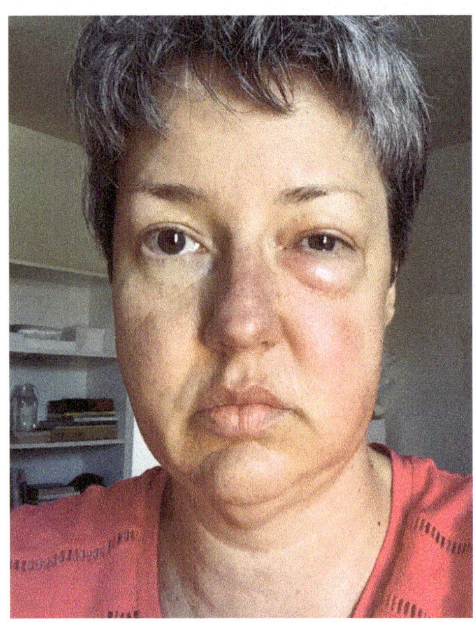

I went to the dentist, had conscious sedation.
No recollection of anything that happened.
My neck hurt terribly .
Crackly noises when touching my face.
Blurred vision.
Hardly able to talk.
Looked beaten up.

Emergency Room
CT scans
High pressure air went into the tissue of my face
under the skin
into the throat
behind the trachea and esophagus
into the chest
around the heart
behind the left eye.

A sense of disconnect.

"You are at risk for cardiac arrest and going blind in your left eye."

"The chopper is on the way to take you to closest big hospital."

"We'll be flying at low altitude to prevent damage to your eye."

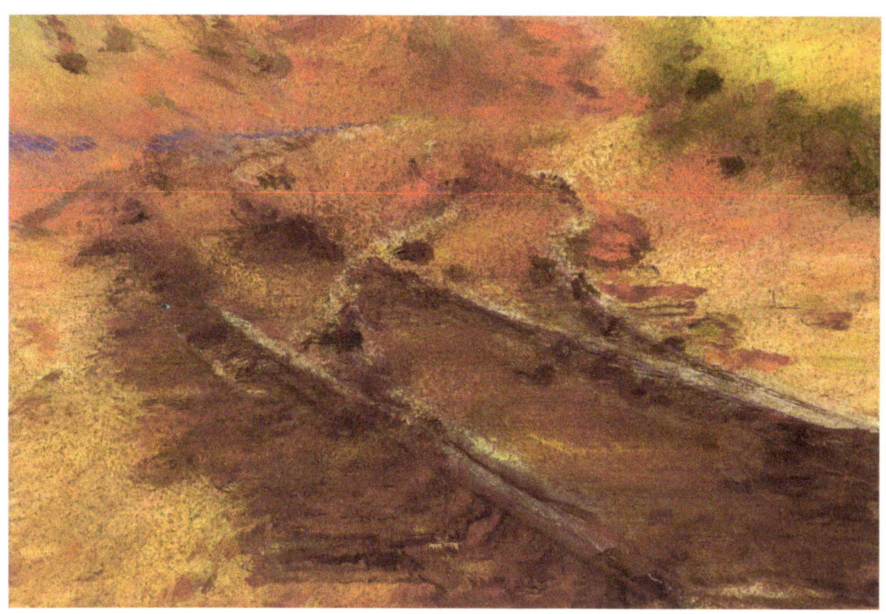

What the hell happened?

I feel and look like a battlefield.

Widespread destruction.

Stunned. Shocked. Bewildered.

The confusion.

What is going on?

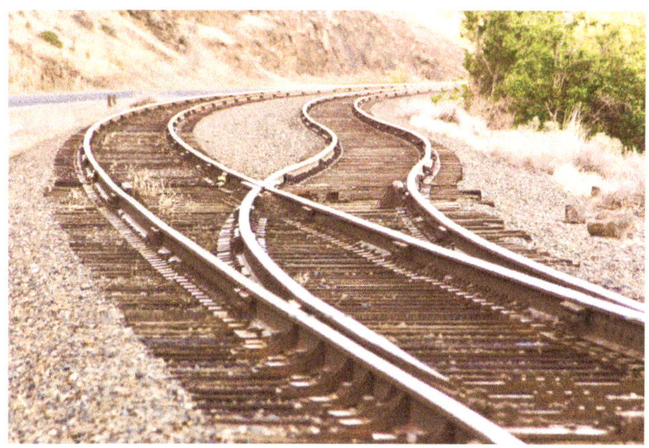

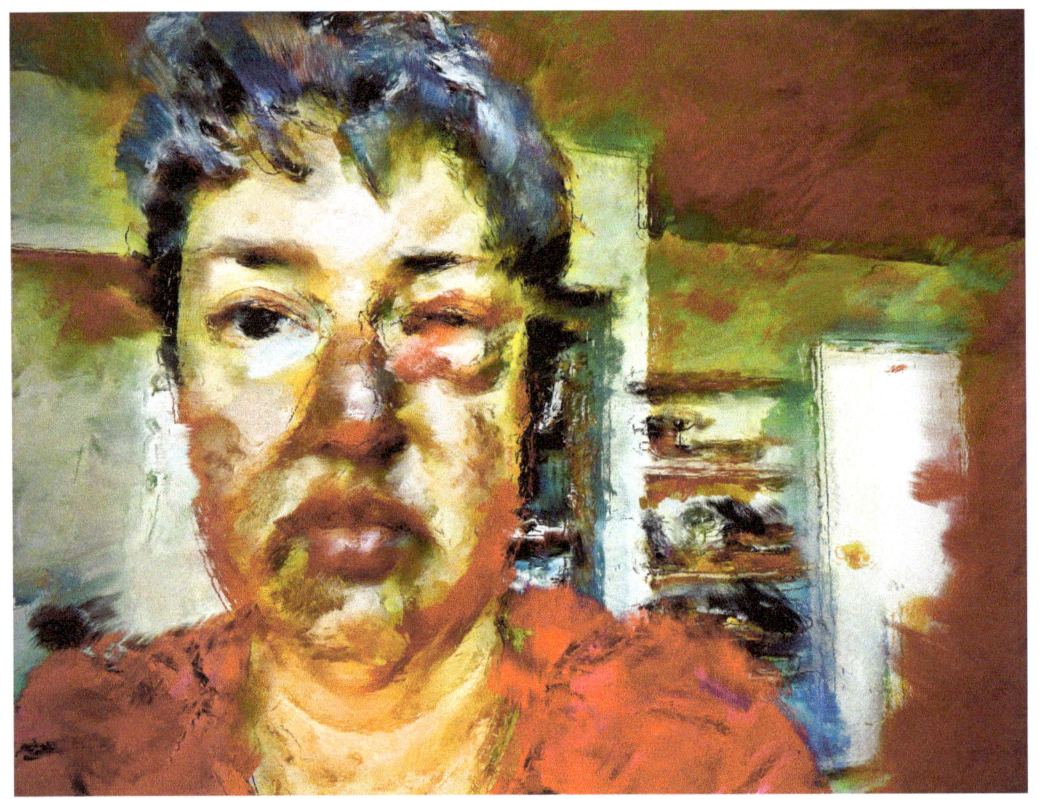

THE FACE OF BRAIN INJURY

Ugly

Mean

Evil

Hideous

Foul

Repulsive

Stripped my life in an instant.

Ripped it out of my hands
before I could say no.

GRAVEYARD OF MY PROFESSIONAL SKILLS

Mercilessly chopped off

The remainders

visible in short stumps

Ripped

Tossed in a thoughtless pile

Stripped naked

Bare

Reduced to nothing

Looking at the destruction

Incomprehensible.

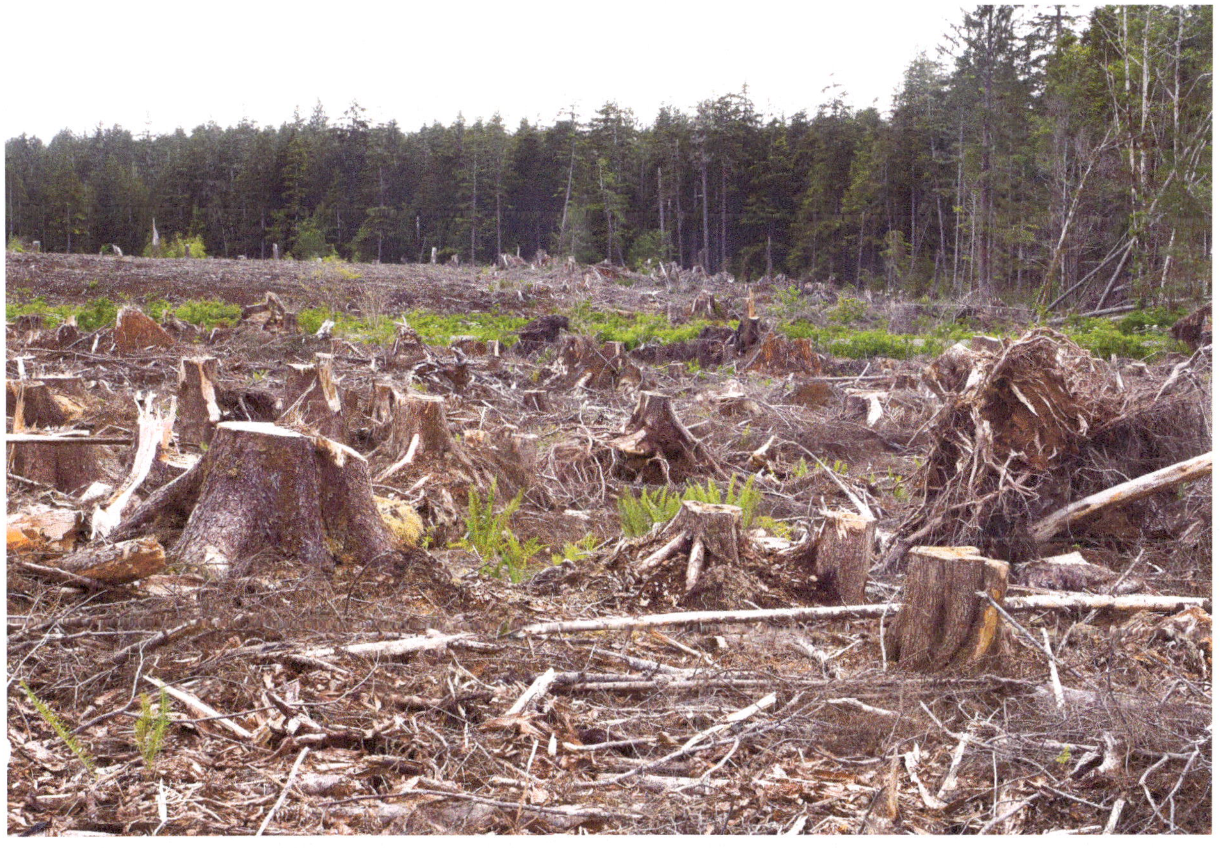

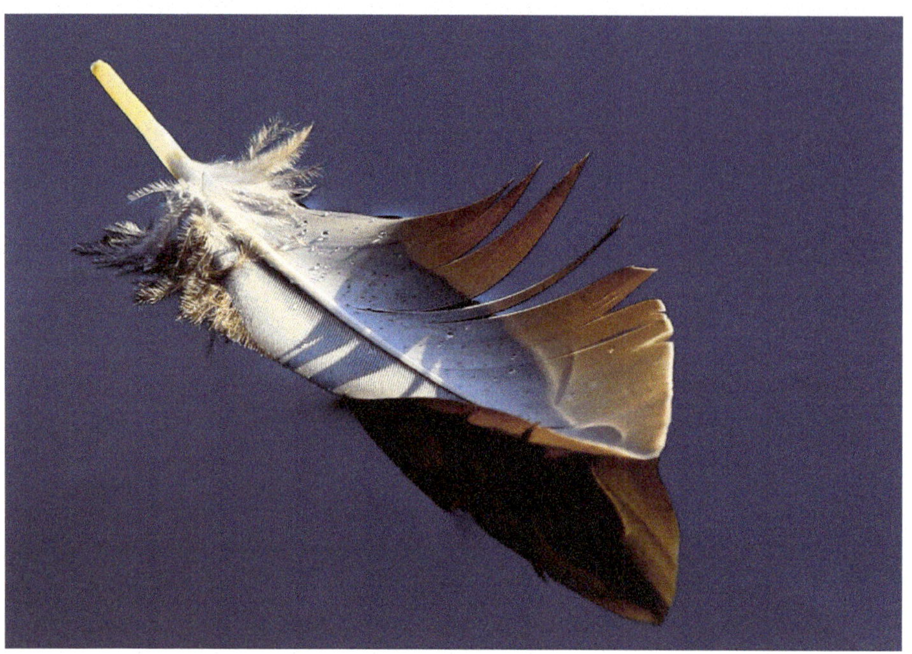

LOOKING FOR WORDS

Why am I looking for words?
Words float on the water
accessible on demand.
Some words, without warning,
sink below the water,
out of sight.
I must wait a few seconds, a minute,
sometimes a few minutes,
sometimes a whole fucking afternoon
to think of a word.
Concentrating on the missing word,
forgetting what I wanted to say.
Talking around it to make up for the forgotten word.
Thinking of a word when writing.
Two seconds later,
the word slips under the water, unusable.
I forget what word I was looking for.

TROUBLE READING

Looking at the words on the page
The font is too small
Too many words
Very hard to look at the swimming words
Starting at the beginning of a paragraph
Slowing down
Looking at every word
Going faster and faster
Skipping over words and lines.
It's too much
too many words
too much effort
I can't find my place
Eye pain
Read a sentence
The words by themselves make sense
Re-reading a sentence, a paragraph
What does it say?
Read it again
And again
The words weigh heavier and heavier
Pulling me under
Drowning the meaning.

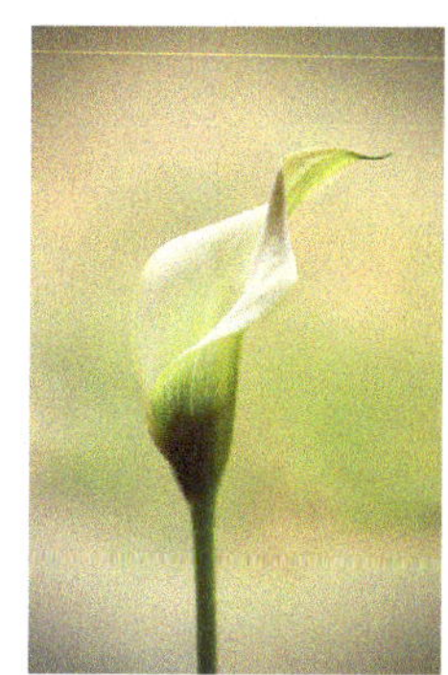

UNDERSTANDING WORDS

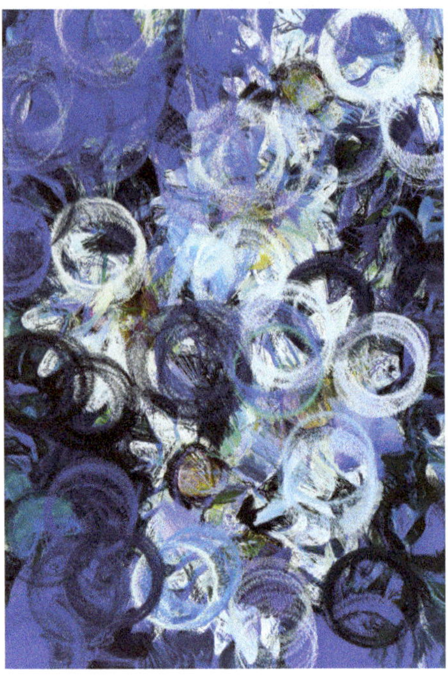

Listening to verbal explanation

Hearing the person talk

Listening to the words

Whizzing by my head

So fast

I can't tell what they are

I see their lips moving

The sound goes away

I know they are talking

I know I don't hear the words

I have no idea what they said.

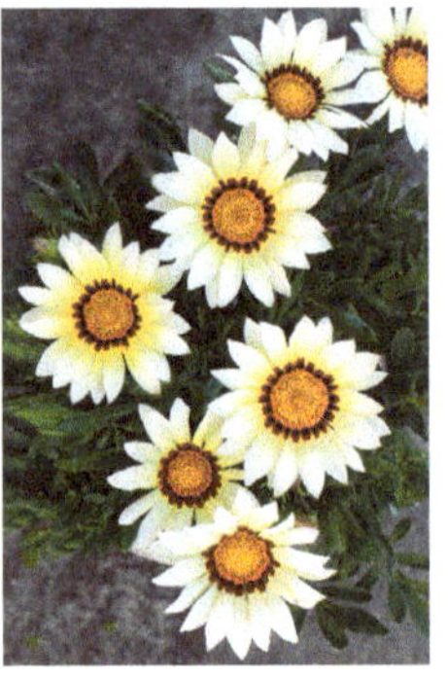

BALANCE AND DIZZINESS

Standing on the sidewalk,
turning my head to look for cars coming.
Losing my balance,
take a step to recover.
Don't fall off the sidewalk.

Relaxing in a chair,
my brain sloshing around in my head.
Sitting in a small boat,
bobbing on the waves of the ocean.

Walking into Walmart,
an assault of lights and noise on my brain.
Lots of people moving around.
Blurred vision,
how long will it take before I find the power strip?
Scanning the shelves, intense dizziness,
holding onto the shopping cart not to fall.

Cars moving in and out of parking spaces.
Unexpectedly, my stationary car feels like
it's moving when it shouldn't.
Feel sick to my stomach,
being propelled into space.
Stepping on the brake hard,
a cold hand grips my heart.

Scrolling on Facebook,
slowly,
not to feel sucked down a tunnel.
A video scrolls by,
followed by a feeling of intense drunkenness.

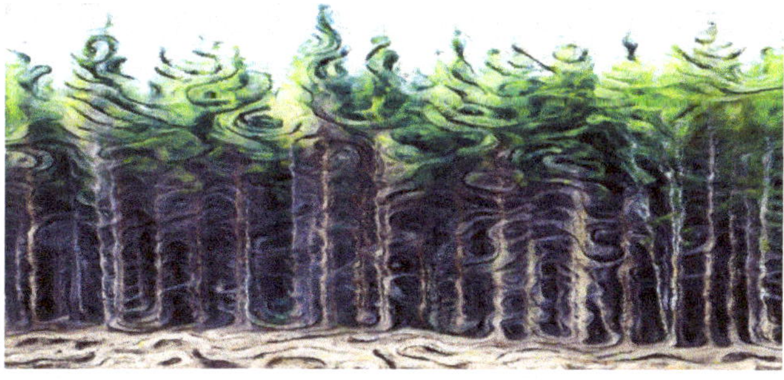

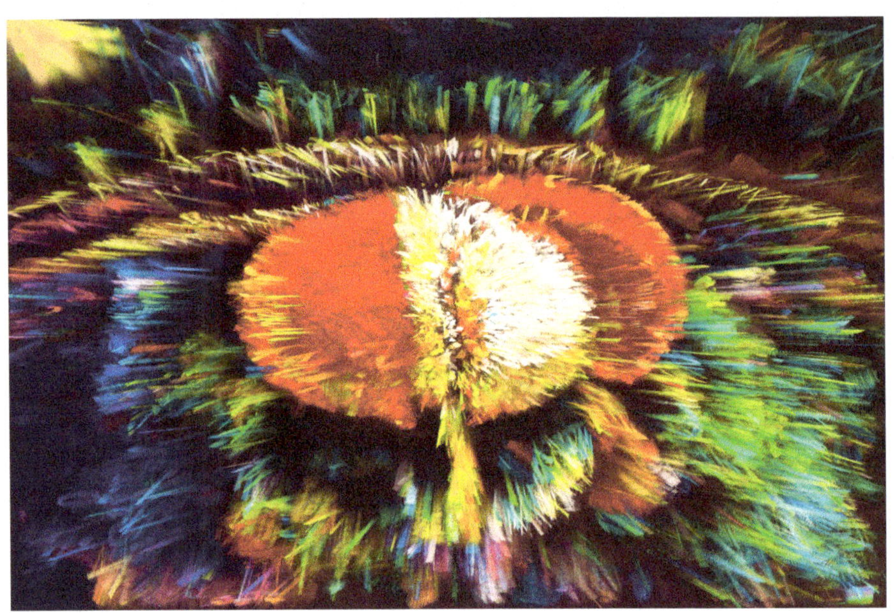

SOUND SENSITIVITY

Sounds hurt
Sharp sounds
Dishes
Coffee cups
Glass bowls
Pots and pans
Cabinet doors slamming
Dogs barking
Children screaming
Toilets flushing
Air dryers
Shopping carts
Music
Cut-off saws

Cuts through nerves.
Ear ache for days.

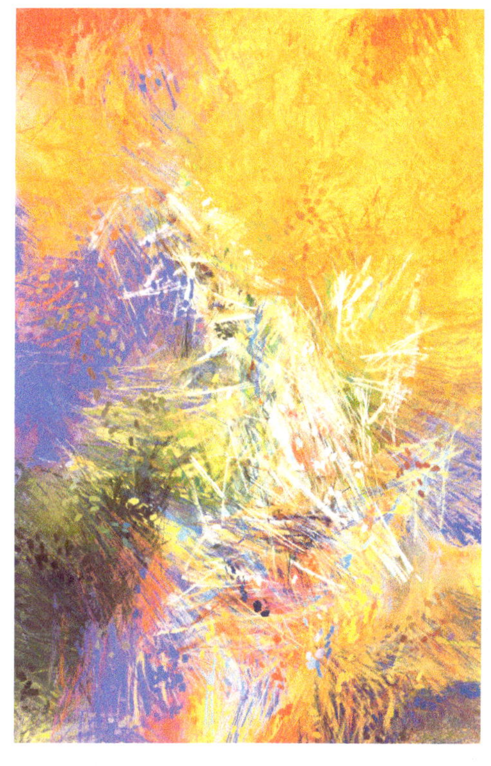

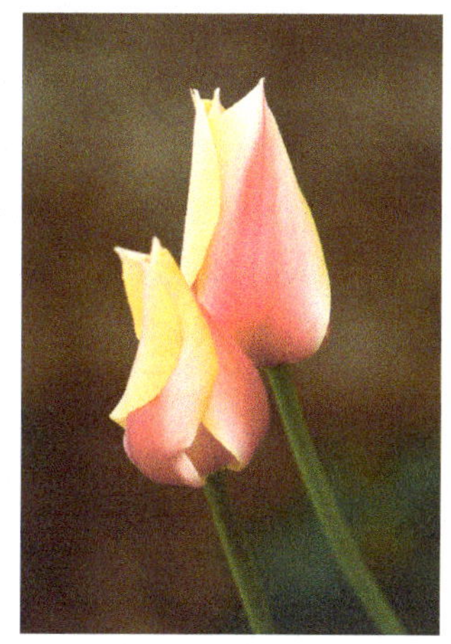

SPEAKING ENGLISH

I'm bilingual.
A blessing or a curse.
Want to write something down,
not a single English word comes to mind.
I'm cringing.
English, my primary language for the last 22 years.

Listening to music with Afrikaans lyrics, reading English.
The Afrikaans music and English words collide in my head,
competing for my attention.
English lost. Afrikaans dominates.
Alarming.

Walk into the living room,
talking to my husband.
My brain pauses,
replaying the words in my head,
checking.
Was I speaking English?
He doesn't understand Afrikaans.

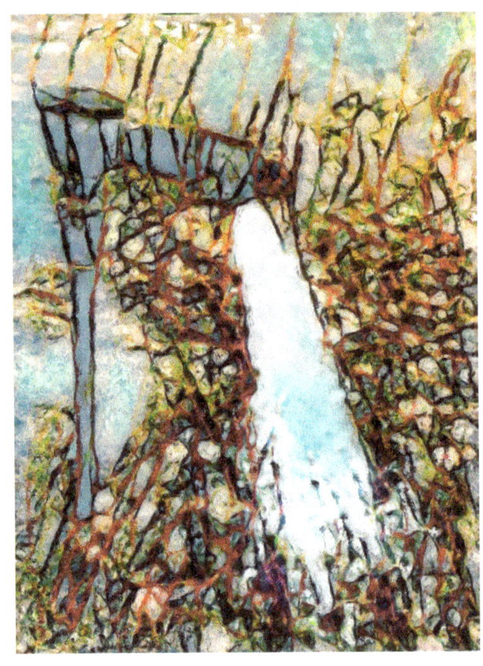

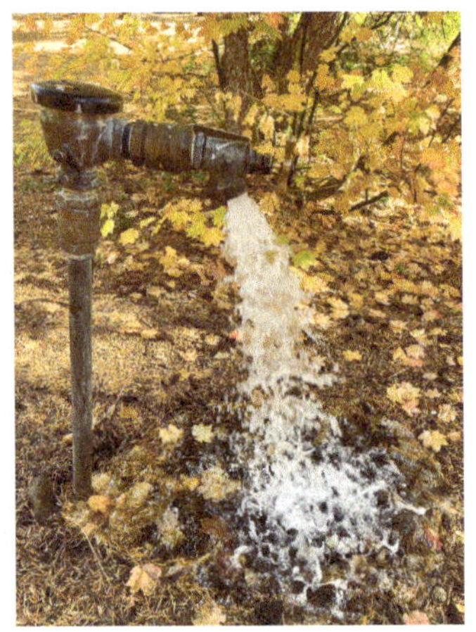

NEUROFATIGUE (BRAIN FATIGUE)

Everything takes so much effort
with an injured brain.
Thinking. Concentrating. Remembering.
Processing everything slower.
Energy runs out full force.
Doing dishes
Vacuuming
Going to the store
Driving
Spending brain energy so fast.

Depleted brain
Going to a birthday party
A friend visiting
Doing laundry
Going to endless therapies
Medical appointments.
Swimming in mud.

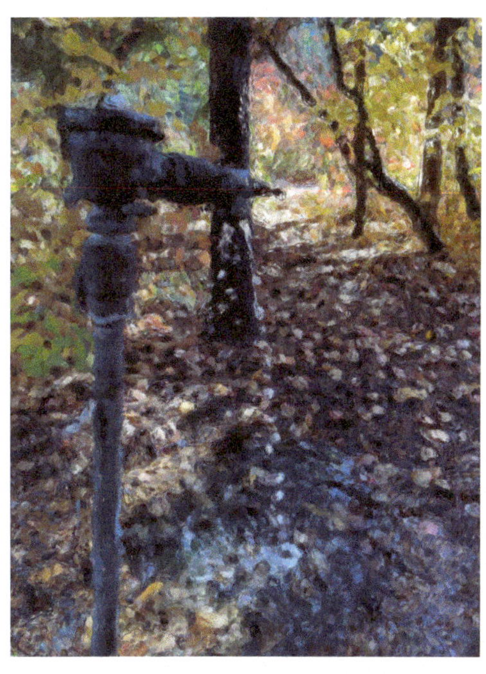

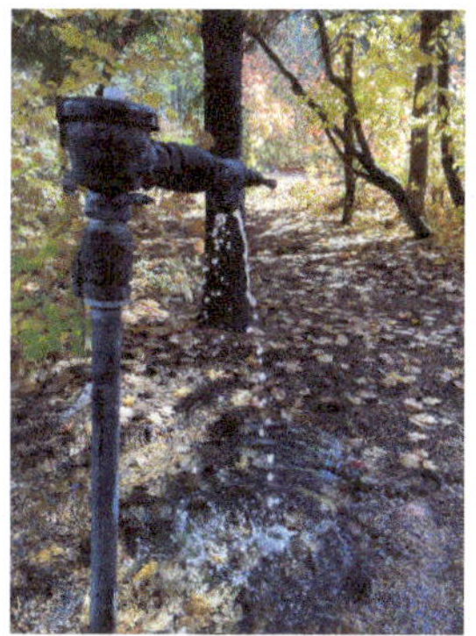

It takes days to recover.
Recharging
Slowly
Drop by drop
Doing nothing
Don't sleep well
The weather changing
Making the fatigue worse
Not feeling refreshed
after a nap
after a night of sleep
after many days
Feeling exhausted
Not getting anything done.

LIGHT SENSITIVITY

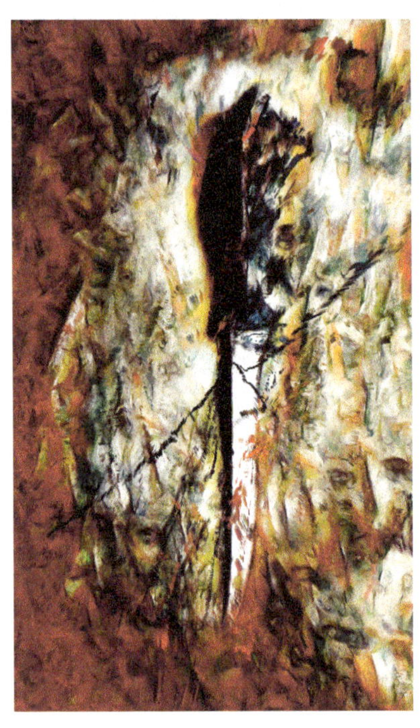

Lights
A sharp knife
in the eyes
into my brain
White pain
Blood exploding
Persistent eye pain

Sunlight
Car lights
Overhead lights
Reflections
Windows
Wet roads
Lights reflecting off raindrops
Shiny trim on the van dashboard
Mirrors
Shiny floors
Store lights

Wear a hat, sunglasses
Tinted van windows
to escape the lights.
The pain.

DRIVING

Cars moving
People moving
Sick feeling in my stomach
Am I moving?
Or not?

Car lights
too sharp
too much

Pay attention
Don't space out

Poles, shadows, fences, trees
flashing by
Exhausting to block out

Dizziness
Feeling disconnected
Off balance after driving

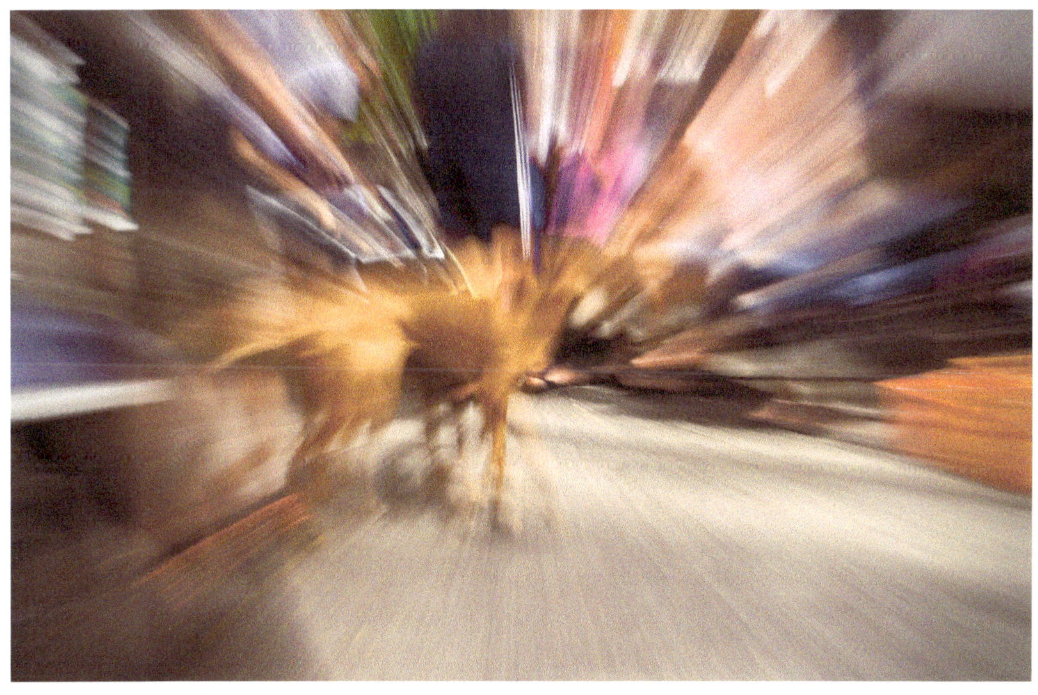

NEW DRIVING RULES

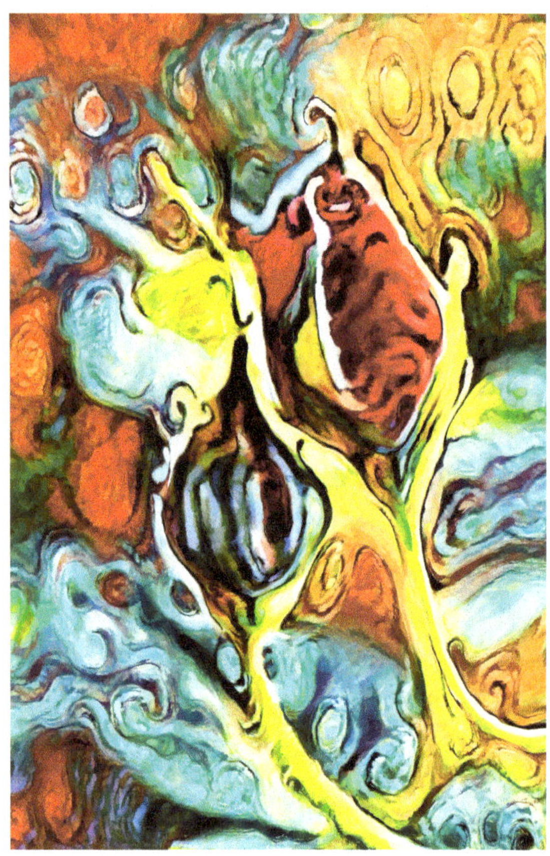

Avoid busy intersections

Use traffic lights to turn left on busy roads

No driving in the rain
Wipers moving continuously
make me dizzy, spaced out.

No driving in the snow
Too much white
Nowhere to focus

No driving in the dark
Getting lost
Too many car lights
Difficult to pay attention

No interstate driving
Too much, too fast
Use back roads
Quiet roads
Don't drive when tired
Don't make mistakes
Ask husband to take me to the store
Or stay home

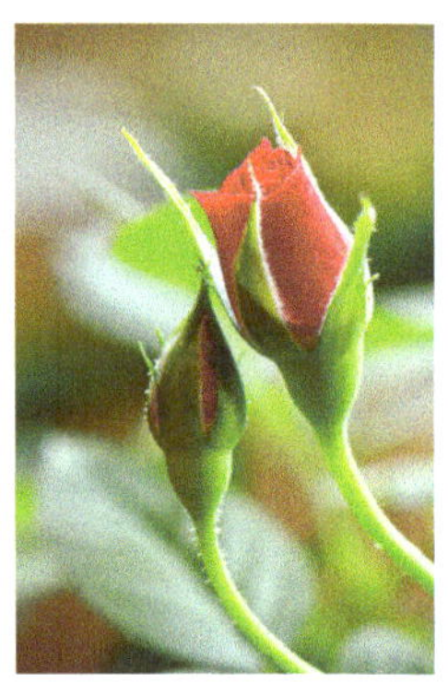

BASIC DAILY STUFF

Found money in the fridge
Found dishes in the garbage can
Found the coffee cup in the freezer
Put an empty pot on a burner on high and walked away
Can't find the pot scrubber, my brain doesn't see it.

Put clothes in the washer, but didn't turn it on
A note in the bathroom "brush your teeth"
Forgot to buy dog food
Took the wrong medication
Three Ambien instead of thyroid pills
Got in the car and went to the gym
Lost my earplugs
Have you seen my bra?
Can't find my sunglasses
Where are the van keys?

Need a list of shopping tasks in sequence
I can't plan and sequence on demand.

Frustrated
Angry
Can't read
Irritated
Fuming
Can't find my words
Distractible
Overwhelmed

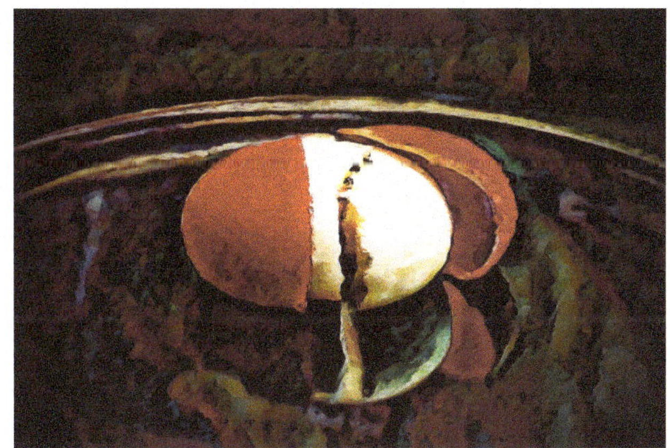

I don't have value
I don't have a job
An income
Who would want to be married to me?

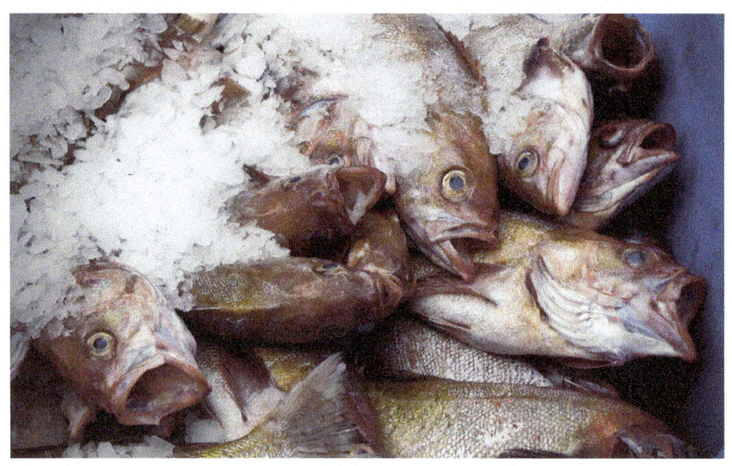

MY CAREER AS AN OCCUPATIONAL THERAPIST

Looking into the cold, dead eyes of

my career

my occupation

my identity

Silent cries of despair

31 years of education, experience, training

Reduced to

Incompetent

Unreliable

Risk to patients

Unable to work

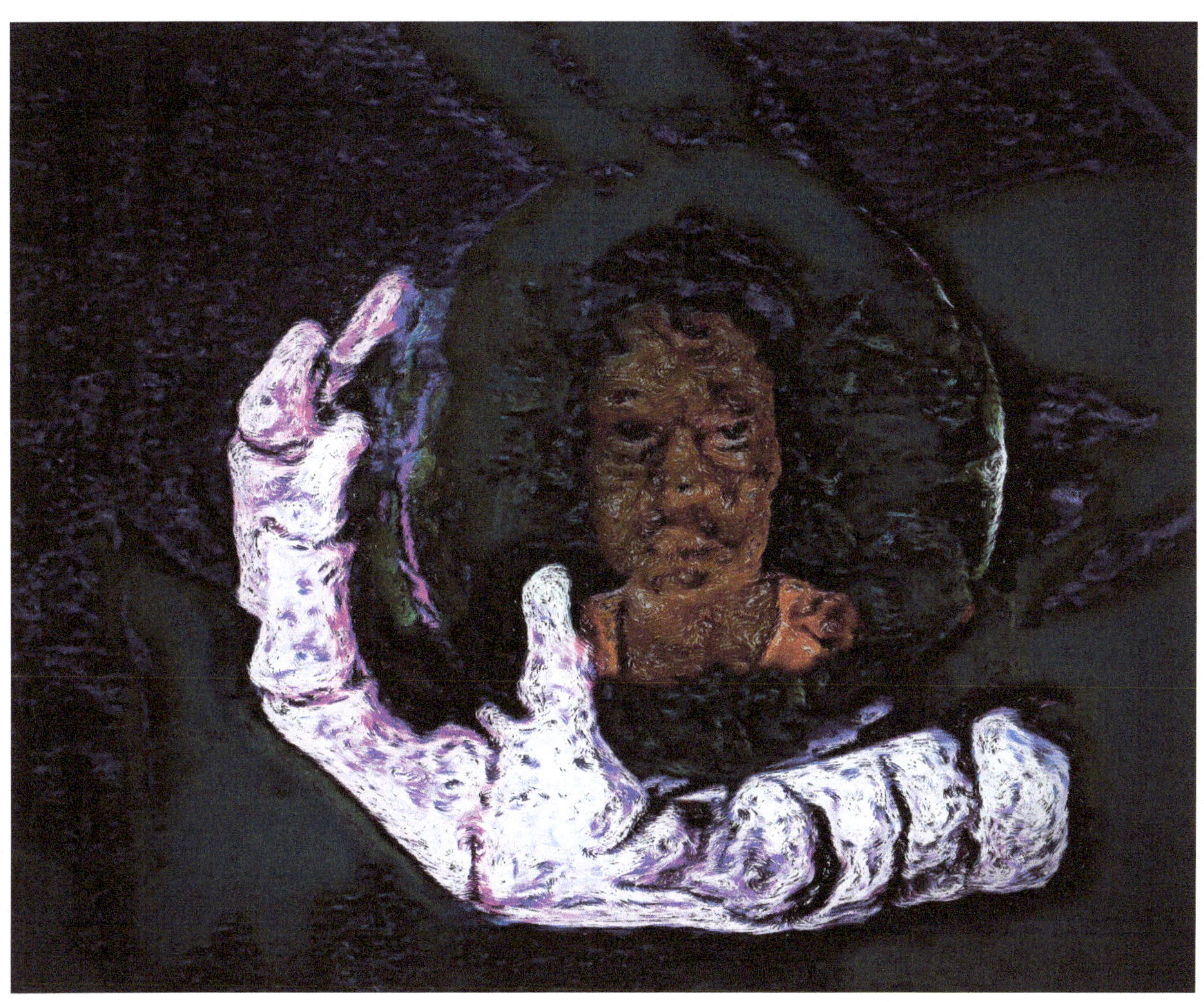

TRAPPED INSIDE A BRAIN INJURY

The Darkness

The Scariness

The Sadness

The Loneliness

The Loss

On May 23, 2018, I suffered a compressed-air accident
at the dentist's office and went home with a brain injury.

It was the beginning of a new life I didn't like.
Multiple complications from the injury.
Severe chest pain, shortness of breath,
swallowing problems, cardiac dysfunction,
dizziness, blurred vision,
poor balance, visual processing problems,
difficulty reading, memory problems,
language processing problems,
and finally, a diagnosis of a brain injury.

I fell out of the sky and landed in Shitville.
A town of trouble
A hellhole
Population: One
I was stuck with all the physical
and cognitive problems.
No way out.
Three years of endless physical, occupational, speech,
and vision therapies, counseling,
multiple medical appointments,
and then the bottom line:

"Your injury is very unusual,
too complicated,
and too expensive to take on for a lawsuit."
No lawyer wanted to take the case.
The statute of limitations ran out.

No compensation for losing the normal life
of a home health occupational therapist
with an excellent income.
Now a disability check every month for 25% of my income.
And life in Shitville.

Living with anger.
Living with grief.
A new person I didn't recognize.
Invisible.
Not valued.
Feeling guilty that my husband goes to work every day.
Feeling guilty for being a financial burden.
Living endless days without a purpose.
A life without motivation.
A life not worth living.

A life I didn't want to live anymore.
The plan was in place.

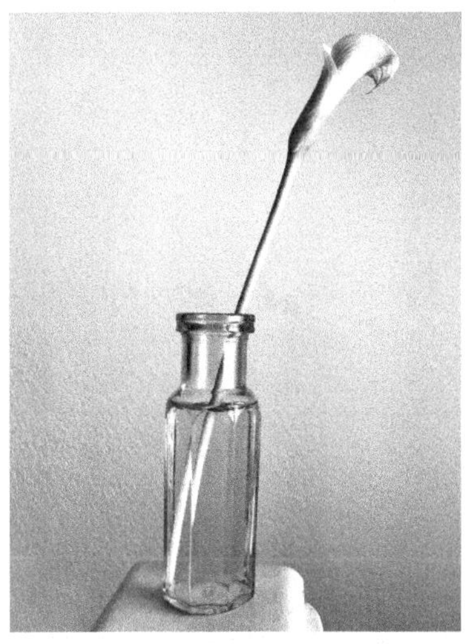

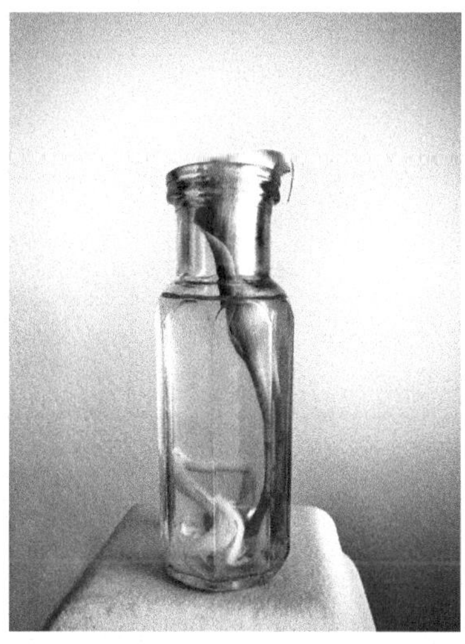

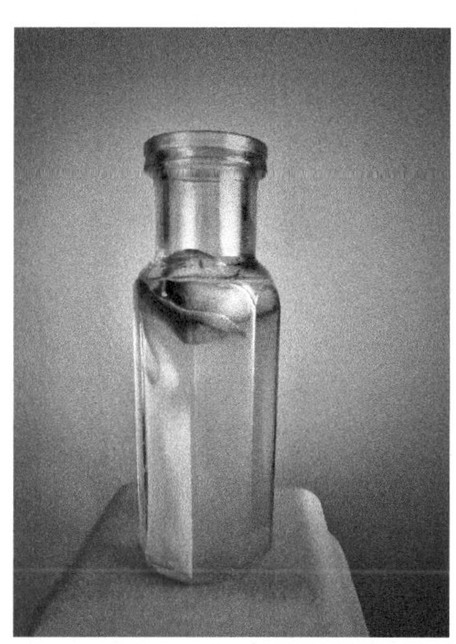

In November of 2021 I made a bucket list of places to see:
photography spots,
things to do.
A list of things to do before I call it good.

My minivan had a bed, a refrigerator and a good spare tire.
I told my husband Mark of my travel plans,
and he was good with the 3-month road trip.
He helped me get the van ready
and installed deep-cycle batteries to power the refrigerator.
It took 3 months to prepare everything.
I would leave in the middle of February 2022.
And end everything when I got back.

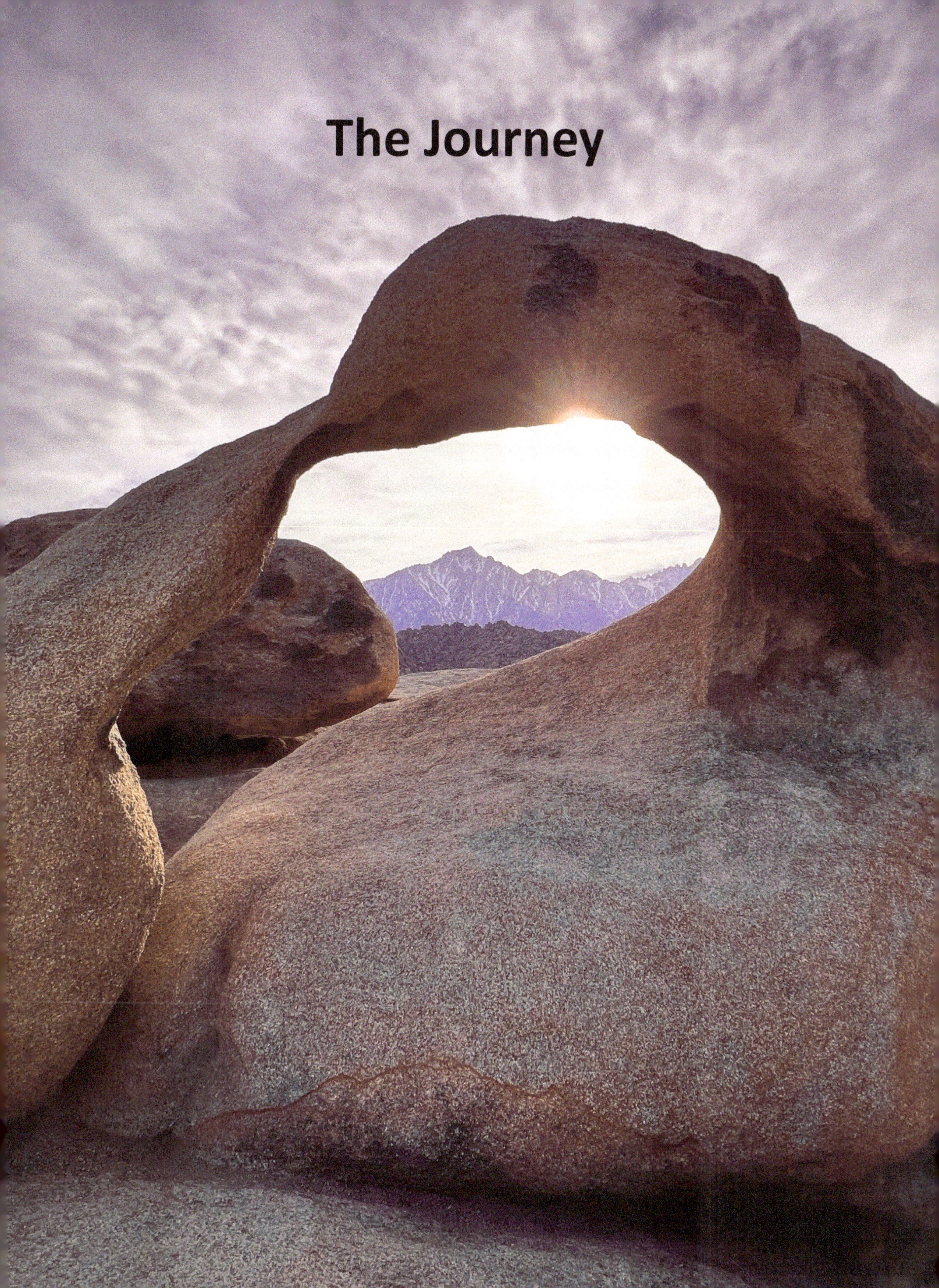
The Journey

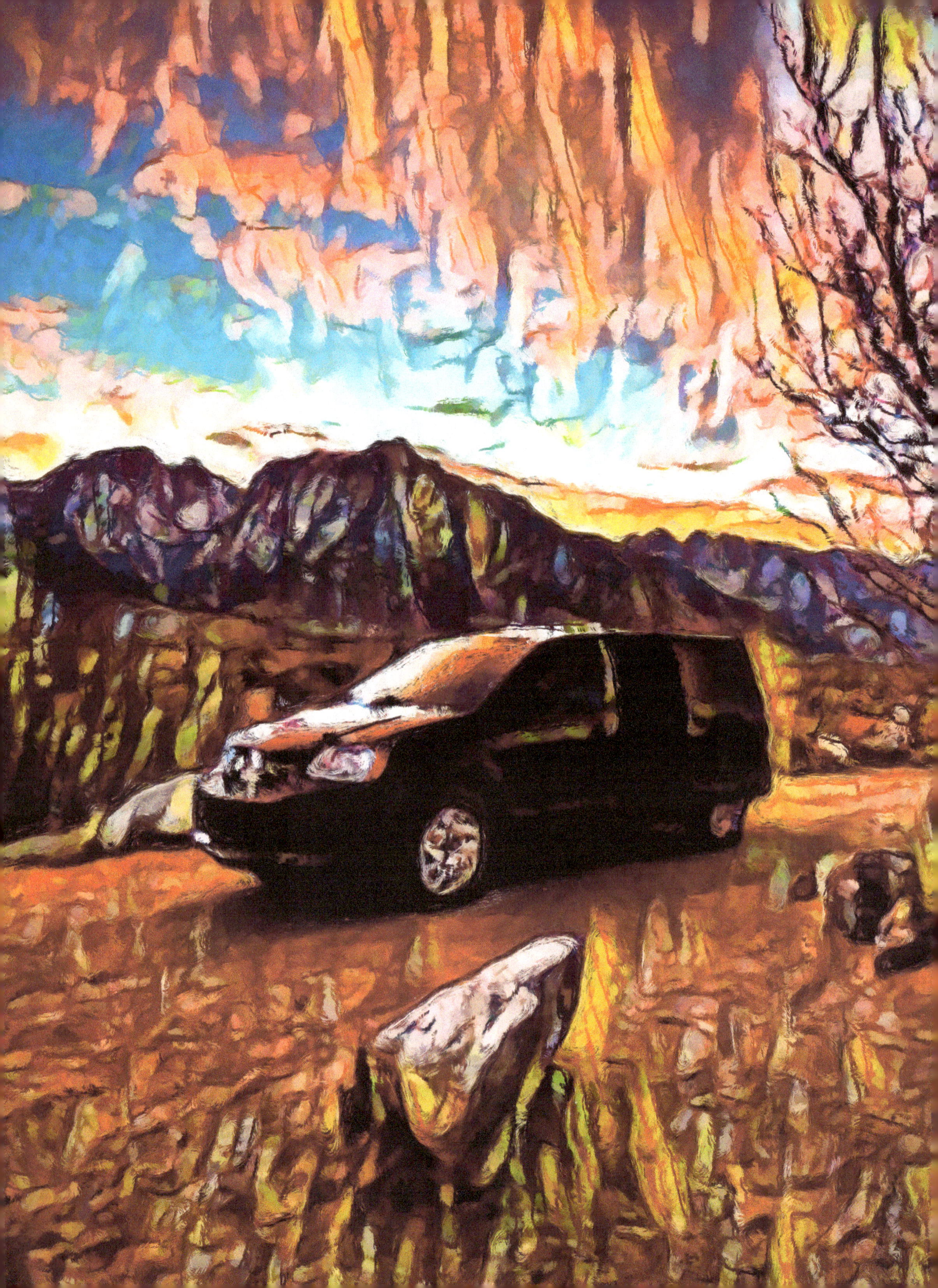

DAY 1 / FEBRUARY 18

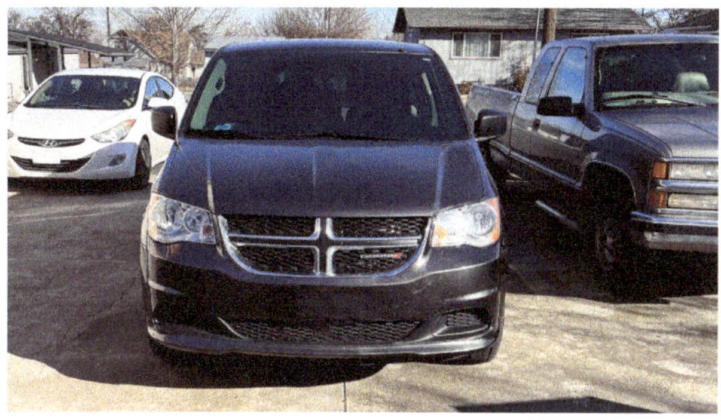

D-day was here.
I was exhausted, and it took until 2pm before
I could get going.
My favorite thing to do.
Back out of the driveway
without damaging any of the vehicles.

My thoughts: "just start driving, leave town."
Driving on the 95 South
Outside town

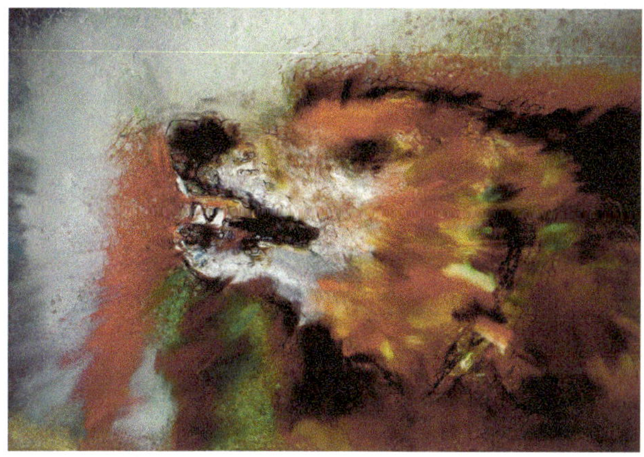

What the hell I was thinking?
Taking on the demon.

Ferocious jaws snapping, savage growling,
wanting to take me down.

Traveling alone with a brain injury.
Panicky thoughts.

Don't wreck the van
Don't set the van on fire
Don't get hurt
Don't fall
Don't lose van keys/glasses/wallet/camera equipment/cell phone
Don't drop the phone into water/river, down a canyon
Don't break the phone, it was expensive
Don't do stupid things
Don't do "nothing"
Don't get lost
Don't cry.

Sickening butterflies in my stomach.

Two hours of driving.
Called Mark from Riggins, Idaho
and he could see my location on the Life360 app.

The plan was to overnight at a rest area south of Riggins.
I forgot where the rest area was,
and was afraid of spacing out while driving
and not "seeing" it.

Big lesson:
enter the destination in Google Maps
and LISTEN/PAY ATTENTION (pick one).

DAY 2 / FEBRUARY 19

Headed down the Payette River area for Boise, Idaho.
Boise was very busy, with lots of traffic.
I went to Sierra Trading Post outdoor store.
The shop was huge, loud, very busy.
Tried to shop, too overwhelming and left.

Had to drive on the interstate,
mercifully for not very long.
Traffic too fast and too busy for me.
Made it to my overnight spot
just south of Jordan Valley, Oregon.
Put the destination in Google Maps
before leaving Boise.
Excellent idea.

A semi-truck was sitting on my bumper.
Making it hard to find the inconspicuous dirt road off the highway.

Arrived as the sun was setting.
A beautiful and fabulous spot by a reservoir.
A clean, well-maintained pit toilet with hotel-standard toilet paper.
I could have stayed there for a week.

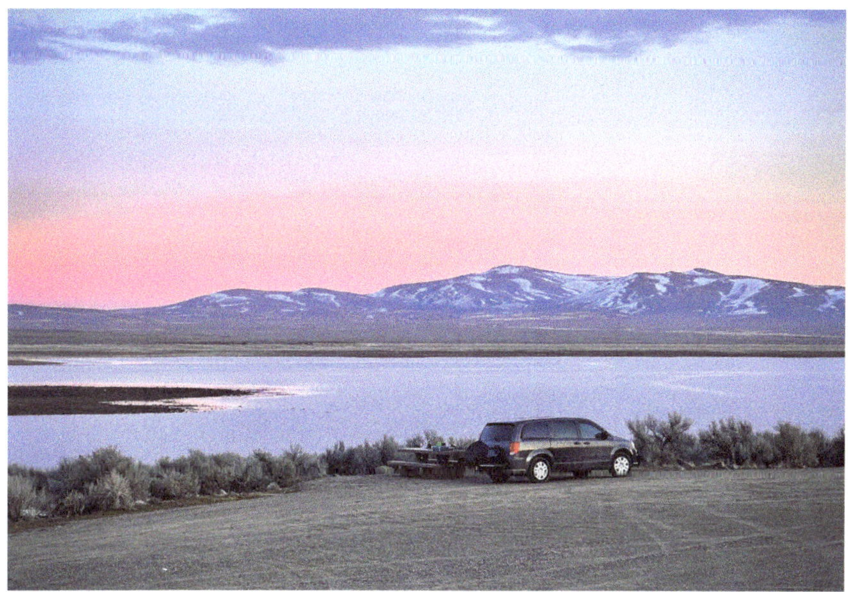

DAY 3 / FEBRUARY 20

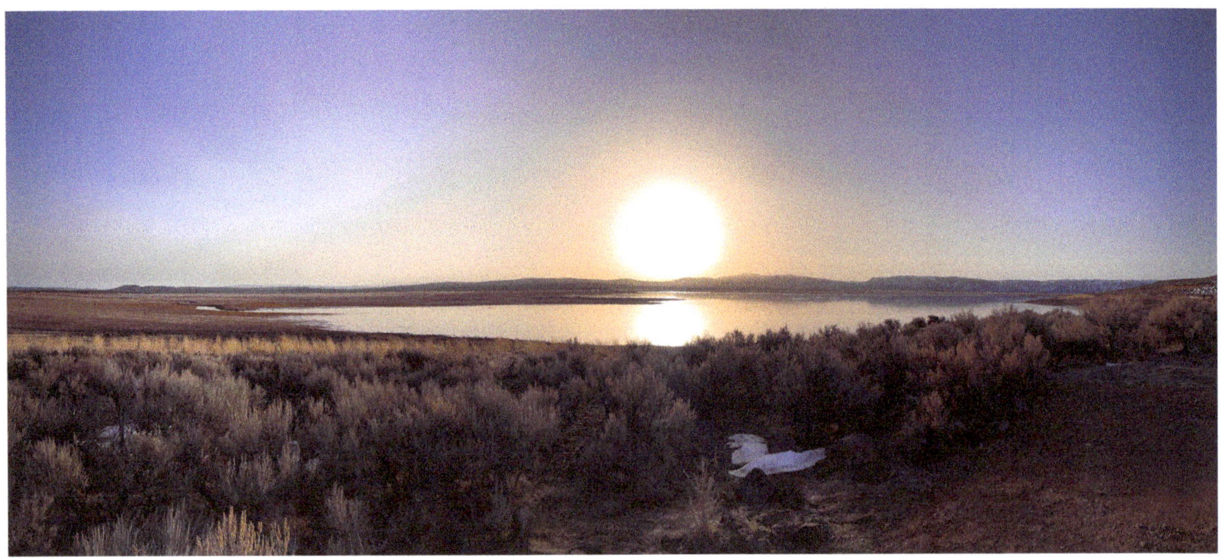

I was the only overnight camper at the reservoir.
No cell service.
Temperature inside the van at sunrise 34F (1C).
Watched the sun rise over a cup of cocoa.

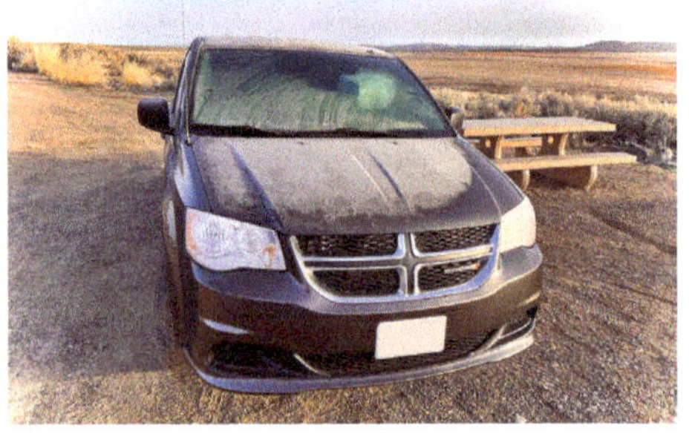

Very windy and cold for the 164-mile drive
to Winnemucca, Nevada.
Drove through rain,
followed by dirt whipping across the highway.

Investigated the overnight options in Winnemucca
on the iOverlander app.
Went by the "vibe" I got from a location.

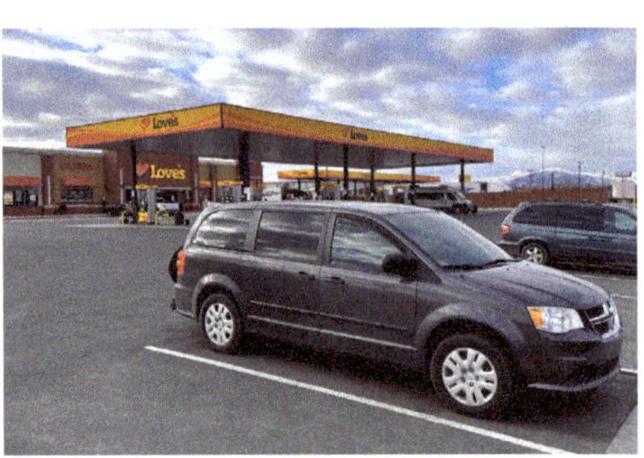

Picked Love's Travel Stop
with their permission.

Spent a lot of time researching
possible routes for the rest of the trip to Death Valley.
Checked the snow forecast,
road conditions and cameras,
weather conditions and overnight options.
Had to avoid high elevations
and time it to stay away from the snowstorms.
Driving in white-out conditions was a no-go.

DAY 4 / FEBRUARY 21

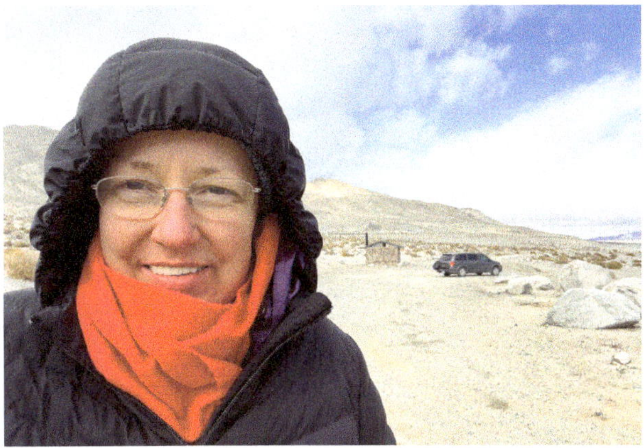

A long day of a gusty and cold drive to Tonopah, Nevada.

Vast nothingness of beautiful open space.
Surrounded by mountain range after range.
Straight roads disappeared into the future.
Dry sagebrush and snow on the ground.

I could not stop looking at the mountains.
Had to control myself to not stop every 5 minutes for pictures.

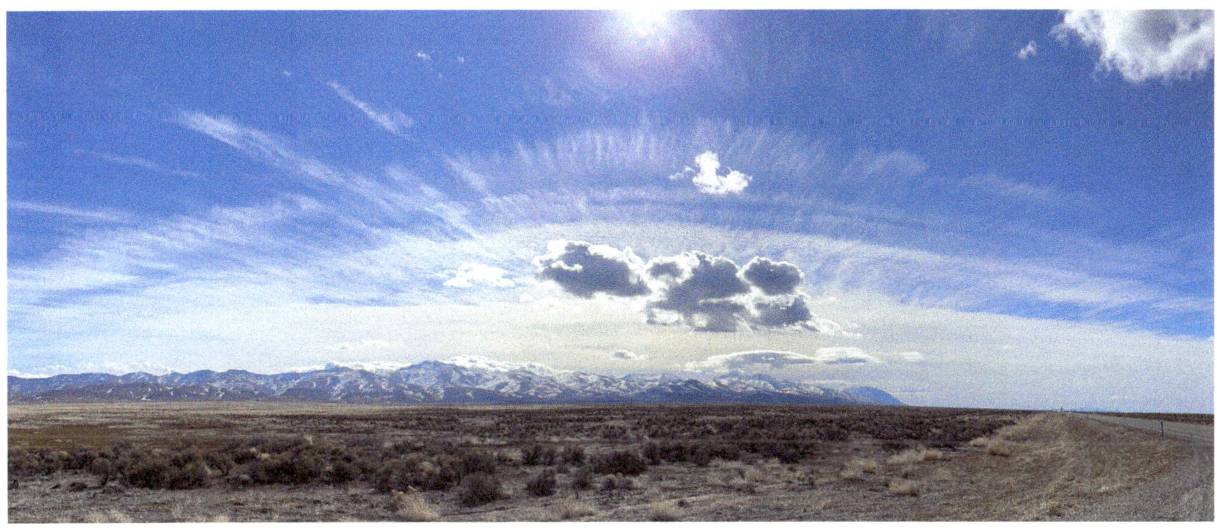

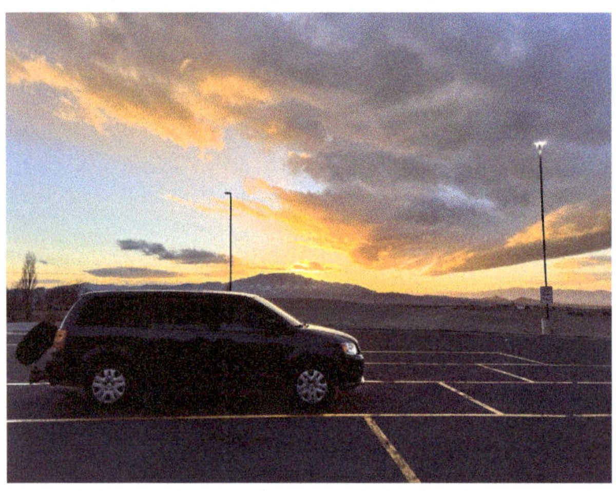

Arrived exhausted during a beautiful sunset
at Tonopah, Nevada.
Overnight parking at the Chevron Station
with permission.

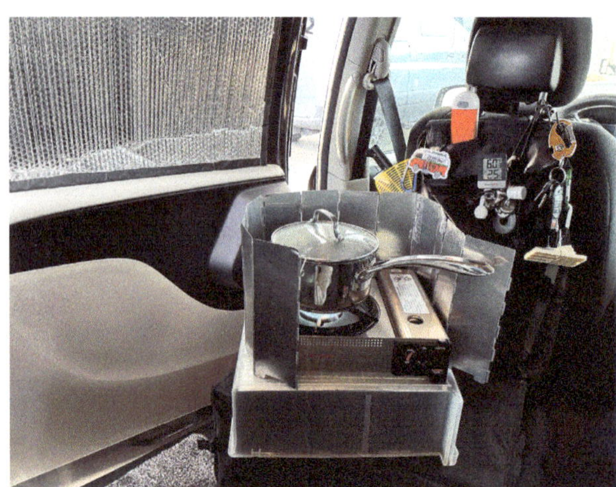

Very cold and windy with indoor cooking.
Set up the -15F (-26C) rated sleeping bag
and king-size blanket folded double.
Hoped I didn't have to pee, it was a production
to get out from under the covers
and then get back covered up.
Passed on the bedtime cocoa.

I woke up during the night,
according to the weather app felt like 11F (-12C).

DAY 5 / FEBRUARY 22

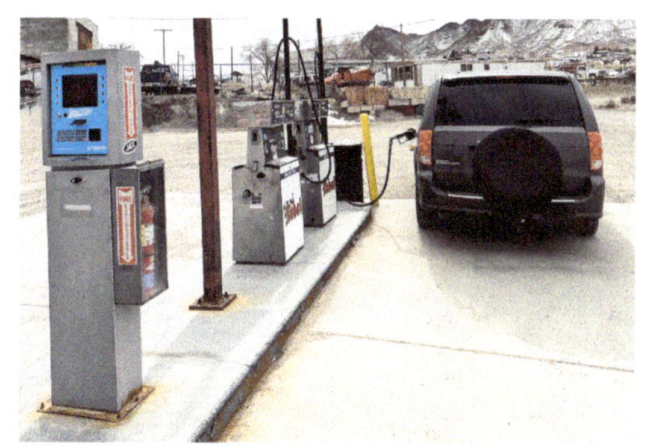

Woke up to 25F (-4C) in the van,
and the outside was heavily frosted.
Drove around town for the best gas price.

It was an old-school gas pump
and a struggle to figure out how to pay.
A lady came by and helped me.
The town had multiple outdoor museums,
featuring mining equipment.

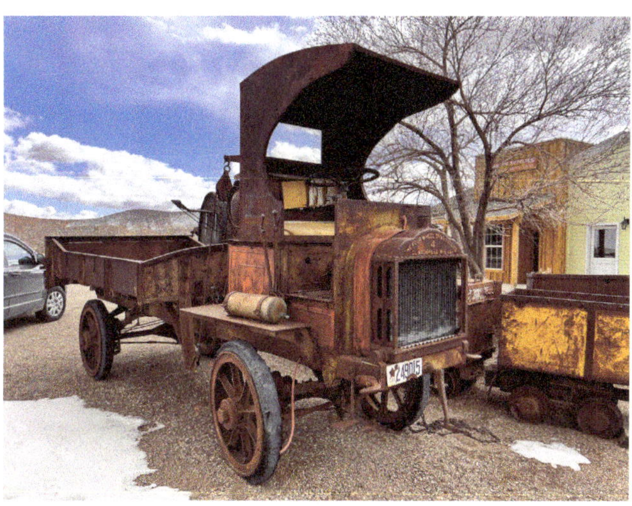

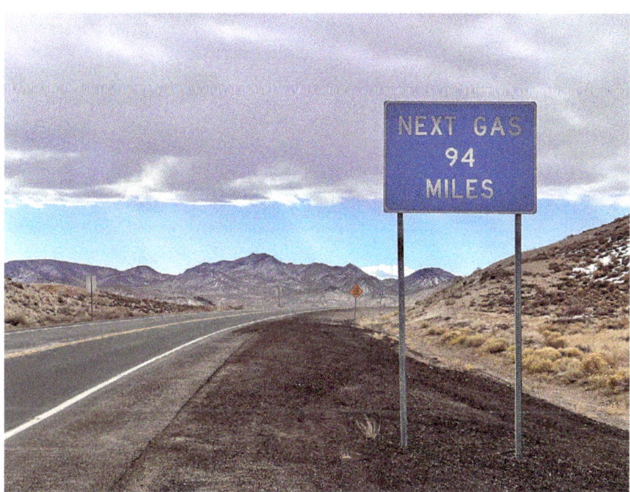

It was essential to take note of gas pump locations
and fill up at every opportunity.
Nevada is vast and wide.

Beatty, Nevada was the last stop before Death Valley.
Filled up, checked out the stores and WIFI options.
Took the van to a car wash.
It was very dirty and difficult to see through the windows.
Went to the library to sync the offline maps between devices.
Did it work?
No.
I did it wrong.

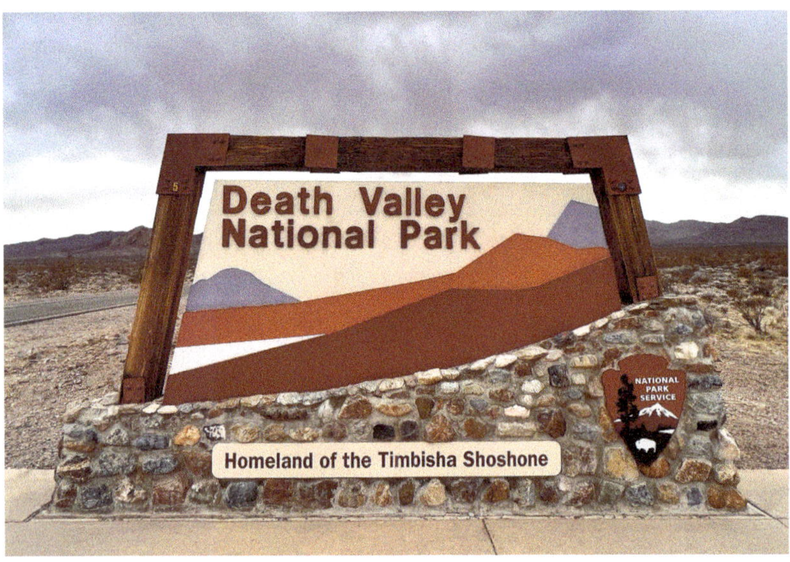

And there it was, the welcome sign to Death Valley National Park.

A 4,000 foot drop from the park entrance to the valley floor.
A beautiful and majestic view of the valley
with a huge windstorm
blowing up sand and dust over the Mesquite Flat Sand Dunes.

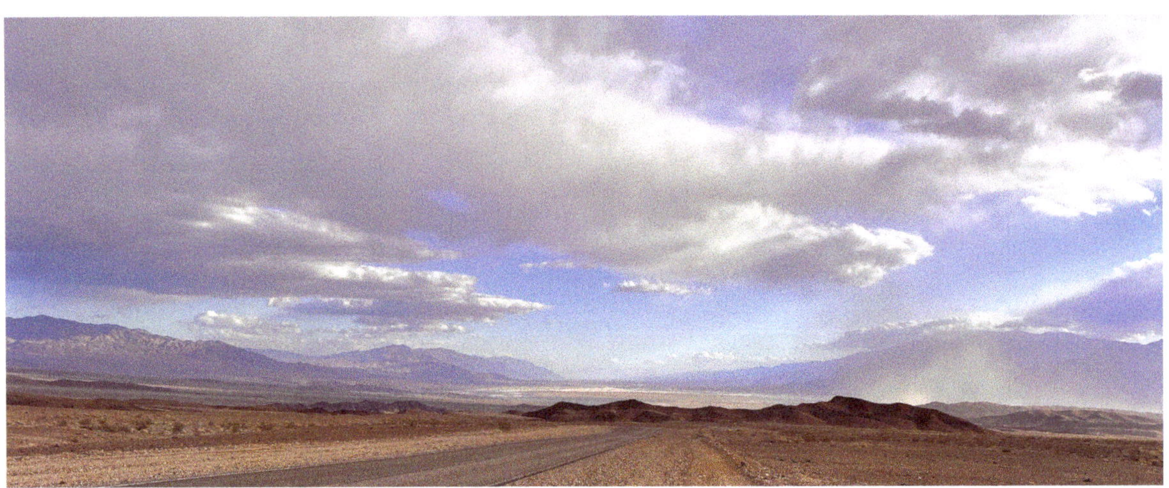

Checked into Sunset Campground at Furnace Creek.
Went to the visitor center to get a pass.
Very busy with overwhelming noise,
lights and people moving around.
Wore earplugs, a baseball hat and sunglasses
to minimize the assault on my brain.

An injured brain lost its ability
to filter incoming information and stimulation.
The gate stays open instead of closing.
Therefore, it fatigues quickly
and takes much longer to recover than healthy brains.
It's like running a car battery dead,
and then it takes a few days of trickle charging to restore the charge.

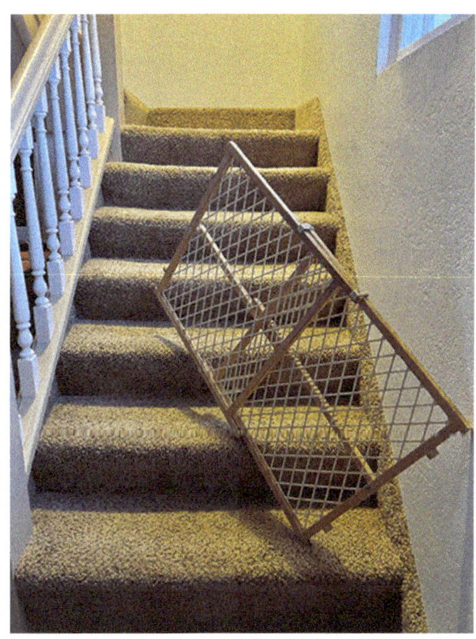

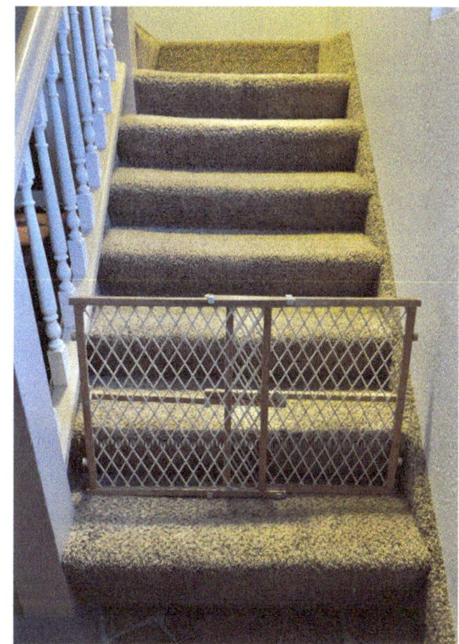

DAY 6 / FEBRUARY 23

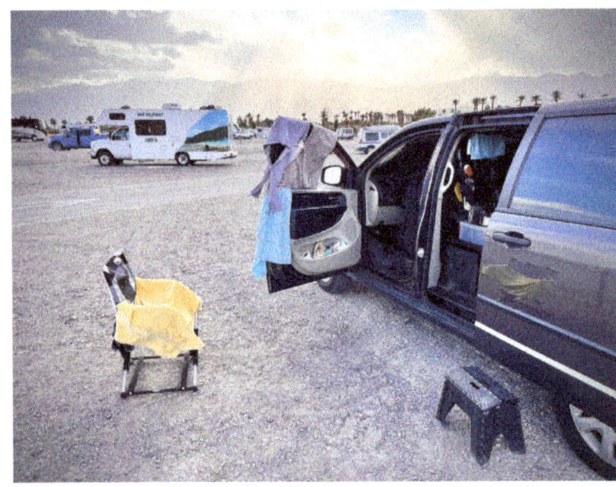

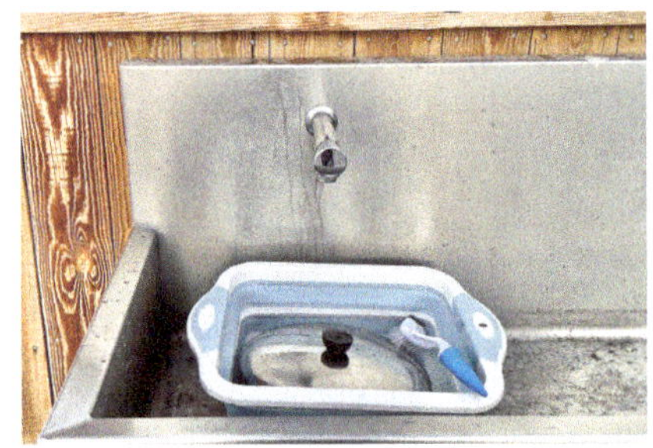

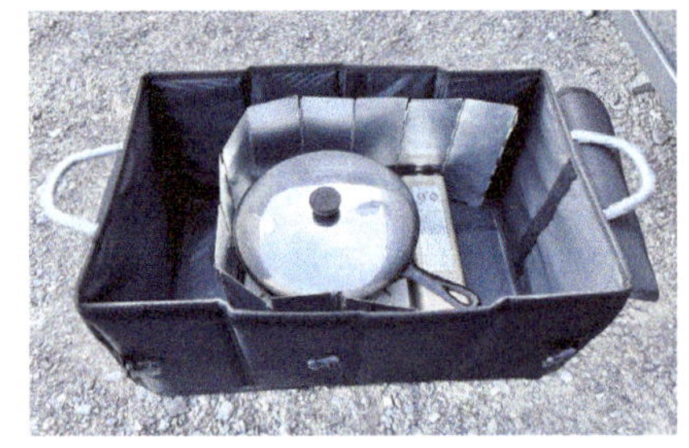

Woke up too exhausted and tired to plan,
sequence or put basic activities together.

Stayed put for the day.
Minimized unnecessary items in the van
and put them away.

With the warm weather,
it was as good a time as any
to do laundry and cook meals
for the next few days.
Made it up as I went.
If you have clothespins,
you could hang laundry on anything.

The campground had a dishwashing station
with fresh drinking water,
flush toilets and garbage collection.
Plenty of water for washing dishes
made it a lot less complicated.

I had to invent ways to cook with propane and butane
while dealing with the wind.
Just a small breeze required ways to block the wind.
Windy weather
changed from almost nothing
to very strong
alternating frequently during the day.

DAY 7 / FEBRUARY 24

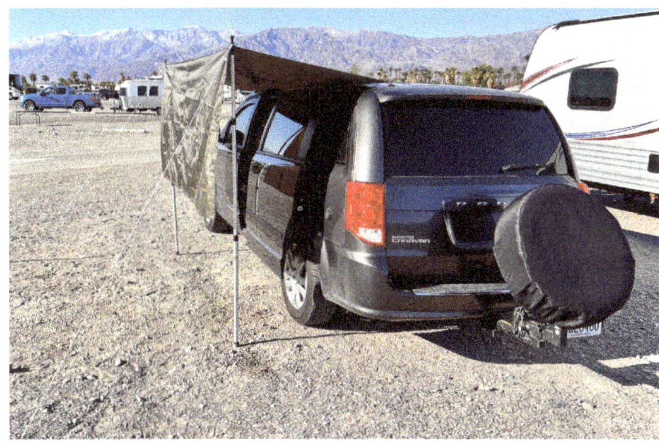

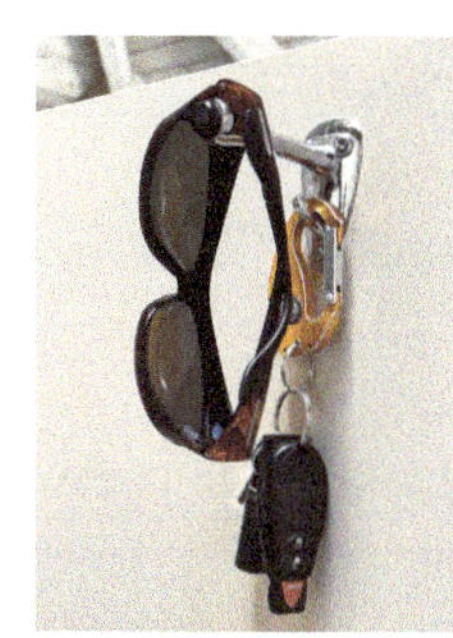

The brightness of the rising sun in the mornings was a shocker.
Challenged my light sensitivity continuously.
Had to be creative with positioning the tarp
to block the light while I was in the van.

I liked the hooks on the bathroom doors.
I didn't always know what my hands were doing (stereognosis)
and dropped things without noticing.
Definitely don't drop stuff around toilets
with automatic flush sensors.

I went to the locations indicated on the park map with public phones.
No public telephones in the park for years.
And no Verizon cell coverage.
Went to the hotel to check options to make a phone call.
The very nice man at the front desk dialed Mark's number.
Talked to him briefly and assured him of my safety.

Went for a drive to charge the batteries
that powered the fridge.
Drove to The Pads Desert Campsite to check it out.
Well-known boondocking (free camping on public land)
spot on YouTube.
Didn't like the vibe,
and it wasn't somewhere I wanted to stay by myself.
Learned to pay attention to what I drove over.
A sharp piece of rusted pipe
stuck out of the cement, could have destroyed a tire.

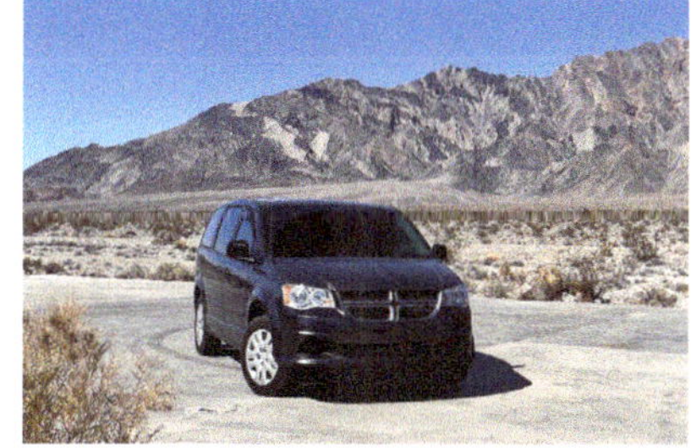

Drove down Twenty Mule Team Canyon.
An otherworldly experience of rock formations and colors.
My first "off-road" experience.
About gave me a heart attack being parked at that angle
after driving over a hump.
Wimp.

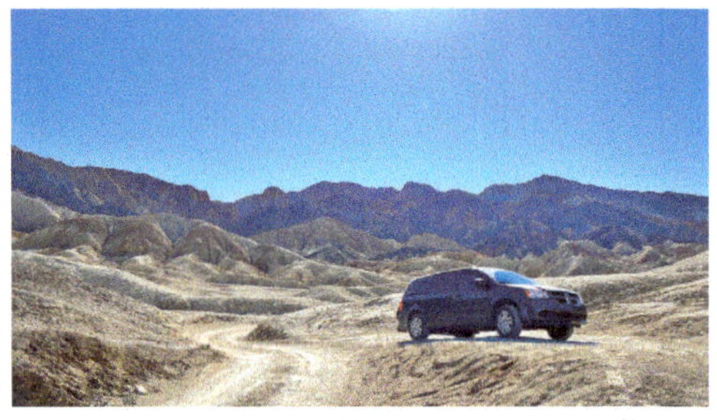

Zabriskie Point,
amazing and unique.
Very photogenic
with many options for abstract photos
Met two Indian women from Atlanta,
also on a road trip.
Took their picture for them.

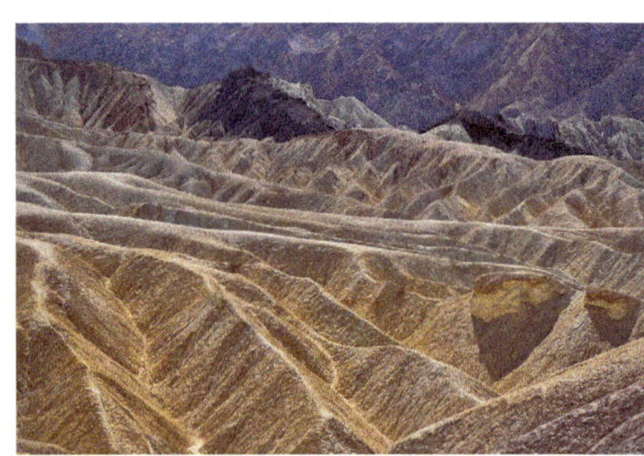

Back at the campground, a man approached me
with questions about the swing-away hitch
for the spare tire carrier.
It felt good to be a source of valuable information.

The refrigerator's temperature was wrong.
Had to pay better attention
to prevent the food from going bad.

DAY 8 / FEBRUARY 25

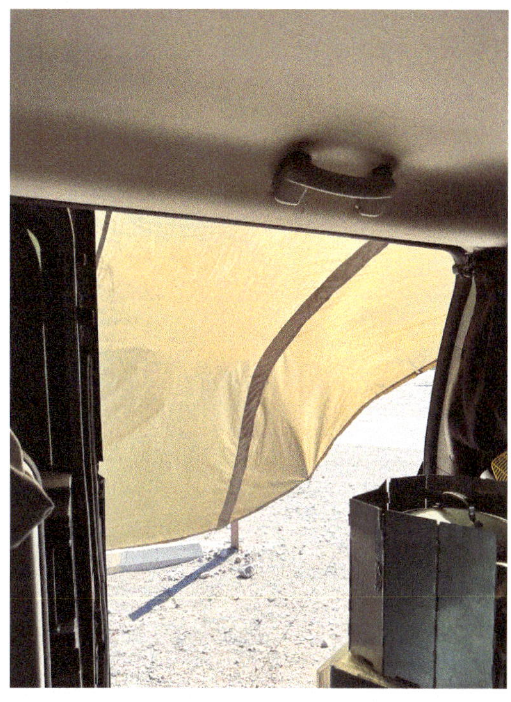

I woke up tired to another windy day.
Drove to Badwater Basin and back.
The batteries relied on daily driving to get charged
to power the refrigerator.

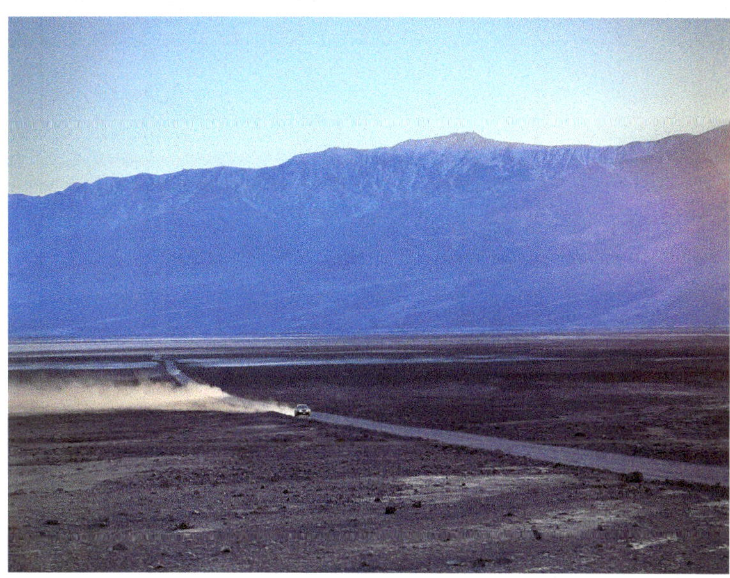

Sunset pictures on the stretch of road by Golden Canyon.

DAY 9 / FEBRUARY 26

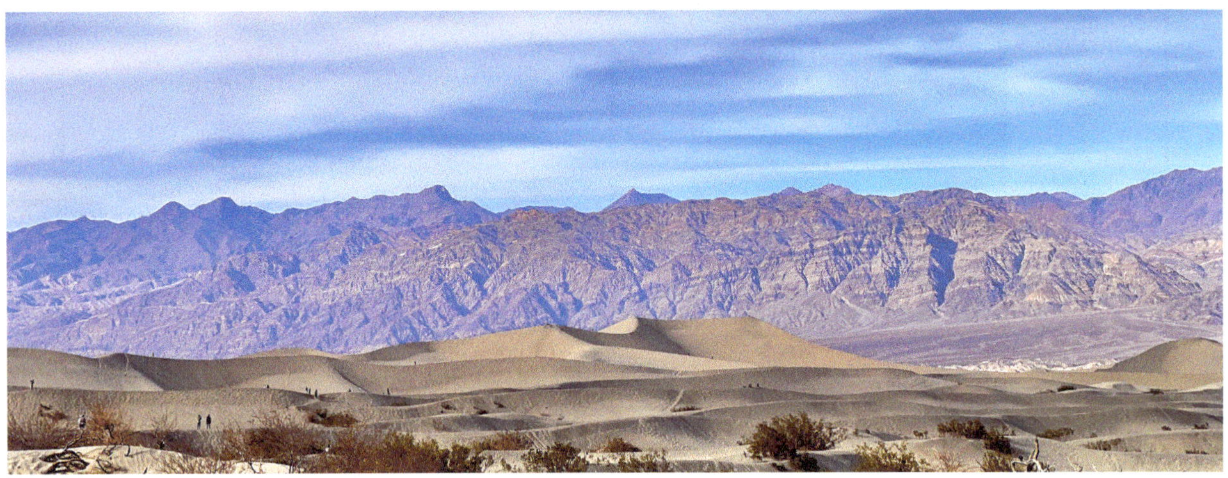

Drove to Stovepipe Wells
and took a shower for $5 at the hotel's pool house.
Met people with a wiener dog puppy.
It felt good to pet a dog after being gone
from home for a while.

The dunes were beautiful.
I wasn't in the mood to struggle to walk in the sand.
Checked out the other national park campgrounds
in the area for future reference.
The General Store sold my favorite wine.

Went back to the Golden Canyon area
for the evening drive.
Found the mud tiles photographers love so much.

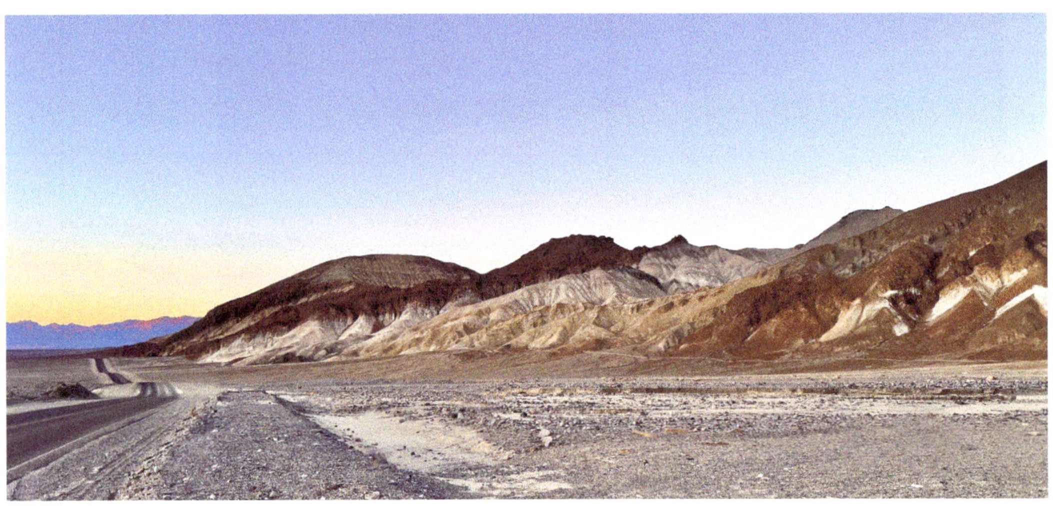

DAY 10 / FEBRUARY 27 / 1,190 MILES

Slept very poorly the night before.
Wanted to get up for a sunrise picture at Zabriskie Point,
the ideal time to be there for photography.
I was too tired and very slow to get going.

A new neighbor moved in next to me
and promptly started his generator.
I moved to a different site.
That neighbor also started his generator.
Hell no.
It would drive my exhausted brain up the wall.

Checked out the Texas Springs campground.
Mostly tents, vans and RVs.
No generators allowed.
Found a level spot close to the bathroom and dishwashing station.

Eventually got moving around 4pm.
Went to Zabriskie Point for a sunset location.
As a photographer I was focused on taking pictures.
It was a new experience to see people
sit and watch the sunset without doing anything else.

Something I should try.

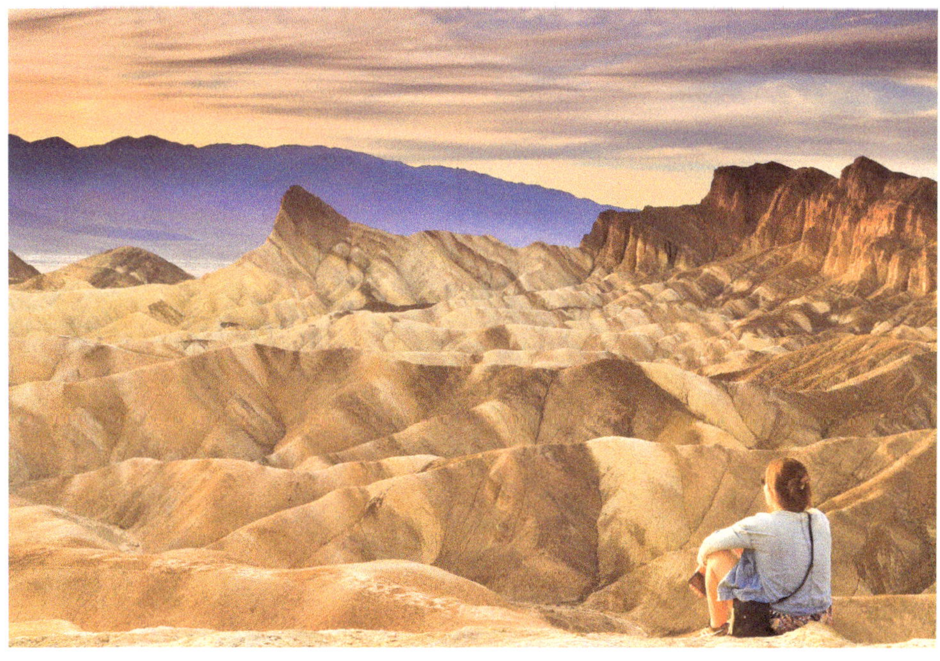

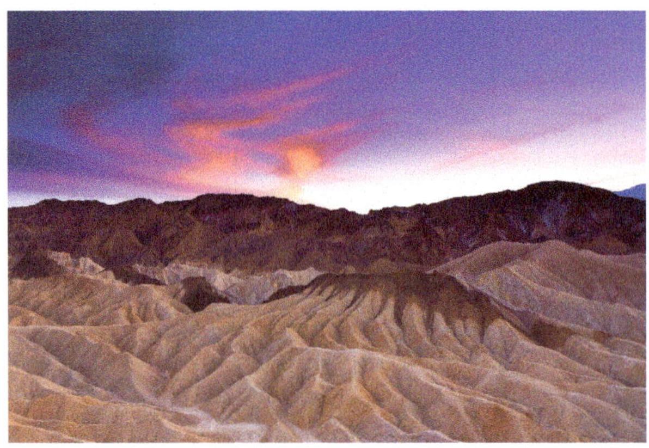

Liked my new camp spot,
a lot quieter.
I also liked the sound of walking on gravel,
I could hear people walking up
without constantly being on the lookout
for what's going on around me.

Used a Jackery power station
in addition to the house batteries
to charge the phone and iPad.

The Jackery had to be charged every day as well.

A huge struggle to keep the charging cords straight.
Each device had a 12-volt and 110-volt cord.
Had to be sure the blue light was on
to indicate it was charging.
And remember to unplug it so it didn't drain
the van battery overnight
and the van wouldn't start.

I was very aware of my deficits caused by the brain injury.

Neurofatigue was such a big deal.
Difficult to recover from daily activities
that drained the brain's energy.
So difficult to get simple activities done.
I forgot where I packed stuff.
The van is not that big.
How hard can it be to find something?

Nothing had changed,
I'm slow.

Ran into people from a 6-day photography class
I would have loved to go to.
Wouldn't be able to participate like everyone else.

Be exhausted after driving to the park.
Get up for daily sunrise pictures.
Driving to all the locations,
morning class,
midday break,
afternoon class,
sunset class,
even a star photography lesson.

The class also included locations
at Alabama Hills, 2 hours from Death Valley.

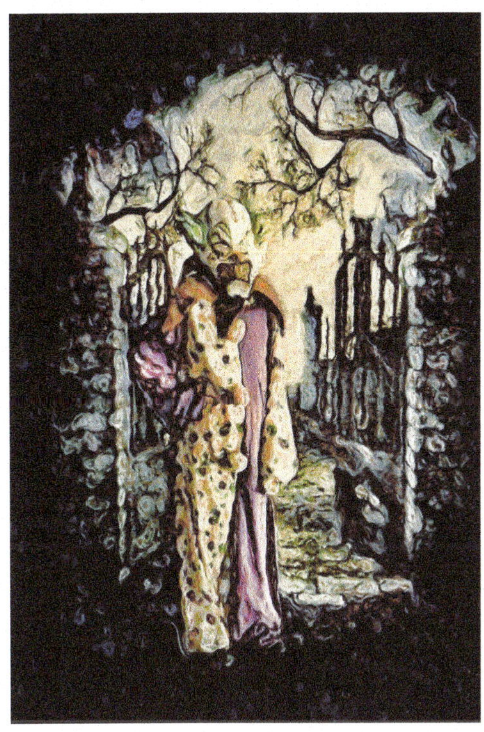

Impossible.
So fucking impossible.
The Guard of Shitville made sure of it.
Wouldn't let me go.

DAY 11 / FEBRUARY 28

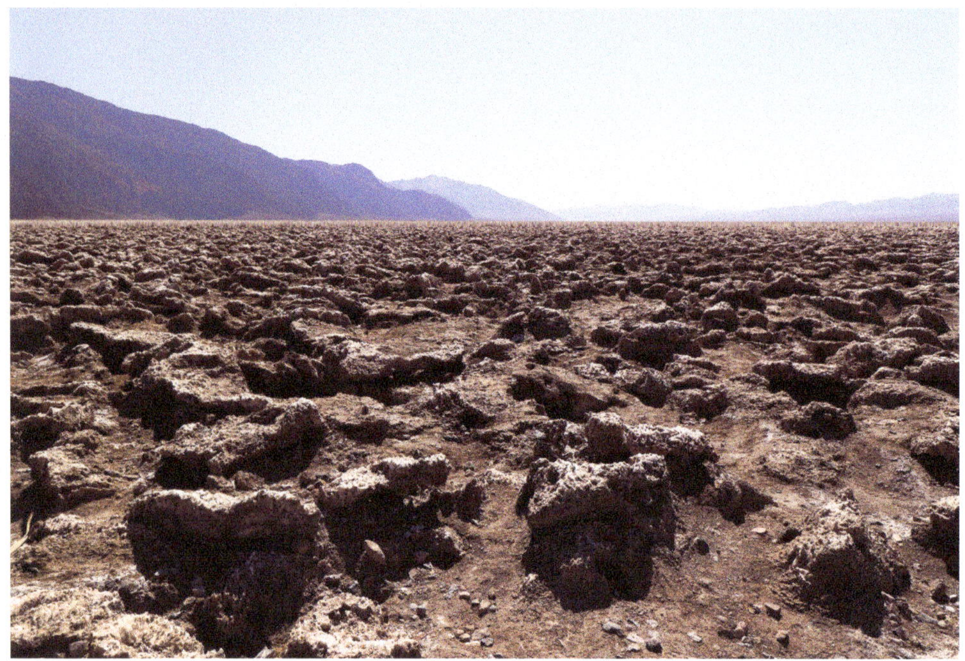

The Devil's Golf Course was very interesting.
It received its name after a 1934 Death Valley guidebook said,
"Only the devil could play golf on this harsh terrain"
and the name stuck.

It's a salt pan with salt spires,
unforgivably hard and jagged with a warning sign,
"Don't fall, you will break bones."

I almost cut my throat
with the sharp kitchen knife.
I forgot I had it in my hand
and reached up to my face.

I couldn't find the van keys to lock the doors.

I looked for my sunglasses for 20 minutes
while wearing them.

What's the per-day word limit for swearing?

The weather was a lot warmer at 87F
and it felt too hot.

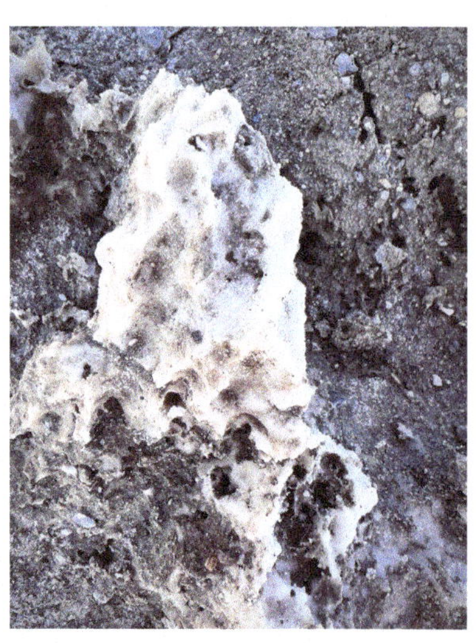

Artist Palette was on a very windy,
narrow, one-way road
with a vehicle length limit of 25 feet.
The true colors were visible after the sun set.

While the sun shone on the rocks,
the colors looked washed out.
I ran into people who recognized me
from a photography class in 2018.
I didn't remember them.

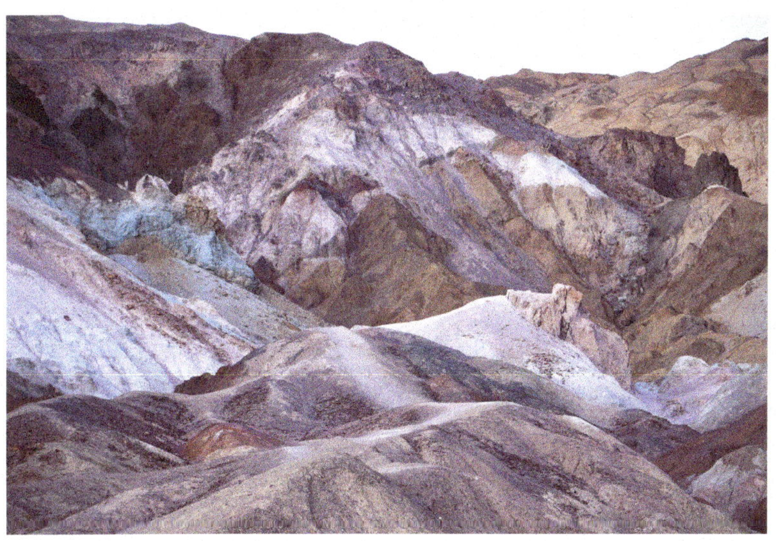

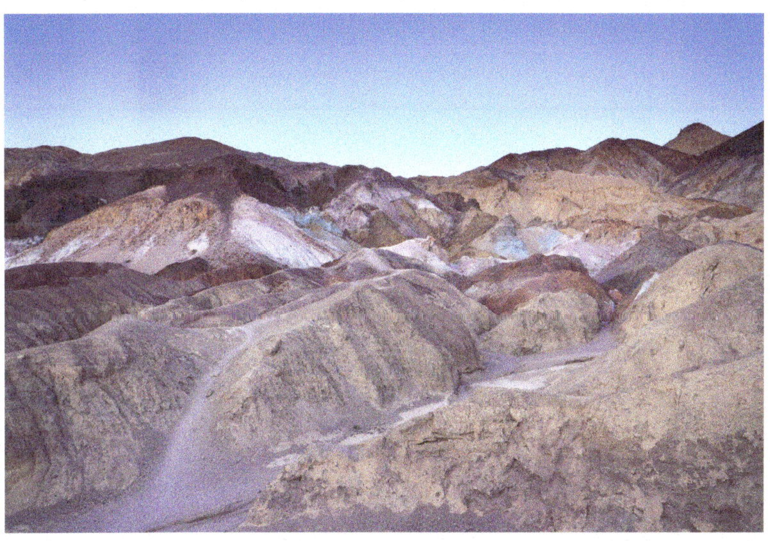

DAY 12 / MARCH 1

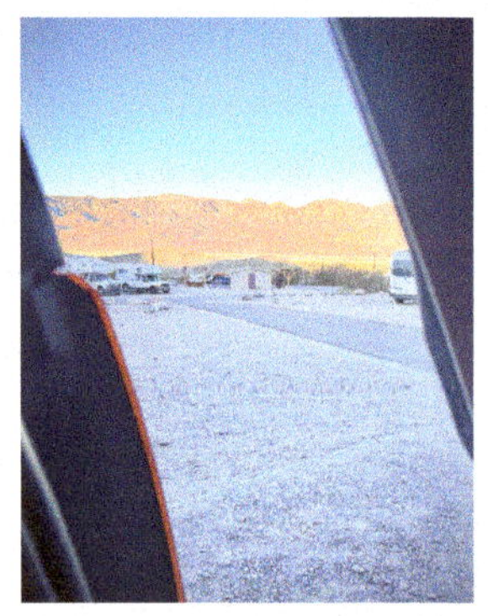

It warmed up at night
and I felt more comfortable in the campground.

I slept with the van's back door partially open.
The spare tire on the hitch blocked the door
from opening any further.
I had to figure a way to keep my pillow from falling out
during the night.

I woke up earlier than usual and could see the sun rising.

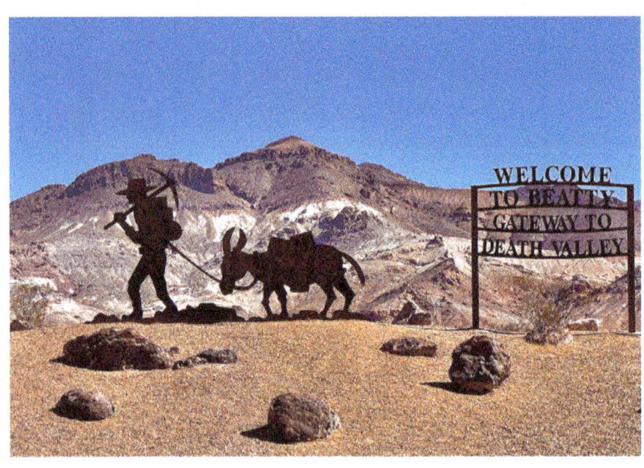

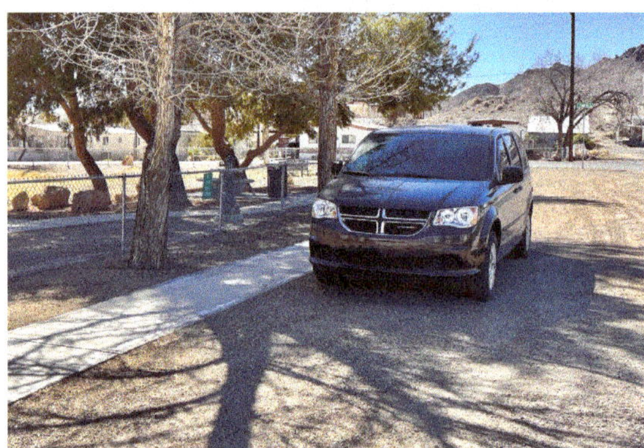

It was the day to go to Beatty, 40 miles outside Death Valley
to call Mark.
I haven't talked to him
since arriving in Death Valley.
And to get gas and a few things from the store.
I even managed to park in shade for a while.
Wanted to download the pictures
from my camera to my iPad.
Couldn't for dear life remember how to do it.
After a while the brain cells must have gotten the message
and I managed to get it right.

A donkey stuck his head in the open sliding door.
Saw a YouTube video about the donkeys
in town being pushy and aggressive.
Didn't know who got the biggest scare,
me or him, when I yelled at him to scare him off.

Called Mark and it was a relief to talk to him.
The stress about the trip rolled off me.
Sent him a few pictures.
I didn't think
we had ever talked on the phone for 1.5 hours.

The agreement was I would call him when I had a signal,
and if he didn't hear from me,
everything was fine.
The police would notify him if something happened to me.
So, until the police showed up,
nothing to worry about.

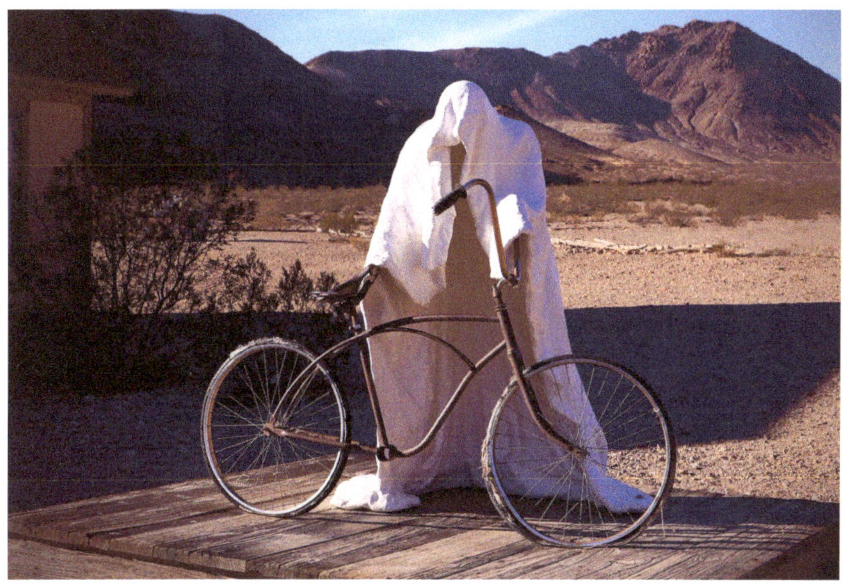

Stopped at the Goldwell Open Air Museum
on the way back to Death Valley.

It was a shock to see the shell
standing by a bicycle with weathered flat tires.
I was looking in a mirror.
I used to ride my bicycle many miles a weekend before the brain injury.

The bike was custom fitted, I'm tall for a woman.
I would take the dogs for a run with the bike,
and they loved It too.

My balance was not good enough to ride the bike
anymore after the injury.
I lost my balance when I turned my head.

It's related to an abnormal vestibulo-ocular reflex,
a complex system that stabilizes the visual field
when you move your head.

It also played a huge role in driving
and dealing with the constant change of the visual field zipping by.
Trees, poles and shadows complicated it.
That's why I was so exhausted
after the 1,000-mile drive from home to Death Valley.

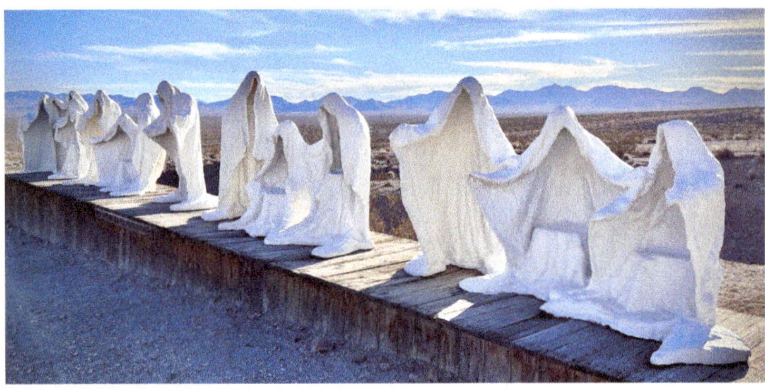

A summary of my life without saying a word.
Displayed on a platform,
the small boundary that my life shrunk into.
The emptiness of the skills I lost.

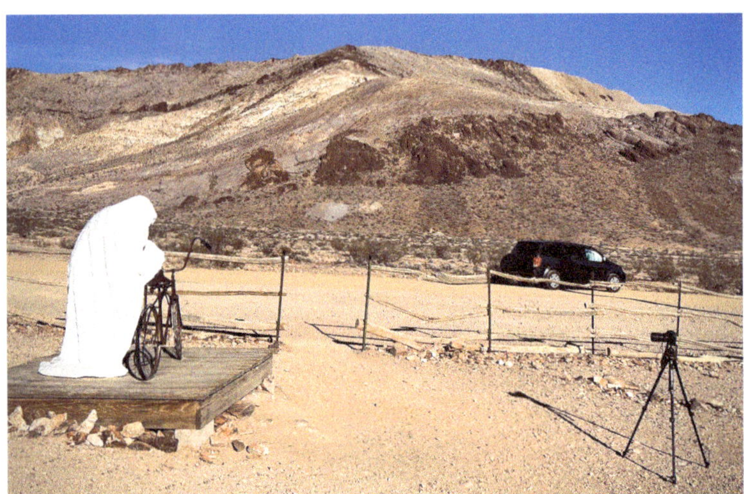

My life summarized in one picture.
The shell of who I used to be
standing with the bicycle I couldn't ride anymore.
The camera on a tripod,
the hobby that disappeared.
And the van.

DAY 13 / MARCH 2

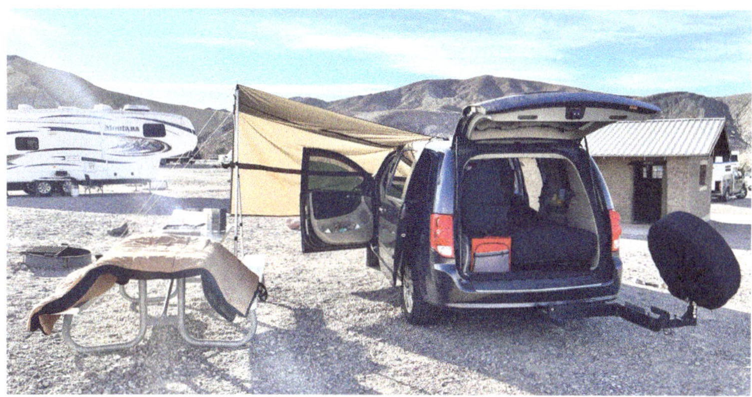

Woke up early and went for a walk
on the hill behind the campground.
I was getting very good at setting up the tarp
to make the right kind of shade.

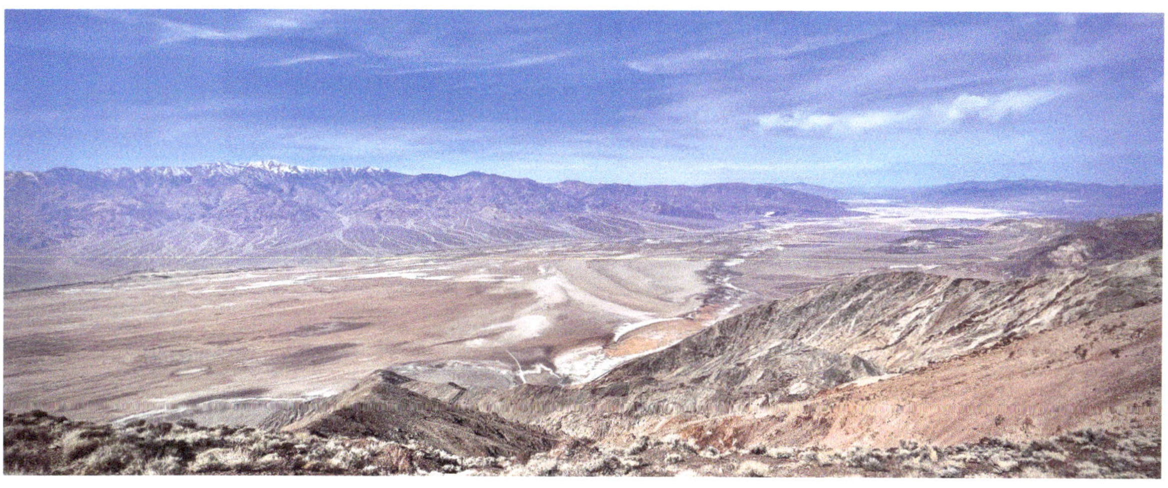

Drove to Dante's View.
5,410 foot elevation.
Beautiful view of Death Valley.

Surprisingly had a cell-phone signal
and called Mark,
but the answering machine picked up.
Left a message.

Plan: Spend the rest of the day at camp
and go back to Dante's View for sunset pictures.

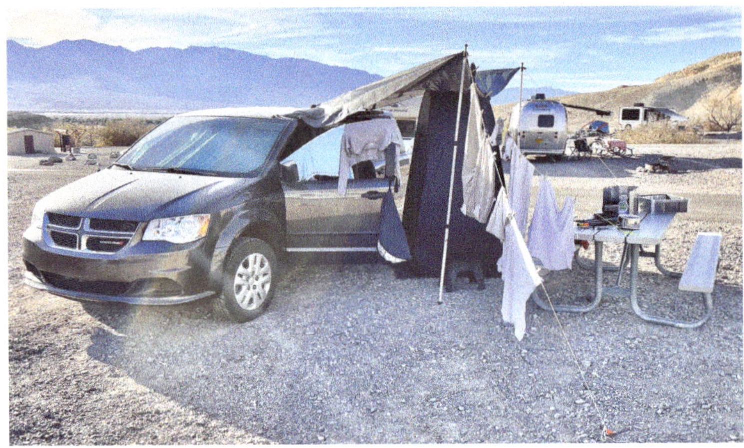

Back at camp I changed my mind.
Did laundry, cooked and took a shower since it was hot.
(It was common to plan something
and change my mind mid-stride.)

It was a good idea.
Unbeknownst to me, a windstorm was coming overnight.
I learned to take advantage of the weather
when opportunity struck.

Since I didn't have a cell signal,
the weather report was nonexistent
unless someone in the campground mentioned something.

Showering in the privacy tent was a new experience.
I needed more water than I thought.
The little pump for the showerhead
needed to be submerged completely to work.
And the collapsible bucket wasn't that deep.
I sat on the foldable stool.
I needed visual input to keep my standing balance.
The uniform color of the inside of the privacy tent
had very little visual feedback
and it was also too close to my face,
throwing off my balance.
Didn't want to fall
and suffer the indignity of taking the tent down.

The dishwashing station was like the water cooler at the office.
A meeting place for people from the campground.

I met Seth and his little boy.
He met his wife in Korea
where they both taught English as a second language.
They traveled in a trailer with their two little ones
while they taught online.

I had many interesting conversations with Seth.
The first time I saw him,
he was carrying water containers uphill
to their site for the children's kiddy pool.

Also met Suzanne and Jonathan,
who were getting married at 64.
Suzanne recognized my South African accent.
She worked in Lesotho 1983–1986 in the Peace Corps.

I hit my head on the door frame
and for good measure did it three more times.
I knew from experience
my balance would be more off than usual
for the next few days.

Extended my stay at the campground.
I picked up on the cultures of the visitors.
When I asked someone where they were from,
they said the state, not the town.
Also, what country they were from.
I was surprised how many international travelers there were
despite the COVID travel restrictions.

Sleeping weather warmed up significantly
and I was sleeping under a blanket
instead of in the sleeping bag.

It was the first day I was not thinking about life
not worth living.

DAY 14 / MARCH 3

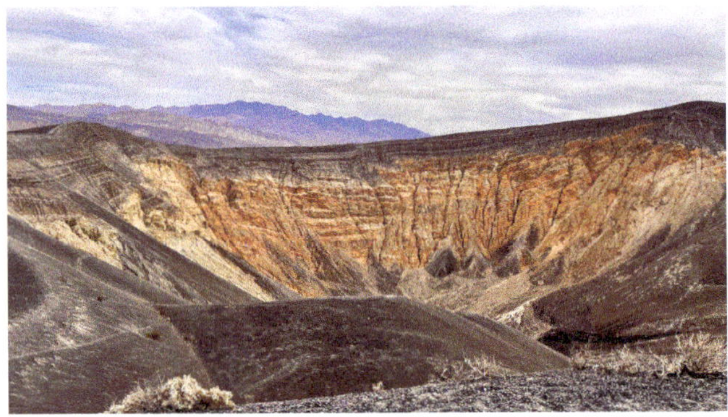

Drove to Ubehebe Crater
and charged the batteries.
Arrived at the crater to hear the beeping noise
of the inverter turn off.

An instant feeling of dread and sick to my stomach.
The beeping was code for trouble.
Trial by fire.

Fought against the wind,
barely able to open the driver's door.
Gave the crater a quick look,
decided to leave
before the wind blew me into the crater.

Drove back two miles to a ranger station with a parking lot.
Bloody hell.
I couldn't call Mark for help.
No cell-phone coverage.
Mark called the van a sardine can for one.
Everything fit tightly
and I had to unpack
and move a lot of stuff.

Moved the fridge sideways
to be able to fold the platform back
to get to the batteries
and other electronics.
What went wrong?
Got the tools out.

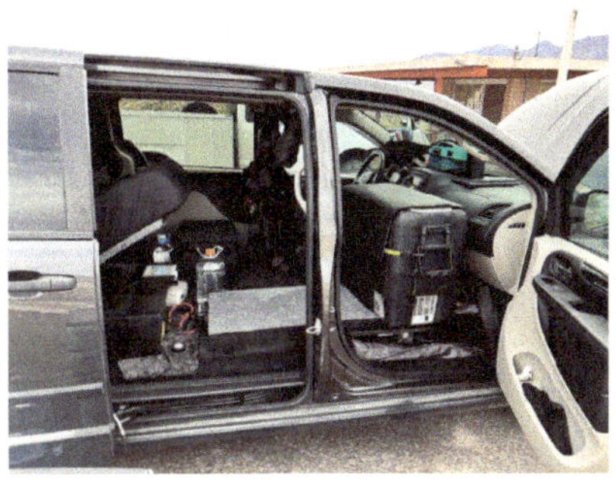

I could see a wire got loose from a fitting.
My automatic reaction was to push it back.
It made a huge sparky shocking noise
scaring the holy bejeebies out of me.
And what possessed me to do it again?
I forgot I was supposed to disconnect a battery terminal
before doing something stupid.

Despite the loud spark,
the inverter and fridge turned back on
after reconnecting the wire.
Tried not to worry about how much
potential damage I did.
And how much of the production
I would confess without worrying Mark.

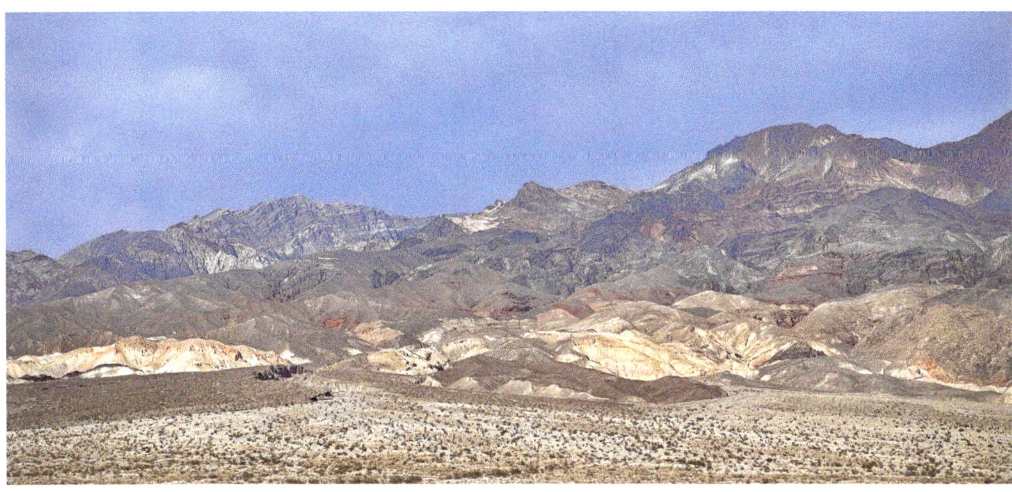

The mountains were beautiful on the drive back to the campground
and I saw Titus Canyon Road.
It's on my wish list to drive one day.

Stopped at the store at Stovepipe Wells
to get some wine to calm the nerves.

Saw the beautiful light in the afternoon
and went to the highway by Golden Canyon
for sunset pictures.

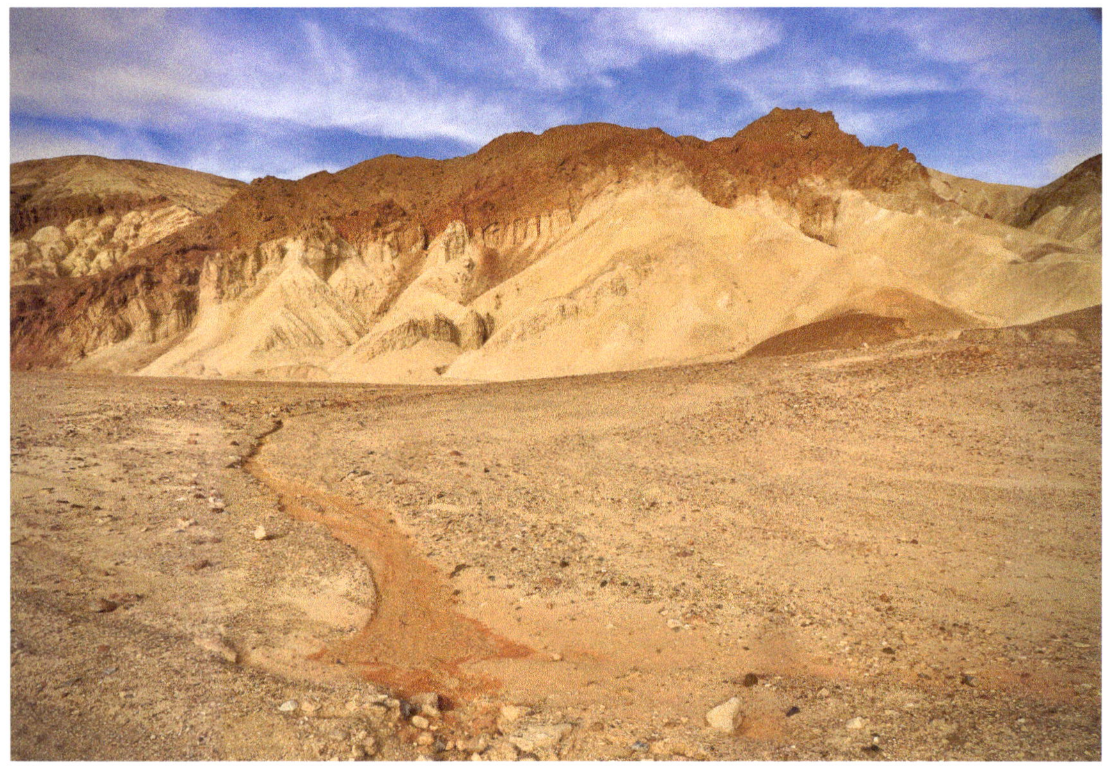

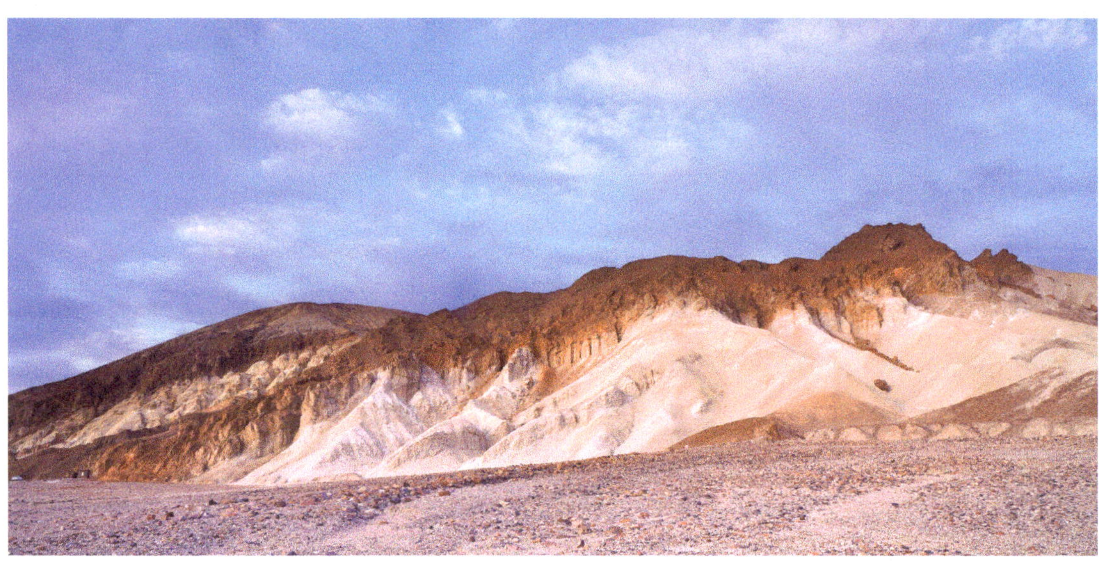

DAY 15 / MARCH 4

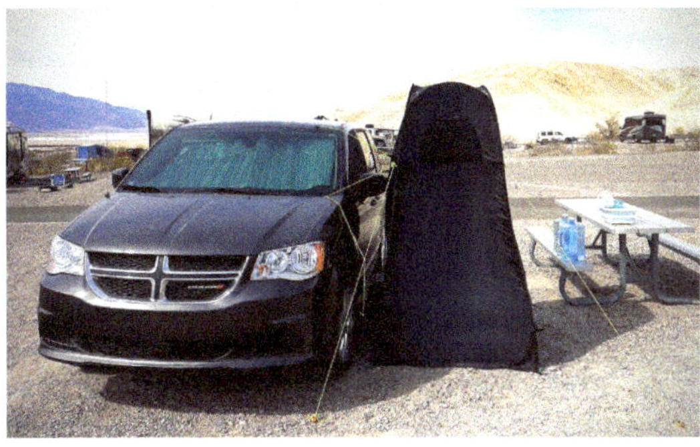

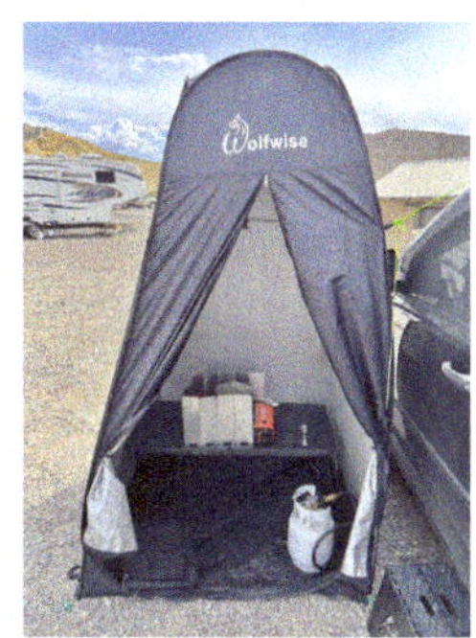

Woke up feeling dizzy and disconnected.
It was very windy
with an overnight windstorm warning
per the camp host.

Cooked a few dinners in the shower tent
as a wind barrier.
Had to stake it down well and
anchored it to a magnet on the van roof.

I met Seth's wife Julia and the two little kids
at the dishwashing station.
They had a travel blog,
and I had the hardest time remembering the name.
It's a sign of language processing issues
after the brain injury.

Went for a drive late afternoon to charge the batteries
and take some pictures.
The wind just about blew me over.

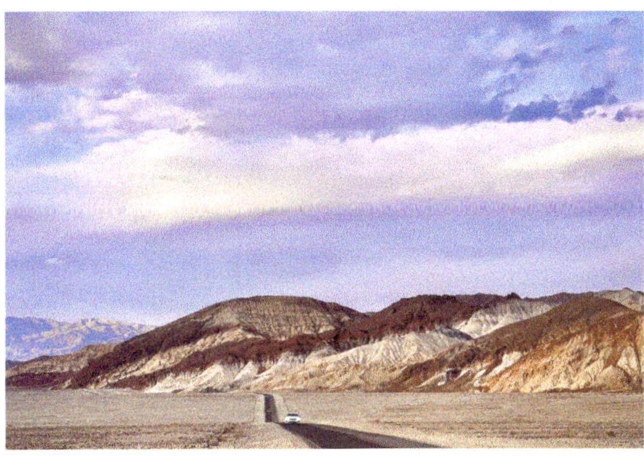

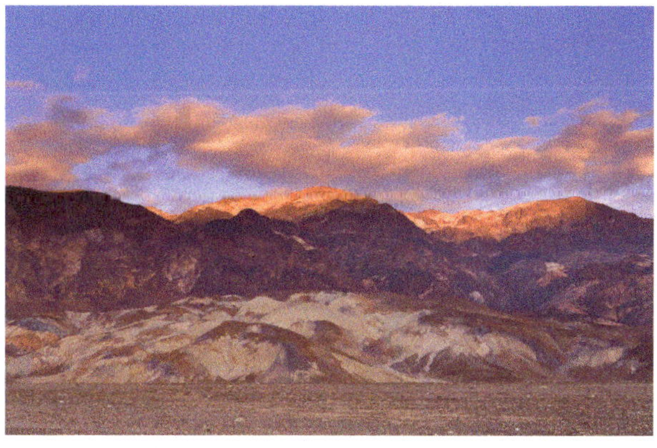

DAY 16 / MARCH 5

Woke up early when the side window reflectix cover
fell out through the window.
Had to get up to retrieve it
before the wind blew it across the campground.
Went back to bed for another two hours.

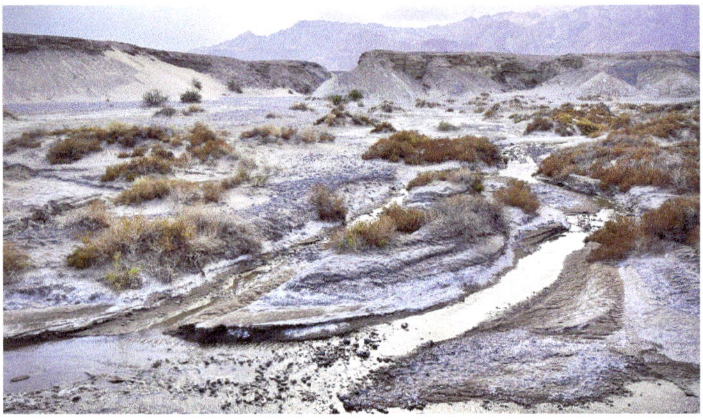

Lee from Walla Walla, Washington State came by
to comment on how stealthy the van was.
It didn't take much to get me talking
about the improvements we have made.

Believe it or not, there was water in Death Valley
at the Salt Creek Interpretive Trail.
Met athletes from Minnesota on a quick road trip to the park.

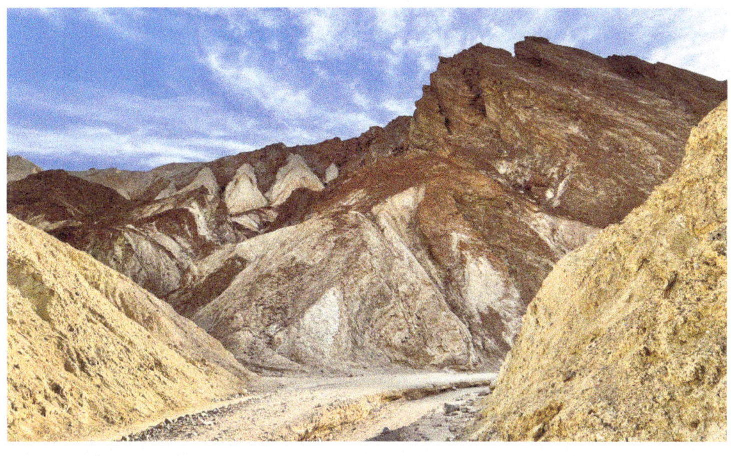

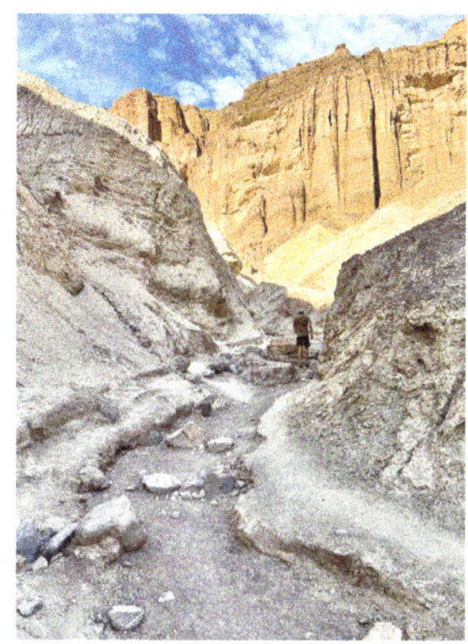

I hiked the Golden Canyon.
2.9 miles.
Got close to the Red Cathedral,
wanted to go back for a sunset shoot.

Went to Artist Drive to watch the sunset.
Met people from London.
Directed them to Artist Palette.
Gave photography tips for good outcomes with pictures.
I took off for Artist Palette.
While I considered my plans,
three men showed up
and I didn't feel comfortable getting gear out.

Took a few cell-phone pictures
and headed back to the campground.
It rained a few drops.

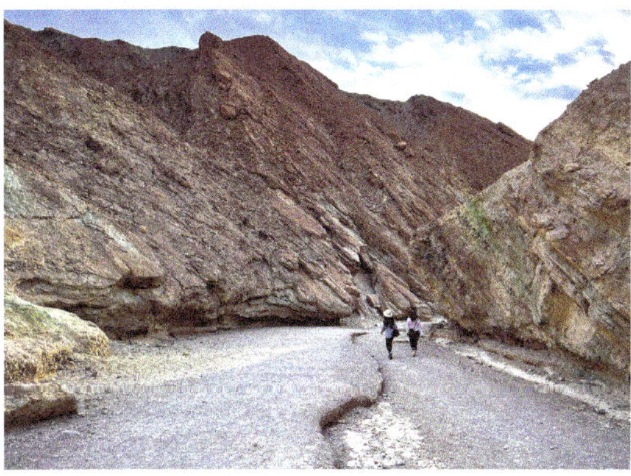

DAY 17 / MARCH 6

Slept like the dead.
Woke up tired.
It's typical to have a decline in function
during weather changes.
The barometric-pressure drop
increases the pressure inside the body and brain.
Increased pressure in the brain
causes more dizziness, tiredness
and a feeling of being disconnected
from the world.
That's why people with arthritis
can tell when it's going to rain.

I extended my stay by 2 days.
Cooked potatoes and lamb chops
for the next few meals.
Perfect flat rocks to level the stove.
Figured a gray-water system with the collapsible bucket.

The plants were green and wildflowers
were out after the little rain from the night before.

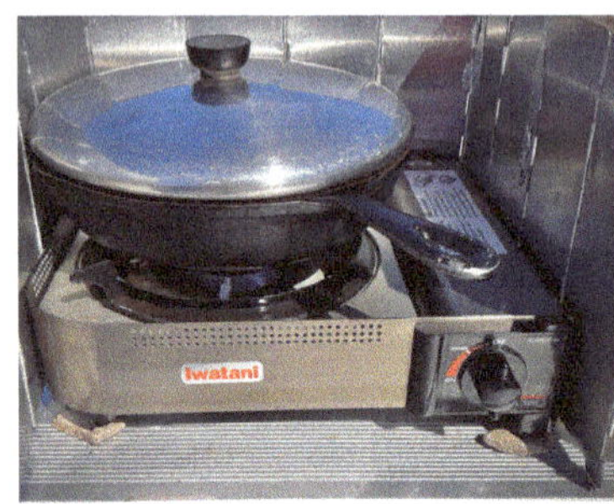

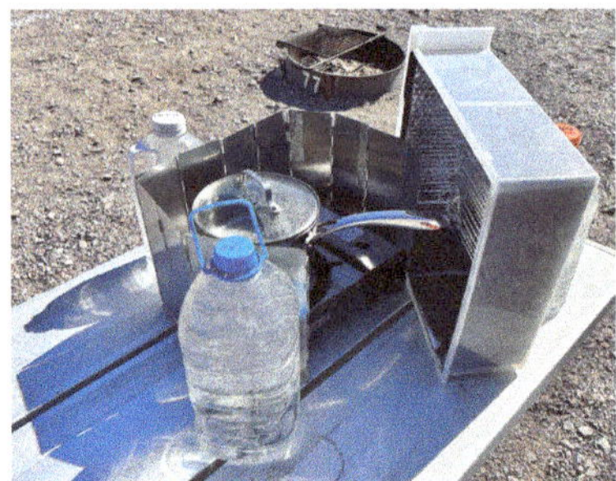

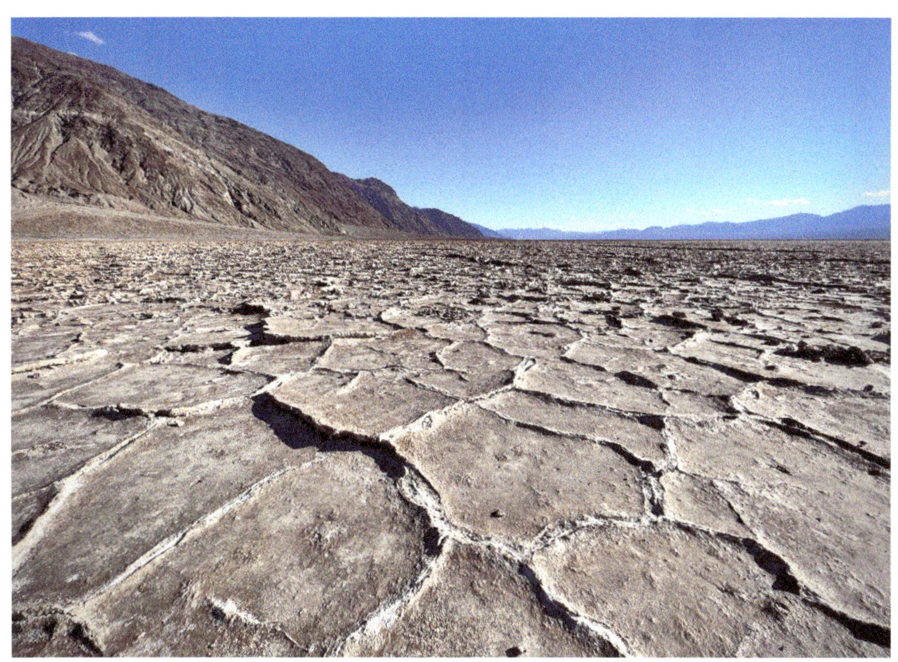

Drove to the salt flats of the Badwater Basin
at 282 feet below sea level.
Walked 2 miles round trip.
Met a group of Indian girls from Texas
who asked me to take their photo.

Found more mud tiles.
Although Death Valley was very dry
and the hottest place on the planet,
it does sometimes rain to form these mud tiles.

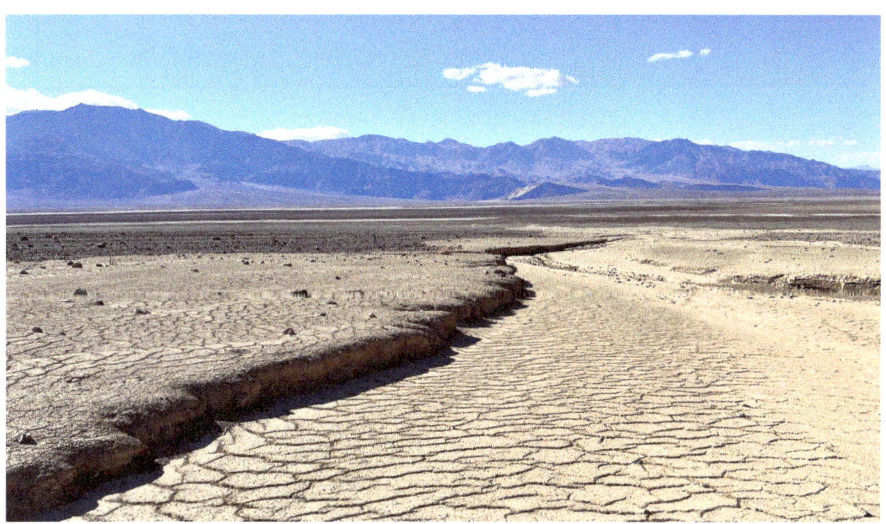

DAY 18 / MARCH 7

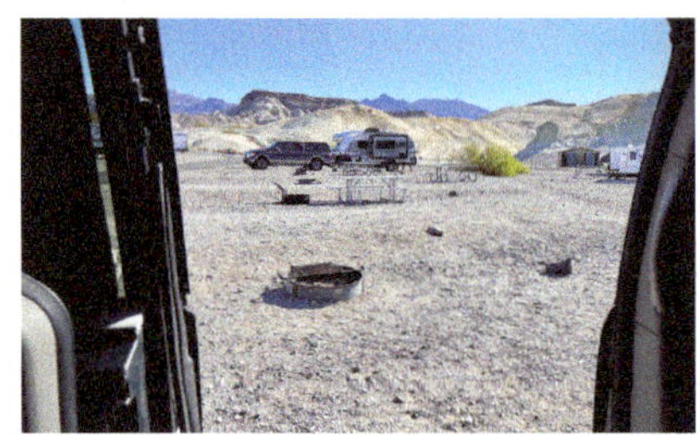

The original plans were
to look for yellow wildflowers,
give the mud tiles another try,
do the Natural Bridge hike
and Dante's View for sunset.
The super-windy conditions changed the plans.
Going to Alabama Hills, 2 hours' drive from Death Valley.
Stopped at Father Crowley Overlook
and the wind about ripped the door off the van.

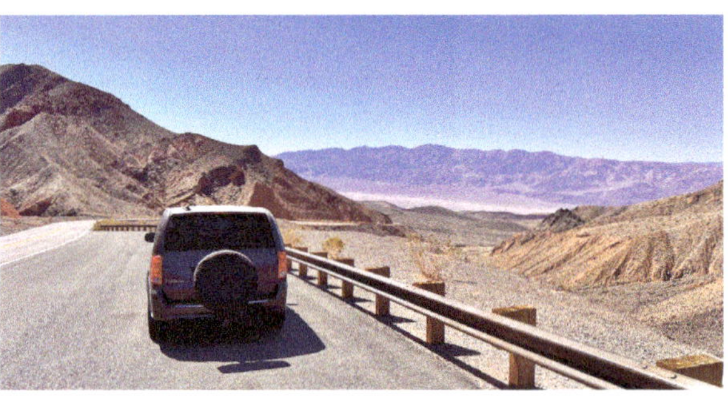

The road was very steep going over
two mountains
destroying gas mileage.
The route was very scenic,
but the wind made it very difficult
to take good pictures.

Checked into Tuttle Creek Campground
on BLM (Bureau of Land Management)
land at $4 per night.
As much as I hate being on disability,
it does have its advantages.

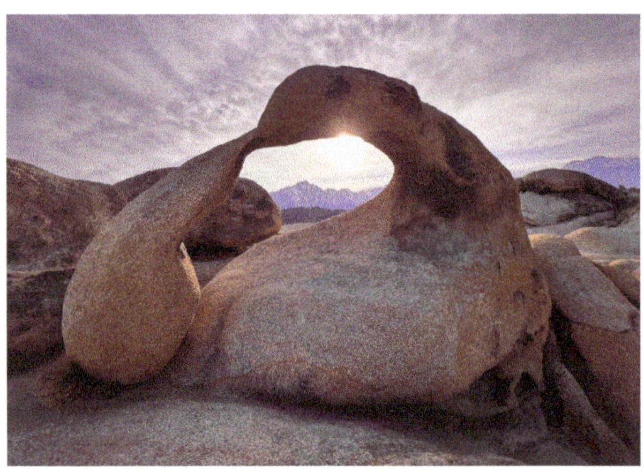

The Access Pass,
available for free to people on disability,
allowed 50% off camping fees
and free entry/day use in
National Parks,
Forest Service,
Fish and Wildlife Service,
BLM, US Corps of Engineers
and Bureau of Reclamation.

It was very cold and windy
but did a drive through Alabama Hills.
Walked the short Mobius Arch trail.
Tried to keep the van in line of sight
so I didn't get lost and couldn't get
back to the van.
It wasn't uncommon to get lost
and struggle to find the van.

I figured out later that I could use
"Navigate" on the *All Trails* app
even if it's not an official trail
to keep track of where I was.

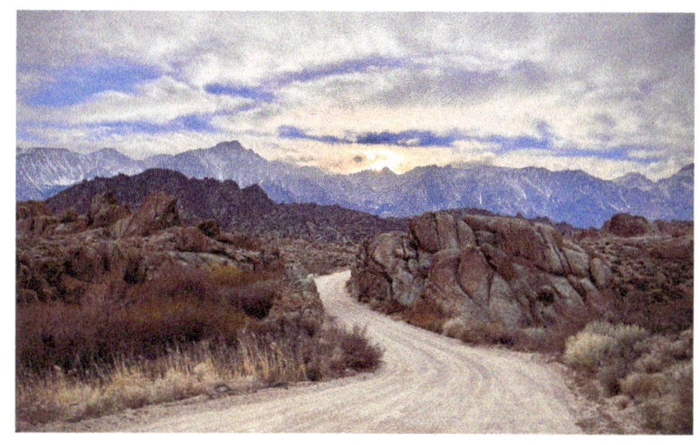

Enjoyed the unusual looking rocks.
Stopped frequently for
cell-phone pictures
from the van.

As I was gunning up a steep washboard dirt road,
I heard the now familiar beeping noise
of the inverter turning off.
It was too cold and windy to address the issue.
Turned all the breakers and the power switch off.
Plugged the fridge into the Jackery.
Worry about the problem the next day.

The campground was very quiet
with no reason to feel concerned about anything.
The outhouse was very clean with lots of toilet paper.
I had a signal and tried to call Mark,
but the call wouldn't go through.

Beautiful sunset with a view of Mount Whitney
covered in snow.

Alabama Hills was on my list for the future.

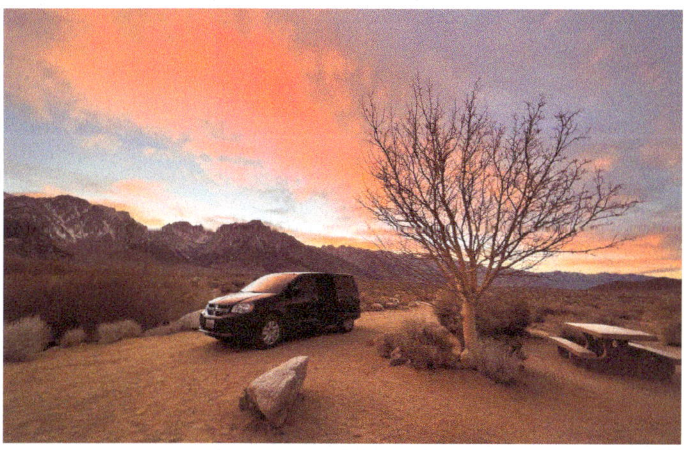

DAY 19 / MARCH 8

A beautiful morning with clear blue skies.
Ready to head back to Death Valley.
Stopped at the Lone Pine Welcome Center
to fix the inverter problem.
It took a lot less time to get the necessary stuff
out of the way to get to the loose wire.
Disconnected the battery terminal.
Put the wire back on without "shocking details."
Stuffed some firmer items behind the smaller battery
to prevent it from having room to slide on rough roads
and pull the wire loose.
Put everything back in the van
and turned the breakers back on.

Nothing.

The inverter was as dead as a doornail.

Well, how about that.
And I was so impressed with myself for "fixing" it.

Well, shit. What now?
Kept driving and thought about it.
Drove about 30 minutes thinking
I blew up the inverter.
Buy a new one?
How would I get it delivered to my location?
What tools would I need to install it?

Maybe I could wait until Mark met me in Texas
and he could fix it?
Should he ship the tools to Texas?
And then

"Oh my God, you dumb shit!"

I never turned the power switch
on the control box back on.
Reached down, flipped the switch, the inverter beeped.
The sound I have been waiting to hear.

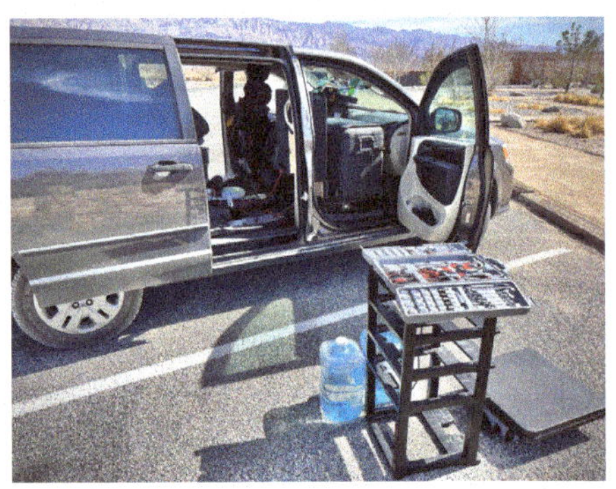

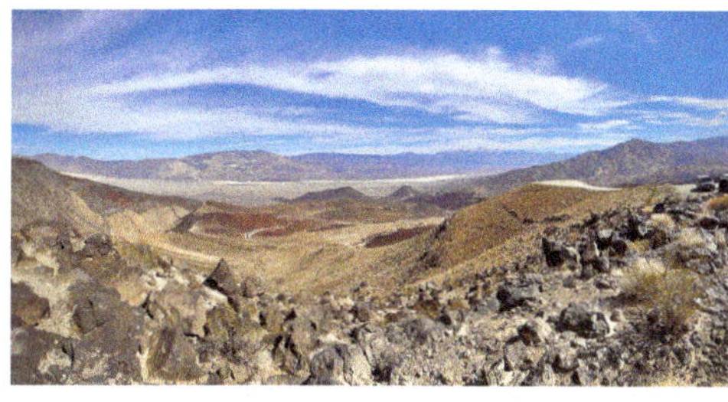
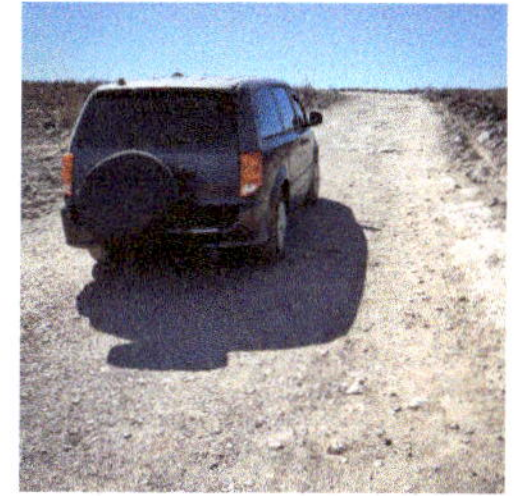
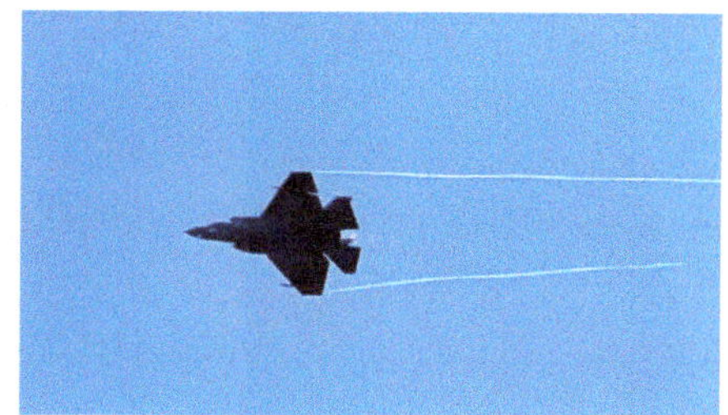

Pulled over at Father Crowley Overlook,
plugged the fridge back into the inverter,
and walked around enjoying Rainbow Canyon.
The area was famous for the Air Force jet fighters
practicing low-altitude flying.
It was my lucky day to see a jet
flying over sideways for entertainment.
Drove down a rough side road to a level spot
hoping to see more jets.
Just as I got out of the van, I hear a man say,
"Here they come."
Two more jets flew over.

Back at Texas Spring campground
I was lucky to get the same campsite.
Time to clean out the van,
reorganize, and put unnecessary items away.
I cut my finger.
Couldn't for the life of me
remember where I put the first-aid kit.

Spent a half an hour looking for it.
I realized I thought "fuck off"
a lot when I was struggling
and thought people could "see" me struggle.

The neighbor Janice gave me a Band-Aid.
After all the driving of the previous 2 days,
I felt very off-balance
walking to the bathroom in the dark.
Stumbled
and staggered a lot.
No.
I wasn't drunk.

DAY 20 / MARCH 9 / 1,970 MILES

Time to get ready to leave Death Valley.
I spent the day doing laundry
and cooked meals for the next 7 days.
It took most of the day from 8am to 3pm
with many trips to the dishwashing station.
Thank goodness for so much water close by.
Got a great looking tan
being in the sun all day in 90F (32C) weather.

Temperature management in the van was a big deal.
I custom-covered the fridge
with a double layer of reflectix (thermal insulating material)
and black contact paper to insulate it.
Made reflectix window covers
and bug screens before I left home.
It helped keep the van and the fridge cool
to use less power.
Cross-ventilation also helped keep me cool in the heat.

Paul, a 77-year-old Danish man from Seattle,
spent quite a bit a time talking to me
and complimented the food.

Brook from Alaska talked to me about traveling by myself.
He watched me from their campsite during the day.
Want to piss me off, ask what my husband thought
about my solo traveling.
I'm slow, not stupid.
And Mark thought I was capable of independent travel.

I had to plug the fridge into the Jackery
as the batteries were approaching 50%.
Lead acid batteries should not be below 50%
as it causes damage.

After taking a short rest break,
I went back to Golden Canyon at 4 pm
one last time to enjoy the rocks and trail.
Golden Canyon was my favorite of Death Valley.

I had more confidence in my abilities.
Not so scared.
My world was bigger than the 6 feet surrounding me.

Going to Las Vegas the next day.

DAY 21 /MARCH 10

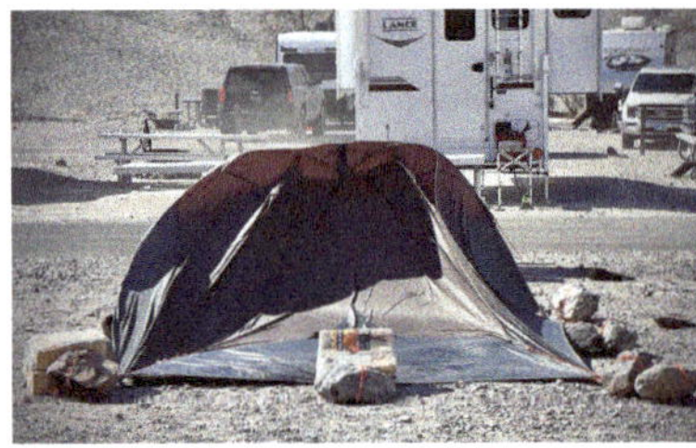

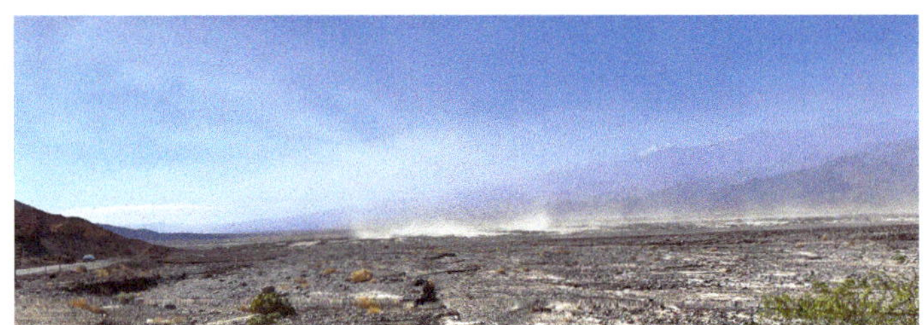

I arrived in a windstorm
and left in a windstorm.
A wind warning for the previous night.
The wind yanked the van around.
Made it hard to sleep peacefully.
Afraid stuff blown around the campground
would hit the van.
Fortunately, no damage.
Struggled to open the sliding door.

I knew then why there were
so many rocks in the campsites.
Securing belongings from being blown away.

Drove to Las Vegas.
Unpleasant discovery in Nevada.
Casino/gas stations allowed smoking inside.
Cigarette smoke made the outside of my brain burn.
Nowhere to use the bathroom
except on the side of the road.
I perfected parking
so traffic couldn't tell what I was up to.

I found a Walmart and Costco close together
on the side of Las Vegas.
I didn't want to drive in traffic more than needed.
My hiking boots needed replacement and found
a REI that had them in stock.
Met a great kid named Dylan
who used to travel in a van.

He offered me an overnight parking spot
in front of their house.
Very kind young man.

It was dark by the time I left REI
and I still had to find a place to stay overnight.
Investigated a few options in the city,
but I didn't feel comfortable with any of them.

An old black man approached me
while pumping gas.
I could tell he was living on the street.
He stayed at a respectful distance.
Didn't make me uncomfortable.
We had quite the conversation.
I asked him to wait for me.
Pulled away in the van so I could retrieve some cash.
Gave him $10 to get something nice to eat.
He was very appreciative
and walked into the convenience store.

Drove to the Petro Travel Center.
They took reservations for overnight parking
and were full.
The Love's Truck Stop on I-15 parking lot
was full as well.
I didn't have much of a choice,
kept driving north on the interstate.
I didn't typically drive in the dark.
Car lights were very bright.
Went right through my brain.

After 45 minutes,
the sign for Valley of Fire State Park came up,
and I took the exit.
Valley of Fire was my next stop anyways.
A casino and a truck stop right by the exit.
A huge relief, it was 11pm.
I found a good spot without interfering with truck parking.
Slept through the night without trouble.

Important lesson learned:
Arrive at the overnight spot before dark,
and have backup plans.

DAY 22 / MARCH 11

I woke up at 7am and left for the state park
around 8am after calling Mark.
Arriving on a Friday morning, didn't matter how early,
with the hope of getting a campsite, was wishful thinking.

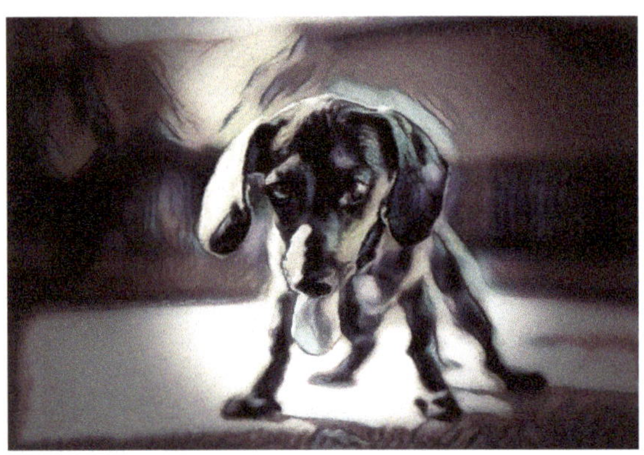

Exhausted and overwhelmed
from the driving, shopping,
and being up late the day before.
And not in a positive frame of mind.
Struggled to cope with the aftermath of the brain injury.
Struggled with how hard simple tasks became.
How much longer it took to get something done,
and the exhaustion that followed.

I found a quiet spot in the wedding area,
hiding behind a very large rock.
Needed somewhere without an audience.
It's hard to not feel watched in public places.
Had to clean up the van,
organize the shopping from the day before,
and get rid of the bulky packaging.
The wedding people showed up
to decorate the area.
I left the space as soon as I could.

Once the van was better organized,
I felt better too.

Started the driving tour
of the park around 12:30 pm.

The rock formations were breathtaking
and jaw-droppingly beautiful.
Hiked the 1.1-mile Dome Trail.
Challenging.
Should have used my hiking poles,
but I underestimated the trail.
Didn't fall, just a few stumbles.
Saw my first slot canyon.
Amazing.
Met two people from Spokane, Washington
who finished the trail with me.

The showers were fantastic.
Very nice to take a warm shower
without a time limit.
Went back to my sunset spot.
The park closed promptly at sunset
and the ranger drove by with a megaphone
to remind everyone.

Many boondocking spots
on the way back to the highway.
I could consider those in future.
I liked overnighting at the truck stop
under a spotlight for safety.
Valley of Fire was on my list
of future trips to the desert.

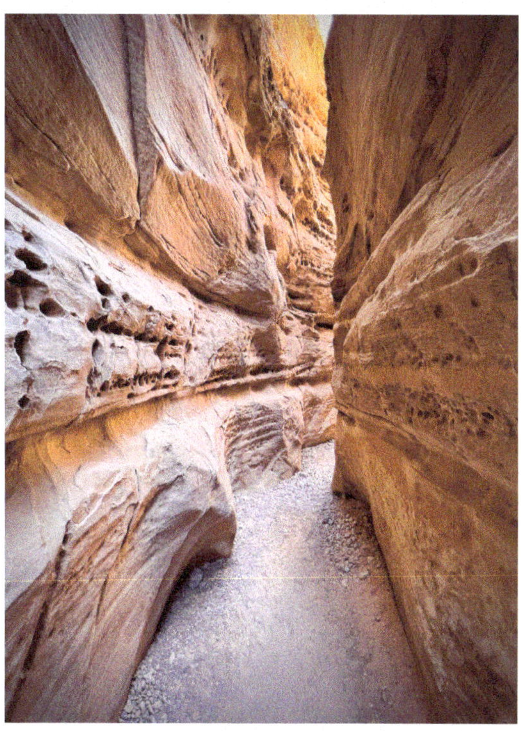

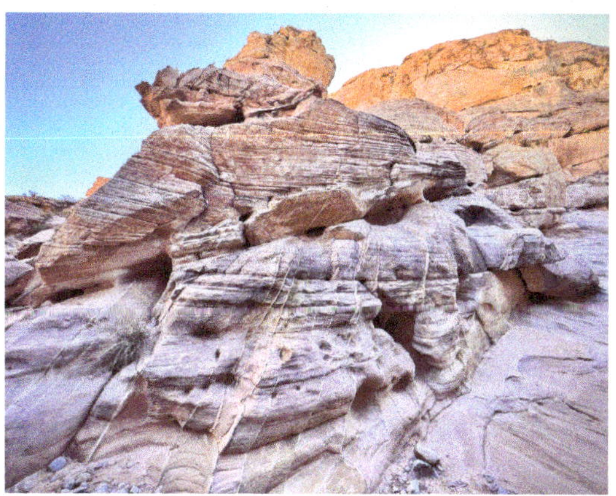

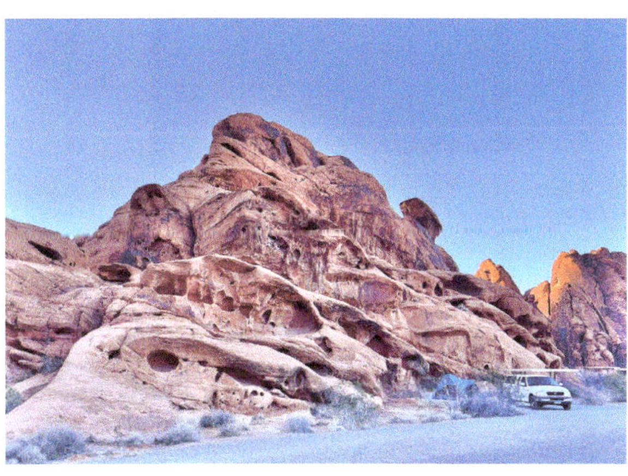

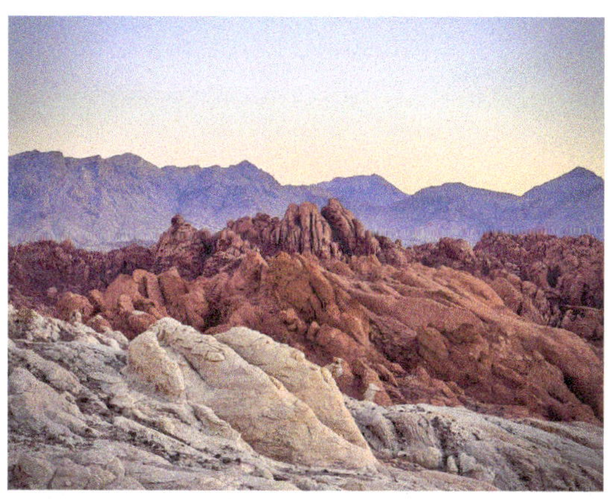

DAY 23 / MARCH 12

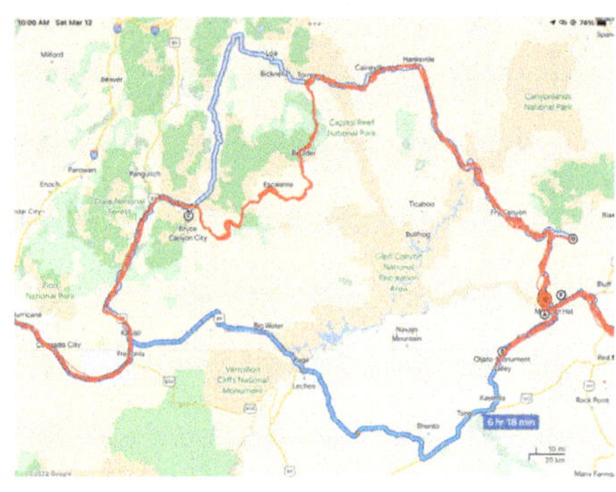

Called my friend Jennie.
Haven't spoken to her since leaving on the trip.

"Where are you going next?"
"I don't know."

I just make it up as I go.
After talking to her for a while
and mentioning my wish list,
I did have some kind of plan.
Screen shot a map.
Drew the route with my Apple Pencil
and started driving.
150 miles of interstate driving on the I-15
80 miles per hour
to 6000 foot elevation.

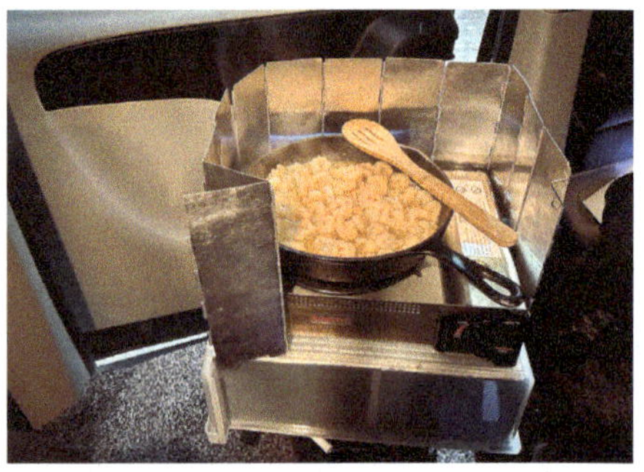

Forgot to refer to my travel plan
and ended up in Cedar City, Utah.
Tired and didn't want to drive anymore.

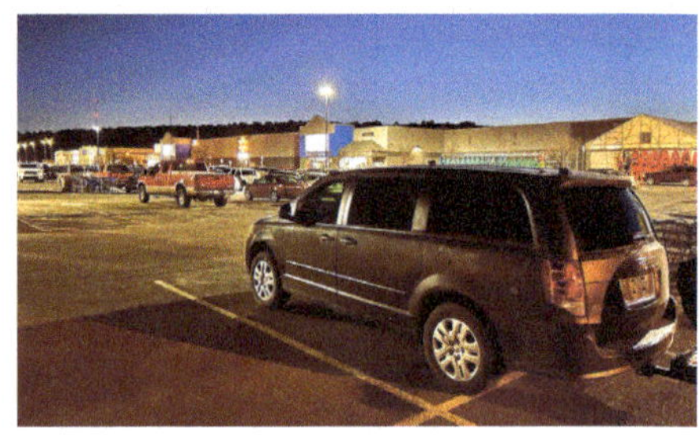

My first overnight parking with permission at Walmart.
A good vibe in the parking lot
and I felt comfortable staying there.
I picked a spot that felt safe,
someone wouldn't collide with the spare tire on the back
by driving too close.
The van was a dark color,
and the spare tire cover was black
and difficult to see in low light.

Shopped at Walmart to support business.
Shrimp for dinner.
Cooked in the van, it was cold and windy outside.

Traveled into Mountain Time.
It was also Daylight Savings Time.
Lost two hours.
Adjusted the clock in the van to reflect time at home.
I wouldn't want to call Mark
after he had gone to bed already.

DAY 24 / MARCH 13

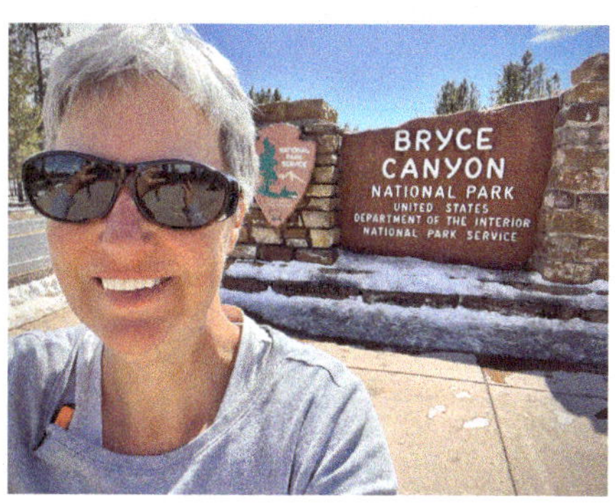

Drove from Cedar City, Utah
to the rest area 3 miles from the
Bryce Canyon National Park entrance.
Made some crazy elevation gains up to 9,870 feet.
Saw lots of snow and it was very cold.

Bryce Canyon was very busy,
making it difficult to find parking in the popular areas.
It was grueling to walk on the ice
on some of the paths and trails.
I was afraid of falling and getting hurt.

Drove all the way to the end of the park
scouting a sunset location.
Met Laura and Benedict from Germany
traveling in a rented RV.
The RV parked across the handicapped parking spots.
He transferred Laura out of the RV.
She had severe cerebral palsy
and relied on him for transfers.
She had a full-time job at a bank in Germany.
They invited me to visit them in Frankfurt.

I watched how much assistance she needed for everything.
And wanted to cry for her.
I could walk and drive,
but couldn't read or think well enough to have a job.
I would take independent mobility any day
over reading,
understanding verbal directions, dizziness
and the neurofatigue.

Changed my mind about the sunset location.
Scrambled to set up the gear.
I had to choose between looking for the gloves
and setting up.
My hands lost feeling.
But I got the shot.
A woman from Salt Lake City looked at my pictures
and helped me get the filter off the camera.

I no longer used the viewfinder to compose pictures.
It was painful to look through
and it caused blinding white lights.
It took a long time to recover from the fatigue
and blurred vision afterwards.

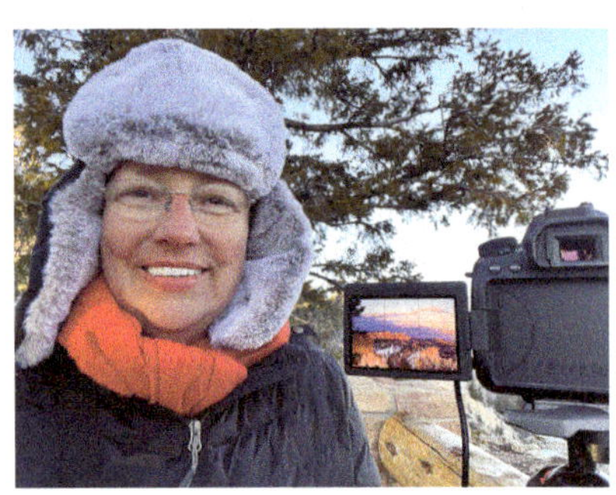

Also, while looking through the viewfinder,
I didn't have visual feedback
from where I was in space
and would lose my balance.
Potentially knocking the camera and tripod over.
And falling.

I used the LCD screen on the back of the camera
to check settings and compose pictures.

Mark's comment on my Facebook post picture:
"You look happy."

I forgot what happy felt like.

I saw everything I wanted at Bryce Canyon.
I didn't really enjoy the scenery.
Visually very busy
and overwhelming to look at,
especially with snow part of the landscape.
Maybe in summer.

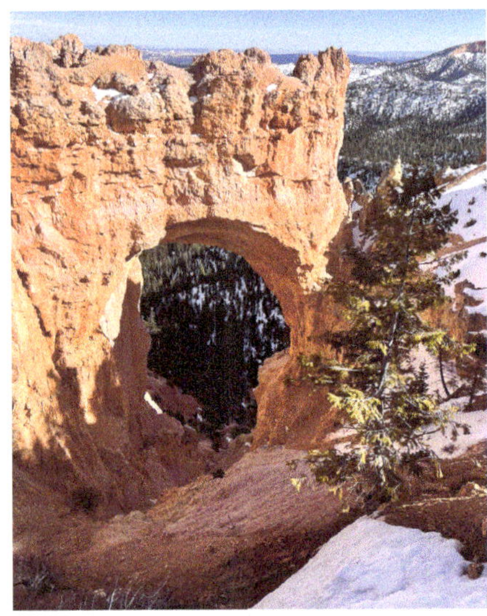

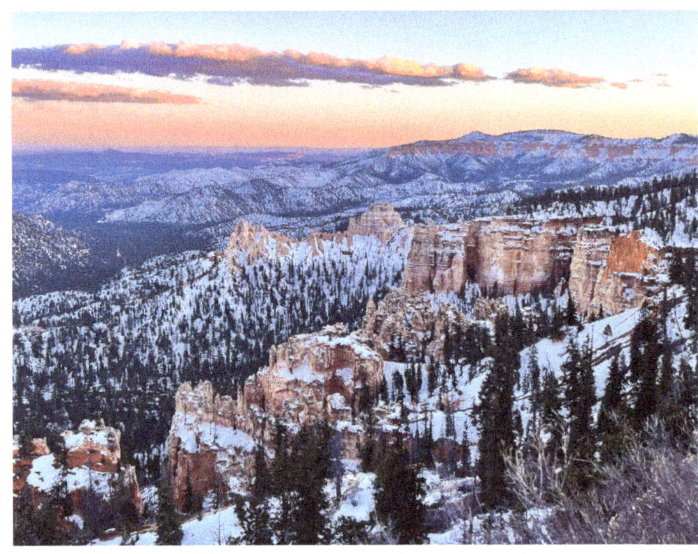

DAY 25 / MARCH 14

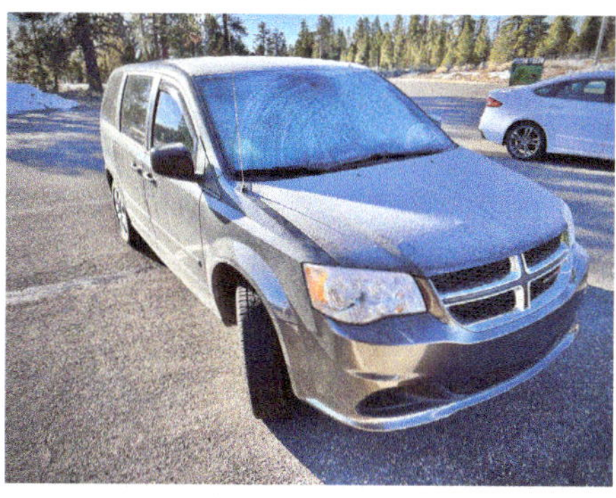

The van was covered
in heavy frost in the morning.
Two girls from Texas in another vehicle spent the night.
I hoped they were warm enough.
I slept in my snow pants and down jacket
in the sleeping bag.

Woke up during the night to put my winter hat on.
That was the only night I slept with the hat on.
It was supposed to be 14F (-10C) overnight
without the wind chill.
It was very windy.
So easily below zero (-18C).

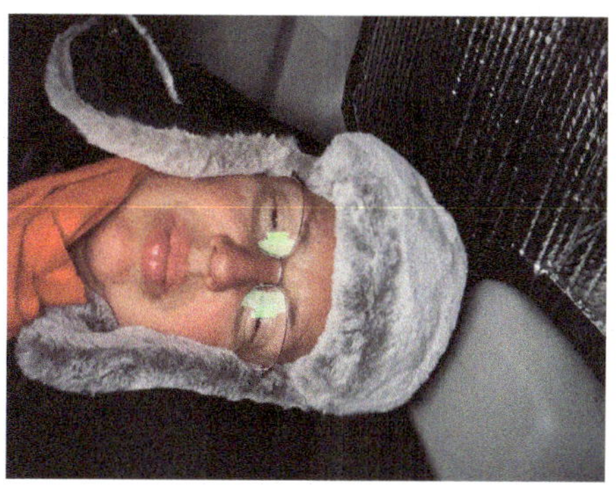

Noticed in one of my selfies
I had a flashlight clipped to my shirt.
Neon orange tape on it so I could "see" it.
Easy access to a flashlight in the dark
without having to look for it first.

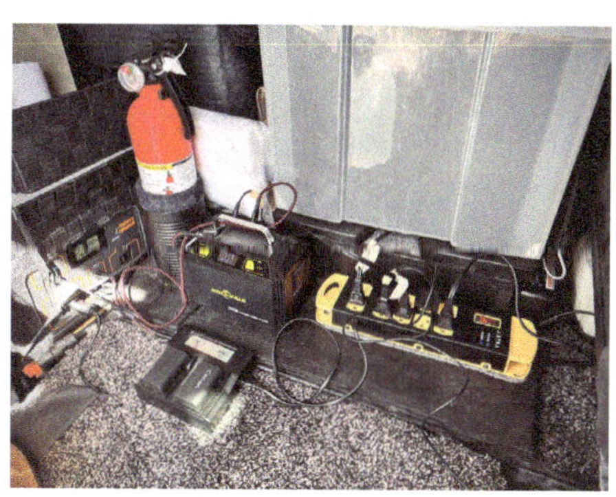

I drove 30 minutes
to Kodachrome State Park and checked in.
I was lucky to get a site with water and electricity.
I could plug into shore power
and charge the deep-cycle batteries,
devices and camera batteries.

Connected the 12-gauge extension cord
from the pedestal
to the shore power 110-volt plug
on the side of the van.

Used the electric kettle to boil water
instead of the butane stove.

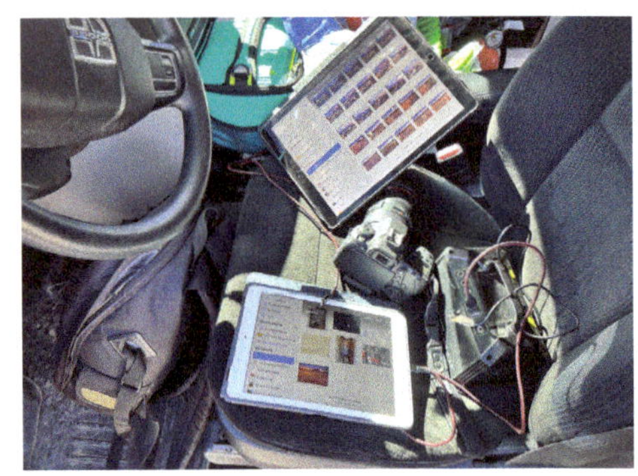

The visitor center had WiFi
and I could download pictures and check emails.
Slowly.
No cell service in the park.
Needed a quiet day to rest.
I didn't feel like driving all day.

Later in the afternoon found a road with deep ruts.
It was dry after the recent mud,
and I followed the road to the end.
Did some serious thinking
about making a judgment error.
Mark said to take time to think about what I'm doing.
Use good judgment.
Translated to "don't do anything stupid."
I thoroughly enjoyed the "off-roading"
and wanted to do more of it.

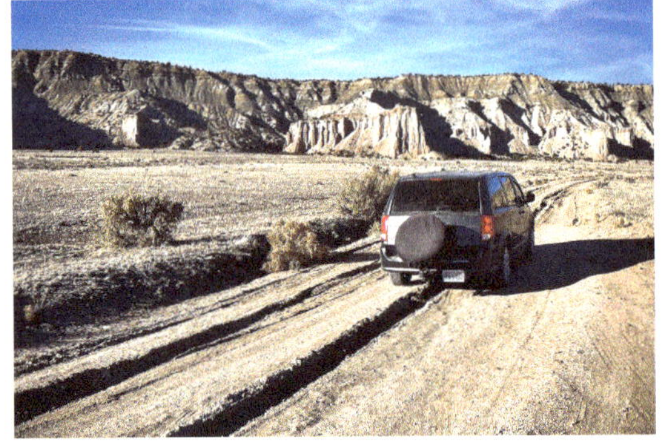

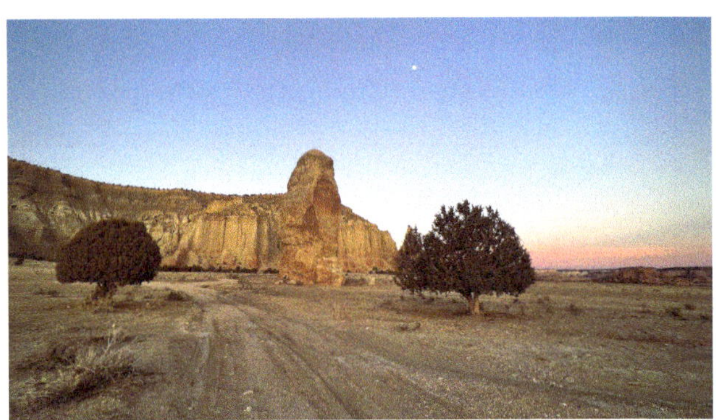

DAY 26 / MARCH 15

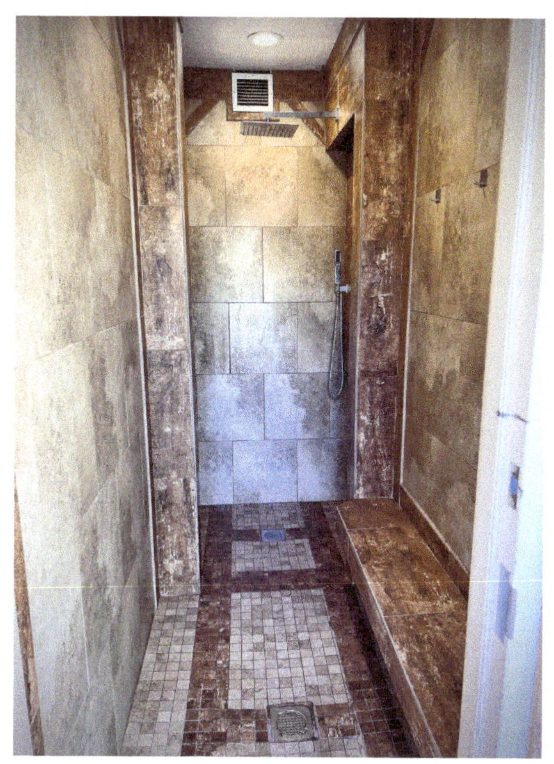

Took a shower in the best
and most modern-looking camp bathroom.

It looked like a bathroom in a luxury hotel.
The advantages of state parks,
showers were included
in day use and camping fees.

Waited at the park visitor center
for emails and photos to download.
Met two cyclist ladies.
They immigrated from Germany in 1998.
They were doing a long cycling route
and looked like professional cyclists.
I arrived in the U.S. in 1997
and became a citizen in 2010.

Drove to Torrey, Utah.
It took 6 hours to complete the 2.5-hour drive.
And I saw Lower Calf Creek Falls Trailhead.
On the list to do on a next trip.
Stopped multiple times
and took many pictures.

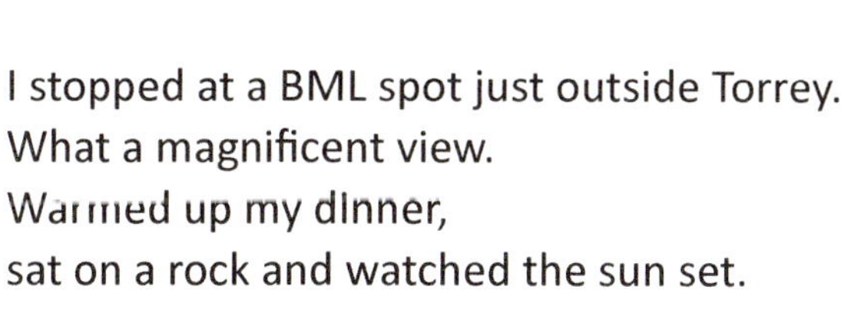

I stopped at a BML spot just outside Torrey.
What a magnificent view.
Warmed up my dinner,
sat on a rock and watched the sun set.

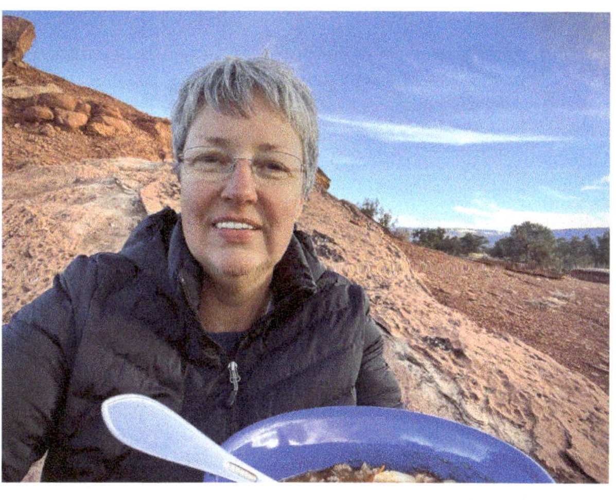

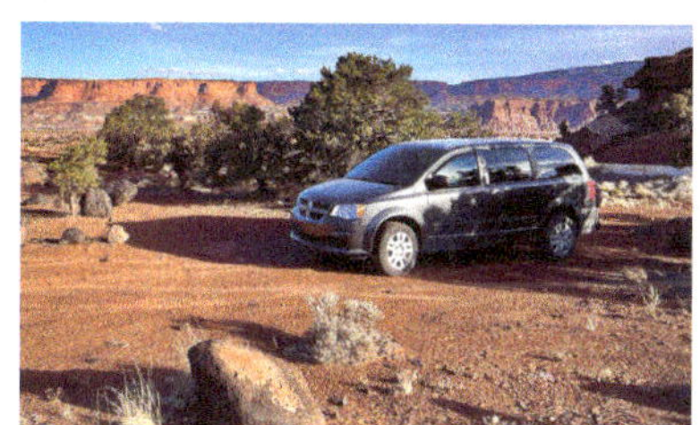

DAY 27 / MARCH 16

Highway 24 from Torrey to the I-70
was unbelievable.
The rock formations and vistas
were magnificent and varied greatly.
I couldn't stop looking
and taking pictures.
I had a cell signal somewhere
and called my brother-in-law Chuck.
He installed the suspension lift kit
and the hitch/spare tire carrier.
Told him how much I was enjoying
the changes he made to the van.
And about my first boondocking experience.

Capitol Reef National Park
was the biggest surprise of the trip.
And I would go back in a heartbeat.

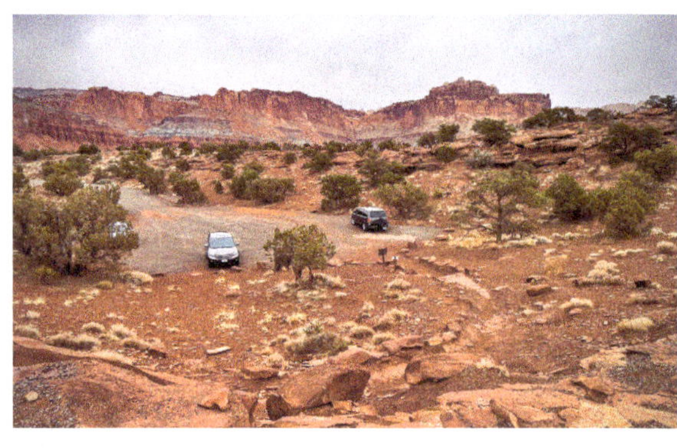

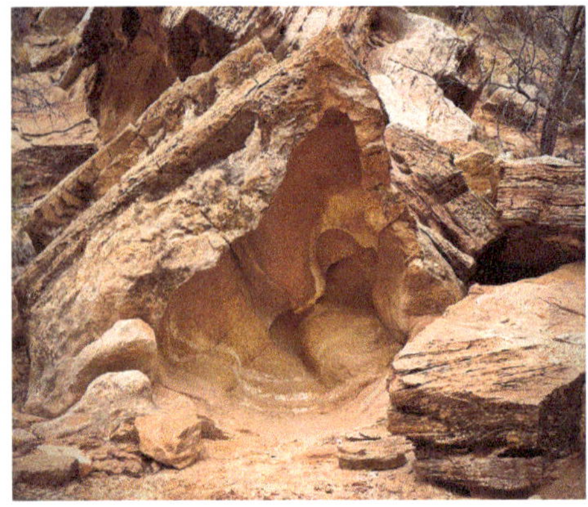

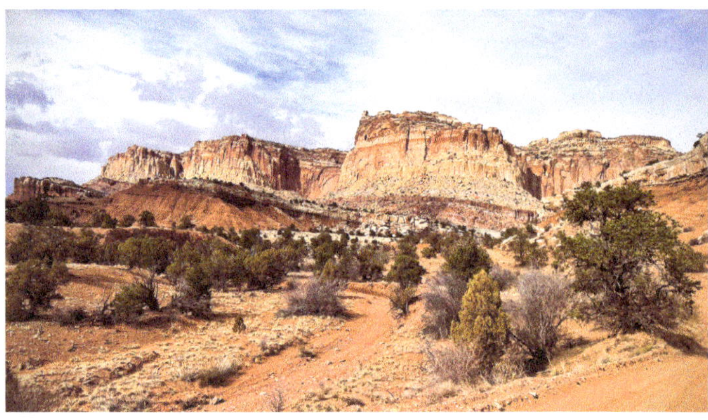

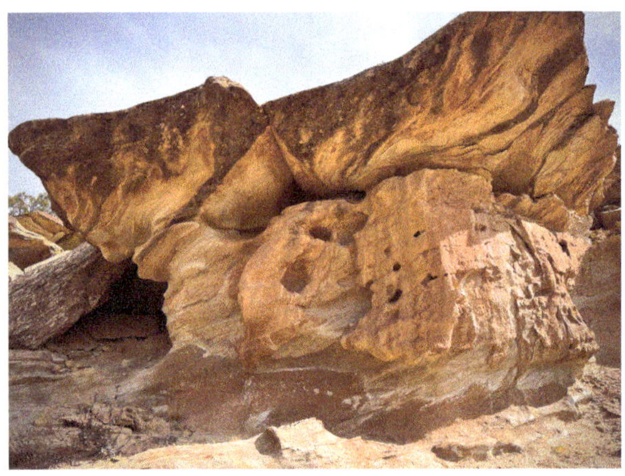

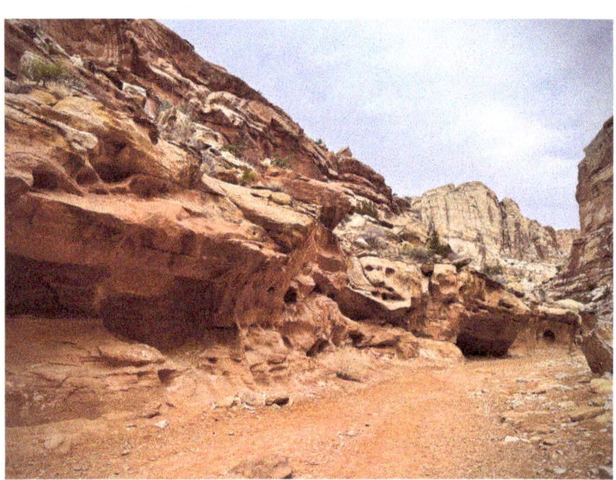

This one was very persistent with the begging,
but he got shooed away.
They were very pushy.
I was afraid they would stand up against the van
and damage the paint.

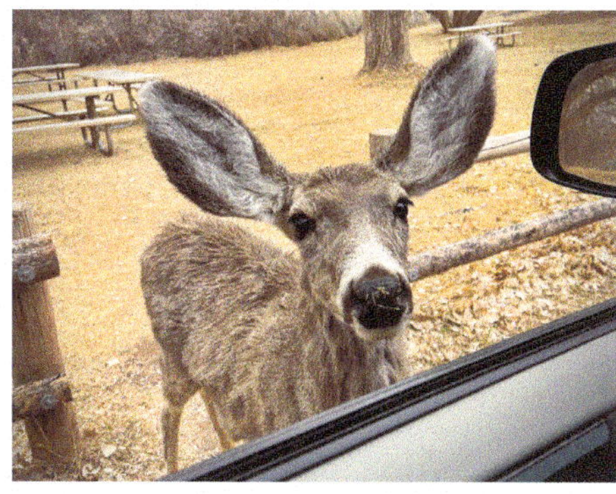

A massive thunderstorm pulled through in the afternoon.
I missed out on the Factory Butte area.
Planned to boondock there,
but when it rained in the desert,
dirt roads became impassable.
And it was better to avoid
expensive tow-truck assistance.

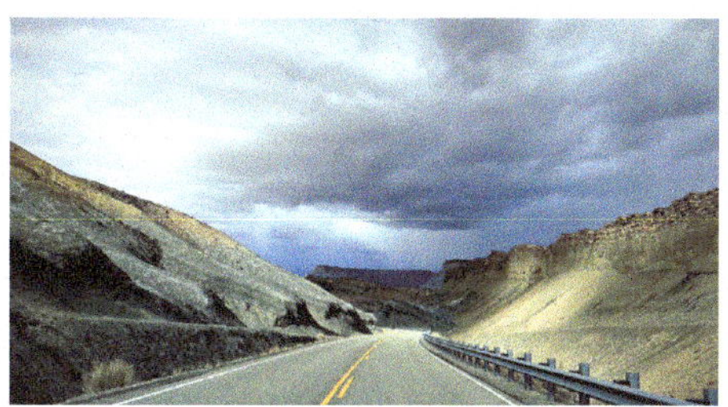

I made it to Green River
and found an overnight parking spot
at Love's truckstop with their permission.

I had newfound respect
for truck drivers on this trip.
They had to find somewhere
to park every night.
We tend not to think about how
the items on the shelves
in the store got there.

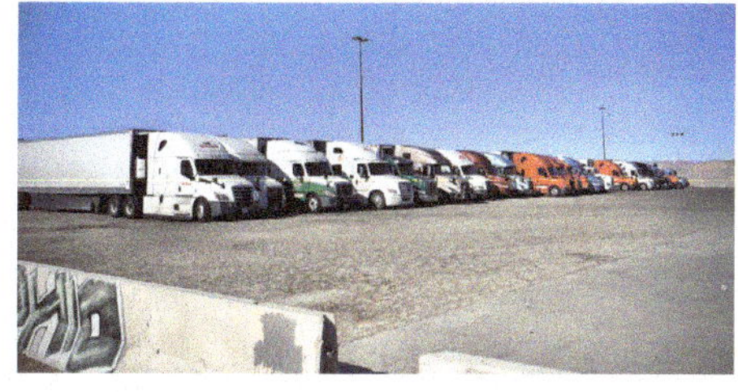

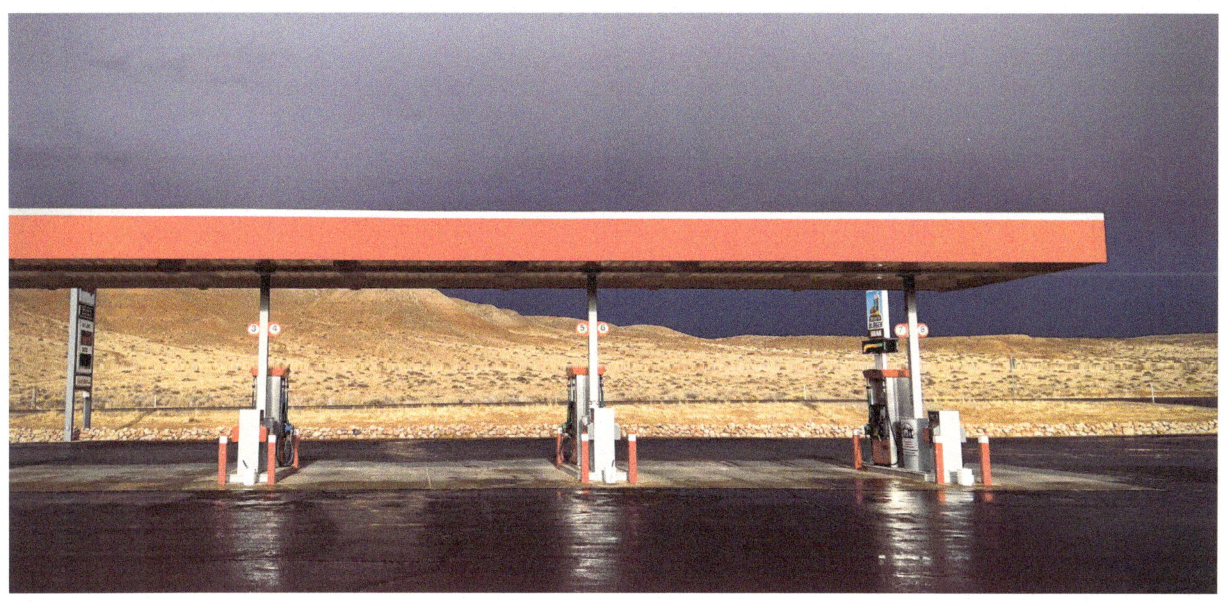

DAY 28 / MARCH 17

I woke up tired
and didn't feel like driving.

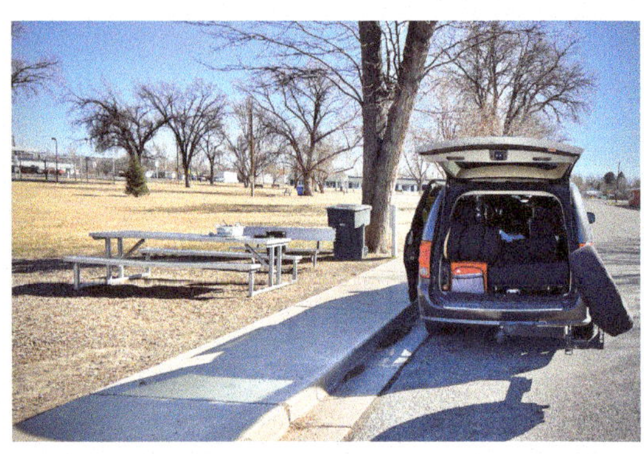

Found a picnic table at the local park.

Spent the day preparing meals,
cleaning fruits and vegetables,
and cleaning/tidying the van.

Amazing how much time cooking,
cleaning and daily tasks took
with no electricity,
running water,
or a washer and dryer.

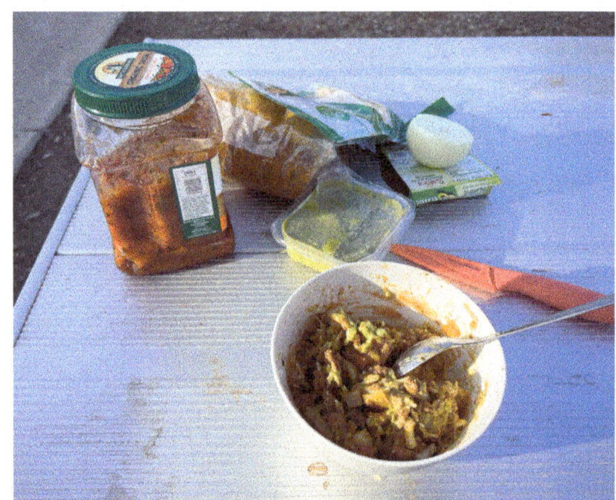

Caught up with friends Jennie, Daniel and Dana.

Took a nap
and shopped at the local store.

Discovered an innovative word.

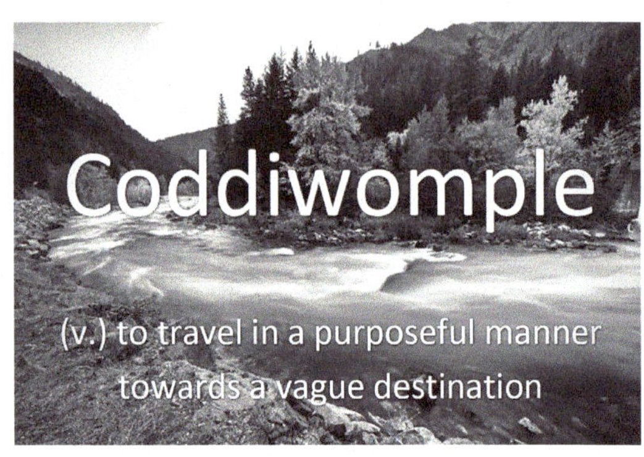

Coddiwomple:
to travel in a purposeful manner
towards a vague destination.

Very applicable to my trip.
Made it up as I went.
And I didn't know where I was going,
except meeting Mark in Corpus Christi.

DAY 29 / MARCH 18

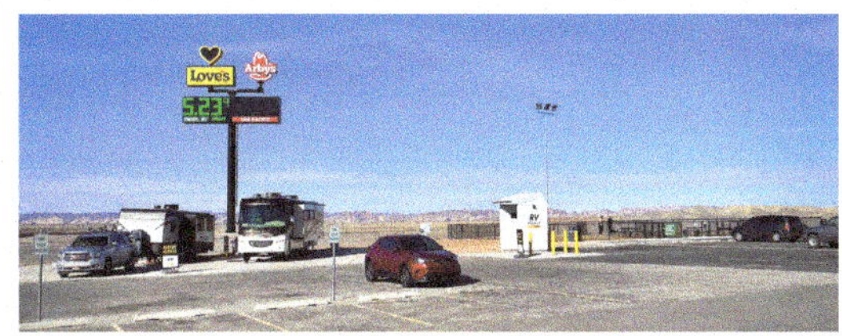

Love's was my favorite overnight spot.
They catered to RV'ers
with water and electricity hookups,
and had a dog park.

I looked out my window
and saw the van next to me
took off after dumping their garbage,
including a used baby diaper,
in the parking lot.
That was the ideal way to act to get
businesses to prohibit overnight parking.
Got gloves and dumped their deposit
in the garbage can.
Some people.

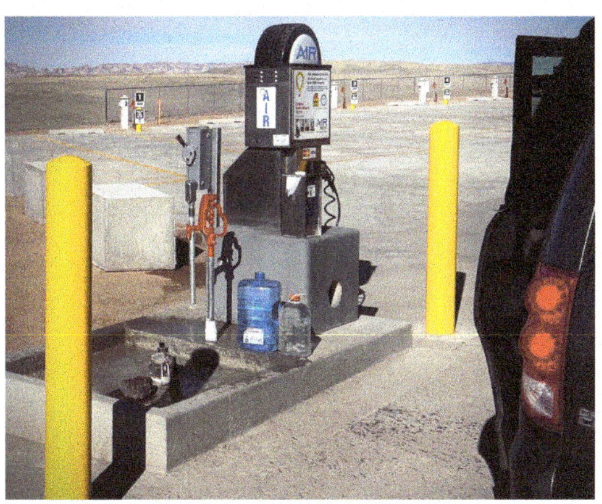

Love's had water spigots with red handles
and drains to dump gray water.
Easy to see,
but they took some getting used to,
and the water came out with a lot of force
if you did it wrong.

Next stop: Canyonlands National Park.

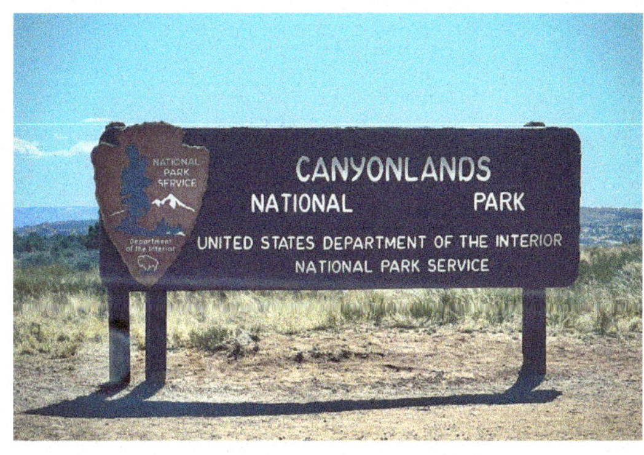

Arrived around noon.
The ranger at the entrance said
I had a remote chance
to get a spot in the campground.
I should drive the 20 minutes and go check.
Well, lo and behold.
As much as I hate the damn disability parking pass,
it saved my ass.

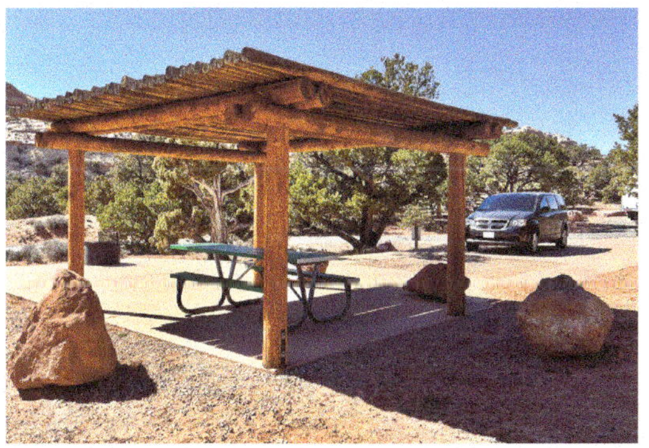

The disability site was still available,
the rest of the small campground was full.
I could walk fairly straight during daylight,
but I had non-existent balance in the dark.
Having a site next to the toilet was a blessing.

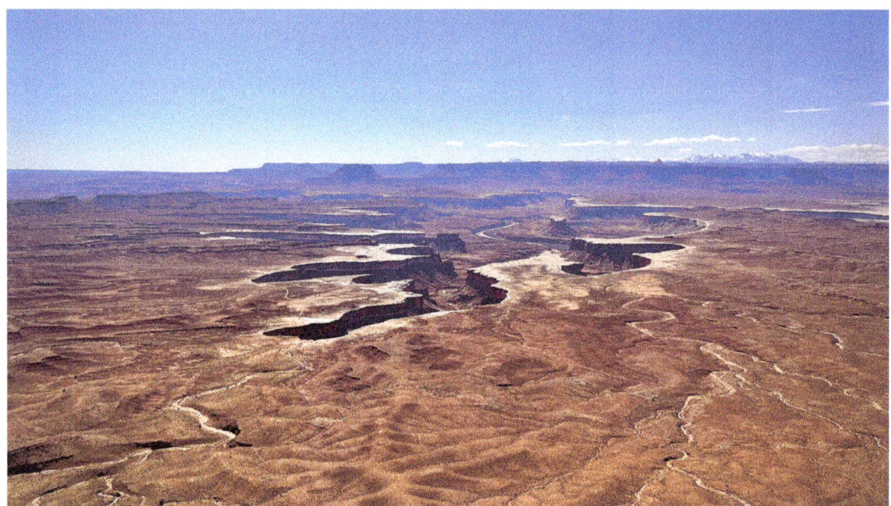

Green River Overlook was right
next to the campground.
I was in AWE of the view.
I saw it on Google Maps
and knew it had to be on my bucket list.
6,000 foot elevation and you could see
a hundred miles.
2,000 foot drop down to the canyon rim.
Unbelievable.
And I drove 2,952 miles to see it.

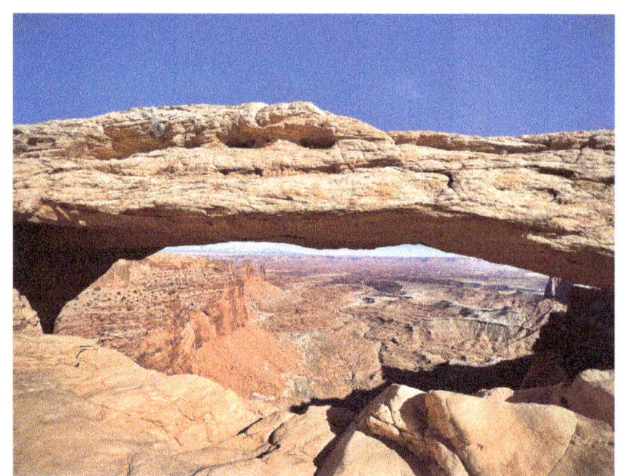

Mesa Arch is well known and too popular
with photographers for sunrise pictures
when the sun reflected inside the arch.
I saw it during the day.
It was difficult to get parking,
and to deal with the line of people waiting
to get a picture of the arch.
Get out of bed at dark, hike the downhill trail
with a big likelihood of falling,
and then elbow-to-elbow it
with 50 photographers to get "the shot"
I don't think so.
Green River Overlook was my scene.

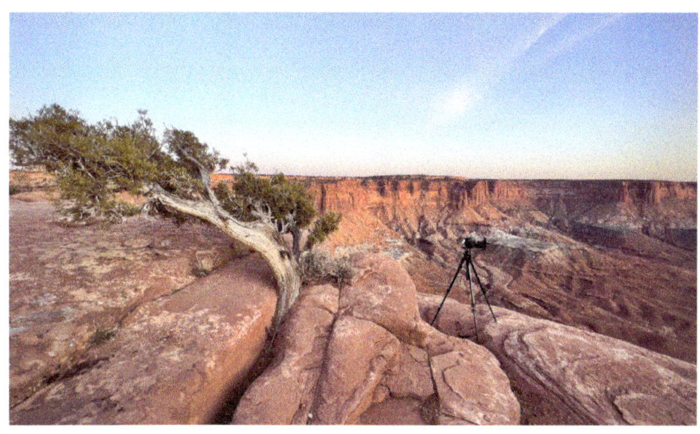

I found my ideal spot for the sunset shoot.
Right on the edge of the canyon.
Sat on the rock and scooted sideways
with my gear until I sat on the edge.
My heart was beating in my throat.
Had to talk myself into staying
and not bailing.
I had my feet spread wide.
I knew that I would have to shift my weight
so far forward
to fall off the cliff,
it wasn't even possible to do it like that
without standing up.
It still didn't take the fear away.
But I got the shot.

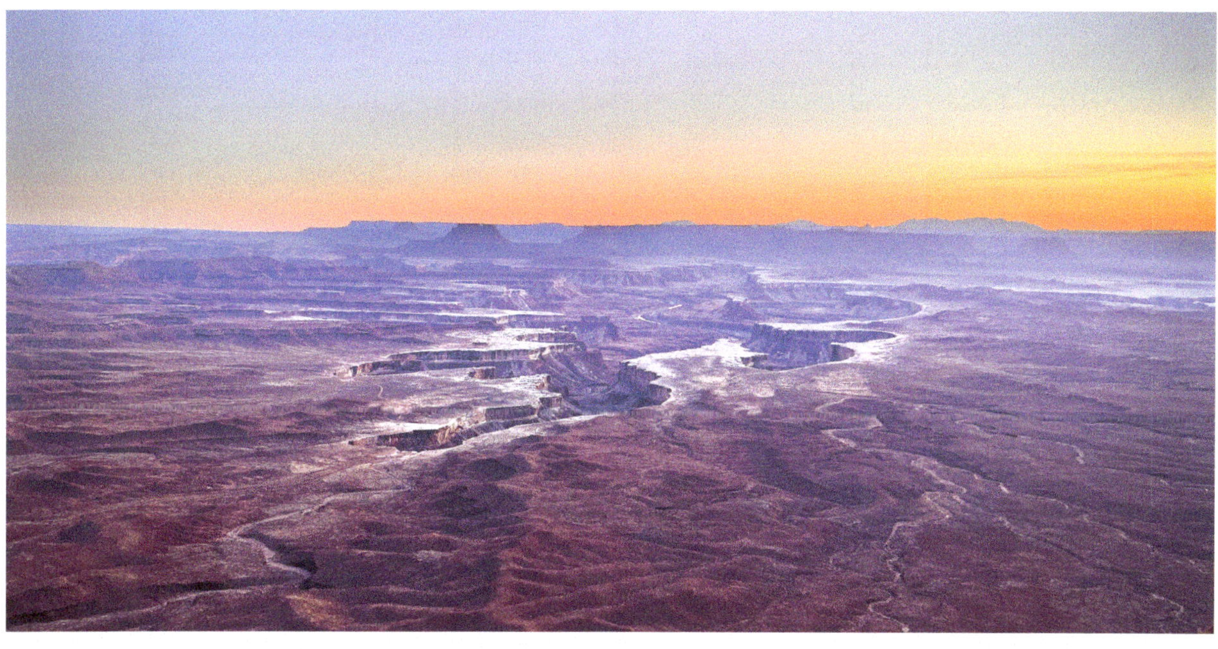

DAY 30 / MARCH 19 / 2,952 MILES

Got out of bed at 6:30am
for a sunrise picture at Buck Canyon Overlook.
It's a miracle.
I don't do mornings.

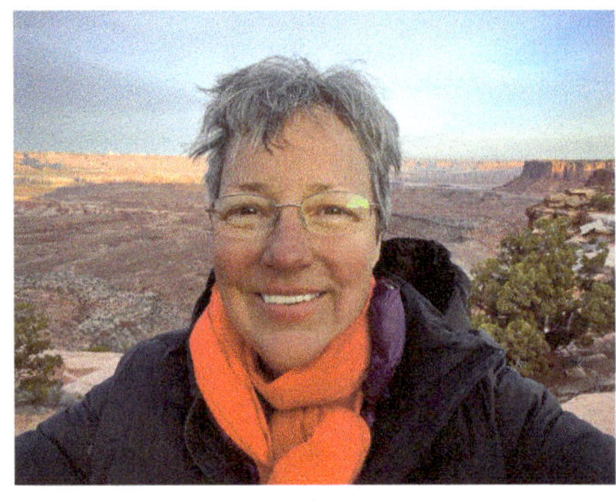

Here comes the sun.
Someone wrote a song about it.
A song about hope.

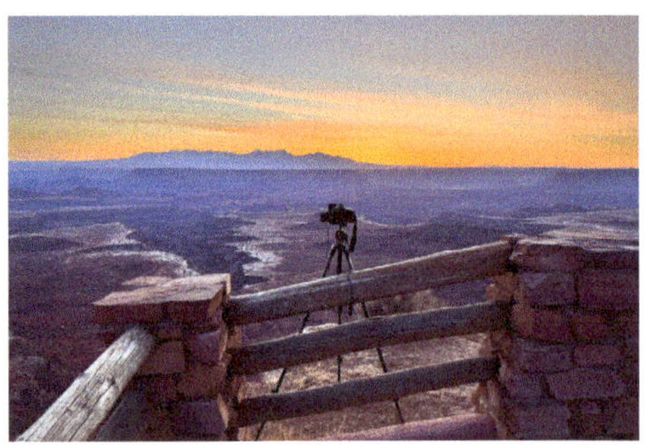

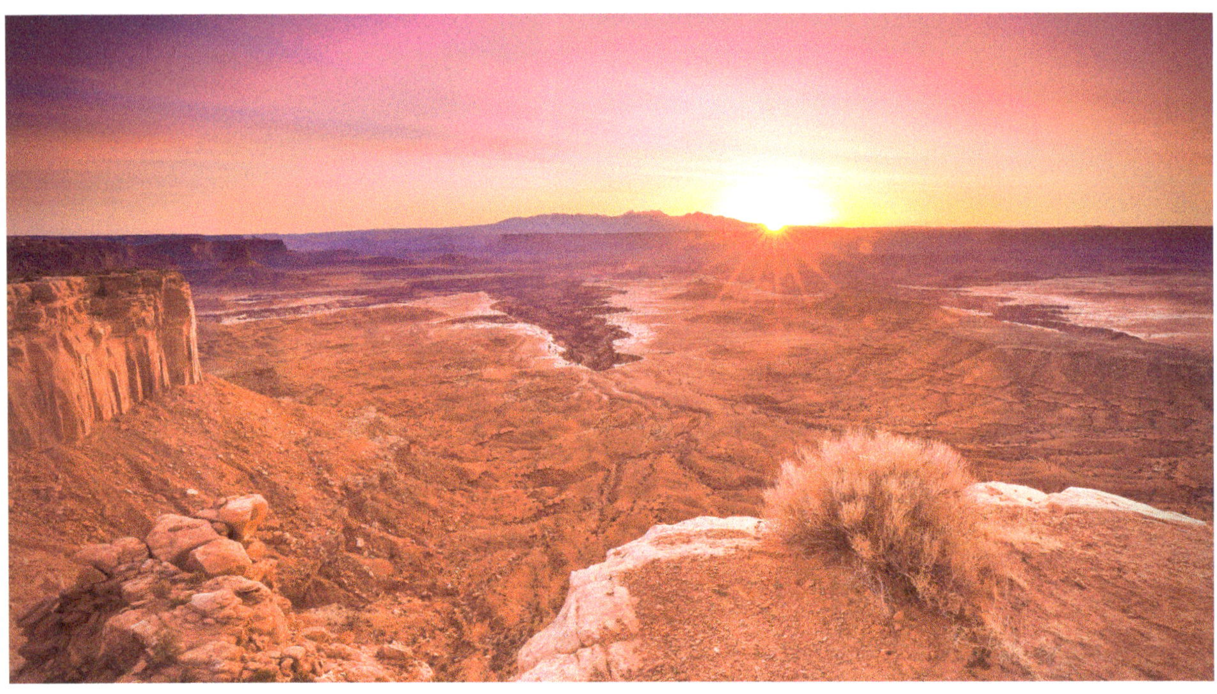

I had to step over the narrow ledge
to get to the edge of the canyon
at Shafer Canyon Overlook.
First, I thought it was too dangerous.
Kids from Wyoming walked by
and casually stepped over.
"Don't hesitate, just do it."
I stepped over.
I am alive to talk about it.

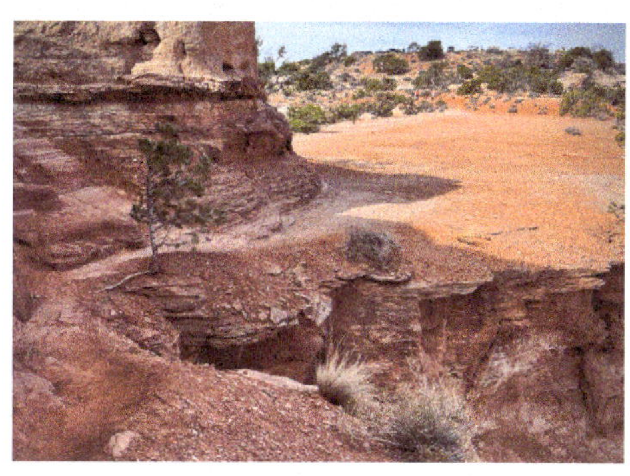

I wanted to lie on my stomach
to look over the edge,
but my butt would look too big in the picture.
I was obligated to sit and scoot closer.
Sliding my heel over the edge
was as much as my heart could stand.

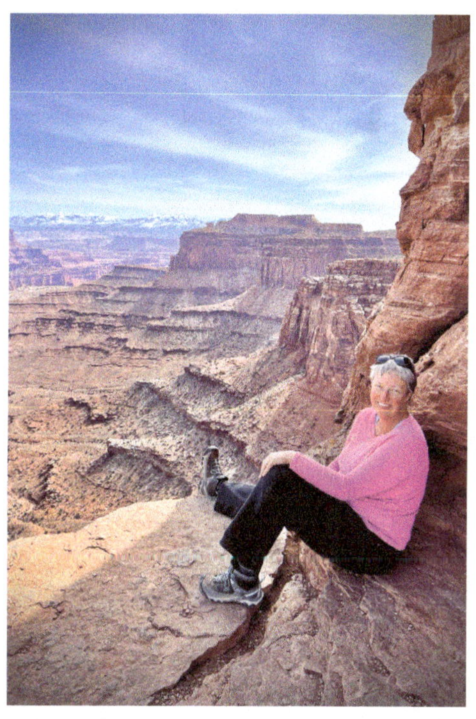

I went to Canyonlands National Park
with the intent of driving down Shafer Canyon
to where it leveled out and back up.
After I watched YouTube videos,
I was sure the van could handle it,
I probably would have a heart attack.

Shafer Canyon is a steep, narrow,
very rough dirt road
with small pullouts
to squeeze past oncoming traffic.
Had to back up to allow vehicles to pass.
The switchbacks were the turning radius of the van.

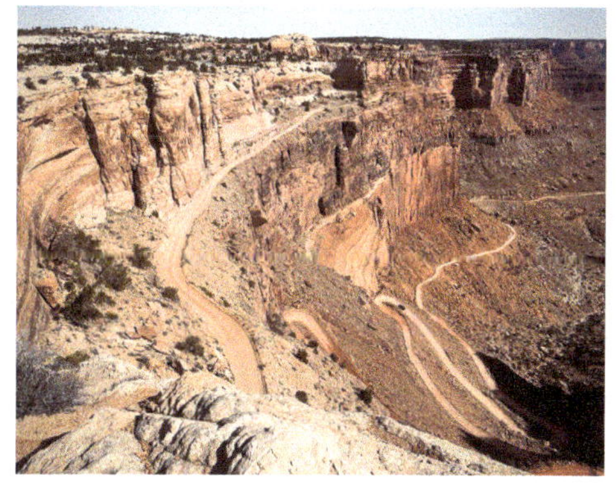

Drove over very nasty stuff
but did not bottom out on anything.

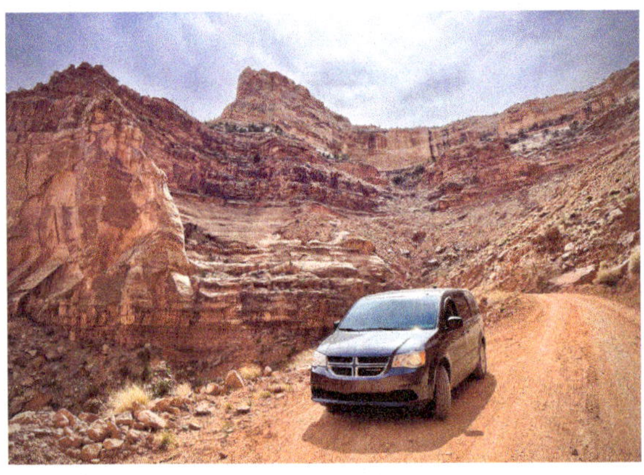

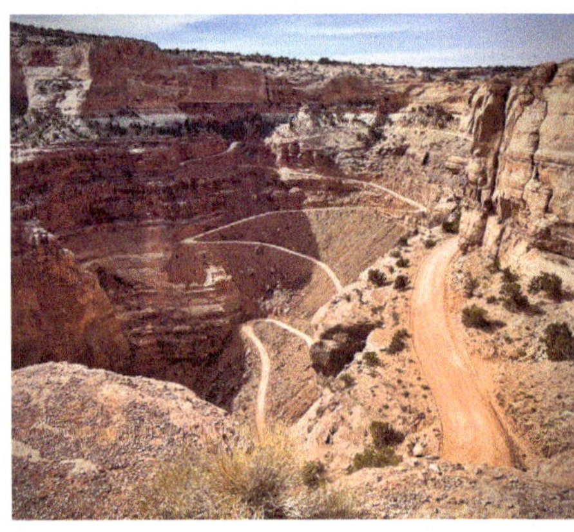

Van ground clearance 9 inches.
No railings anywhere.
I measured the incline, 9%.

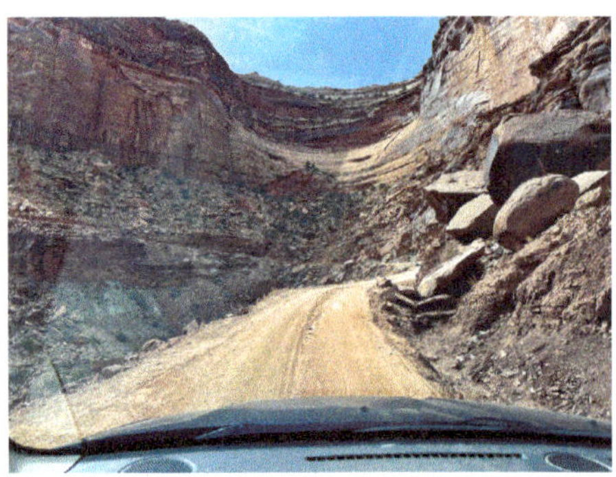

Was it worth it?
Oh, hell yes.
I was the only minivan on the trail.
And scared out of my mind.
Oh, and I shot video with my right hand
while driving back up.

The smile after I got back to the top
and my legs stopped shaking.

More a grimace than a smile.

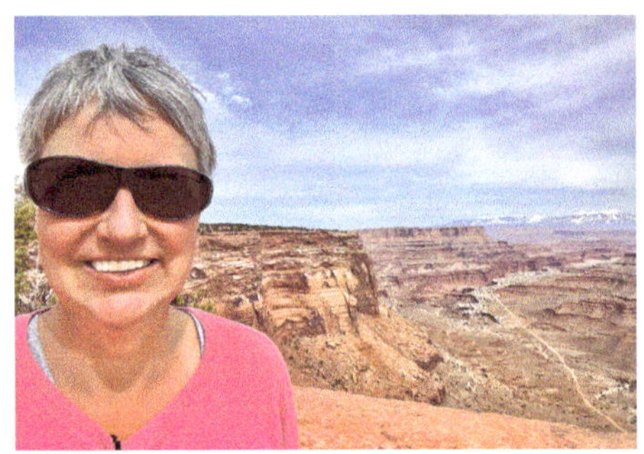

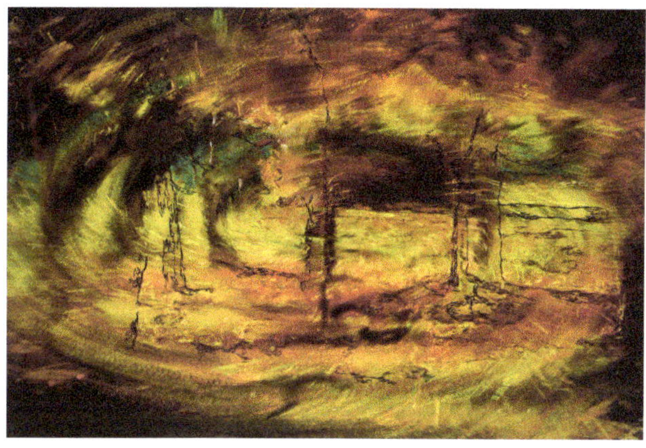

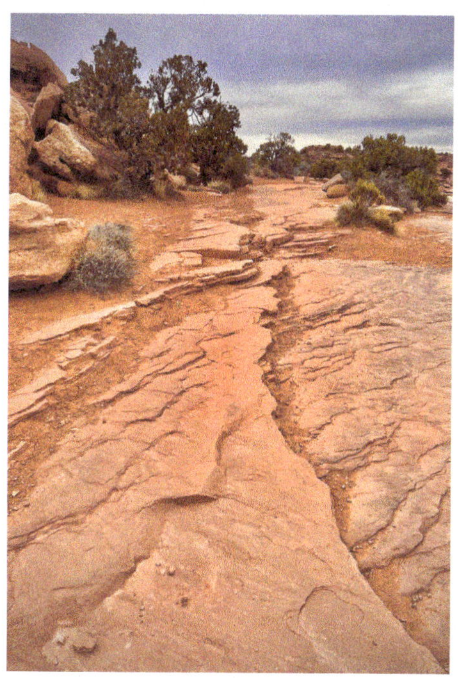

A side effect of brain injury was dysautonomia,
an autonomic nervous system malfunction.
It controlled blood pressure, heart rate,
temperature and pupils.
When my blood pressure dropped,
my heart beat like crazy to get it back up.

Felt dizzy, my heart jumped out of my chest
and I struggled to get air.
Also known as POTS.
Postural Orthostatic Tachycardia Syndrome.
Took a pill to lower heart rate.
Sometimes when hiking uphill, it would be bad.
Or just standing still.

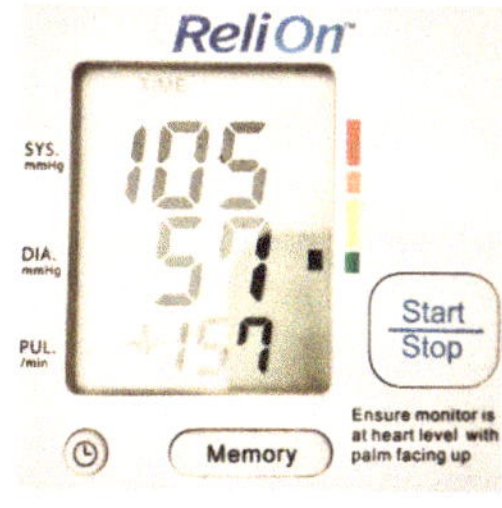

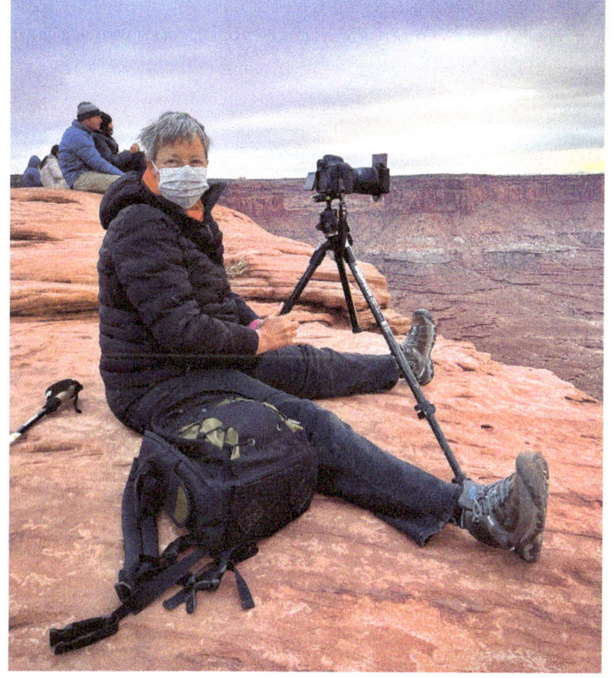

Another sunset picture session
sitting on the edge of the canyon.

After the day's activities,
there wasn't much left to fear.
Hung onto the tripod
in case it got sucked off the edge
by an invisible force.

DAY 31 / MARCH 20

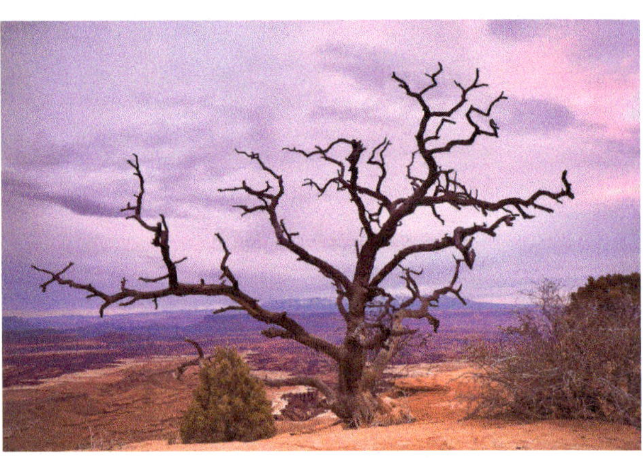

I got out of bed for a sunrise shoot.
Not much of a scenic sunrise.
And nothing new anymore,
standing on the edge of the canyon.

I was tired and unmotivated,
most likely caused by the change in weather
and fatigue from the previous day's activities.

Drove to Dead Horse Point State Park.
The $20 entrance fee
allowed park entrance
for two consecutive days.

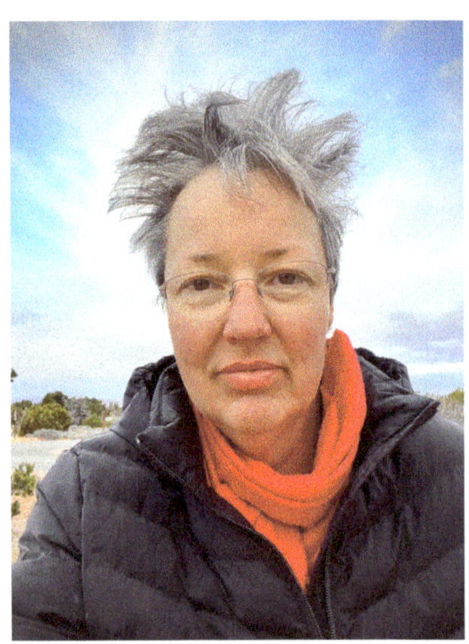

Scouted photo options,
and the park did not disappoint.
The horseshoe bend
in the Colorado River was spectacular.

I sat on a high rock enjoying the view
until the wind came up.
It felt like I could be blown off my rock.

The day didn't have much sunset potential
and I went back to the campground.

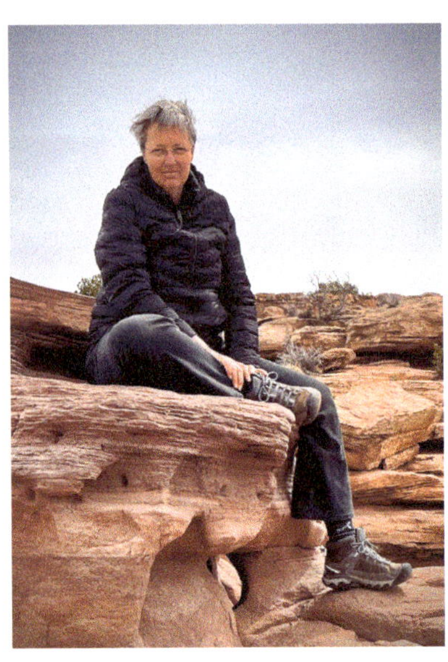

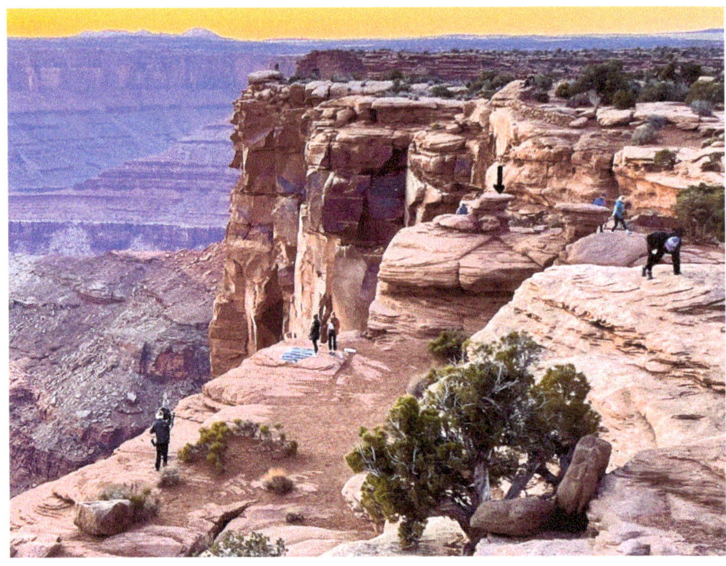

DAY 32 / MARCH 21

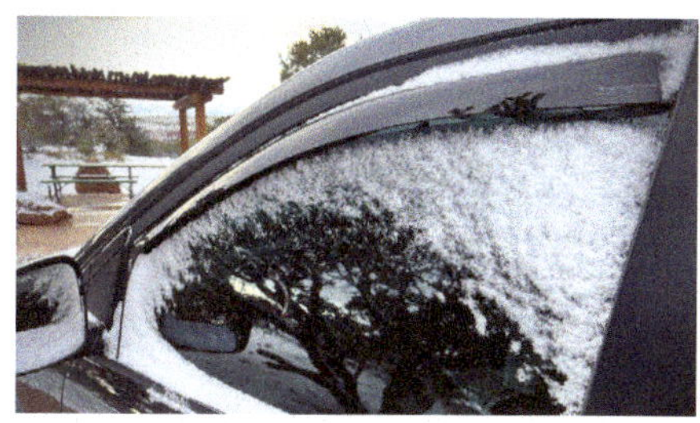

Well, yikadoodles.
It took a while to notice the snow in the van.
The wind must have been very blustery
to blow the snow through the
2-inch window opening
mostly covered by the rain guard.

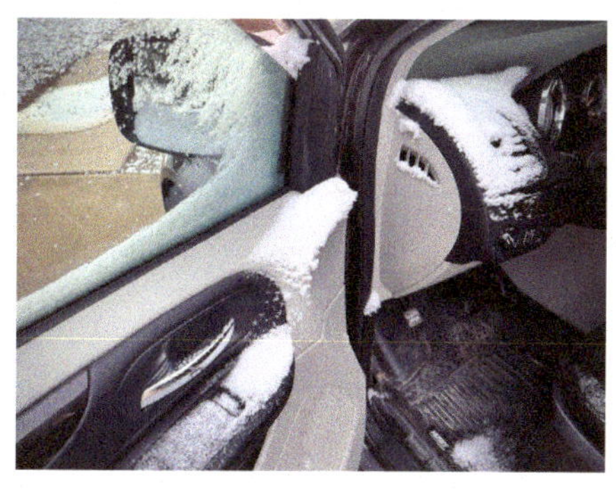

Slept like the dead through the night.
I could tell it was cold when I woke up, 28F (-2C).
It was warmer in the fridge than in the van.
I was very glad to be done with tent camping.

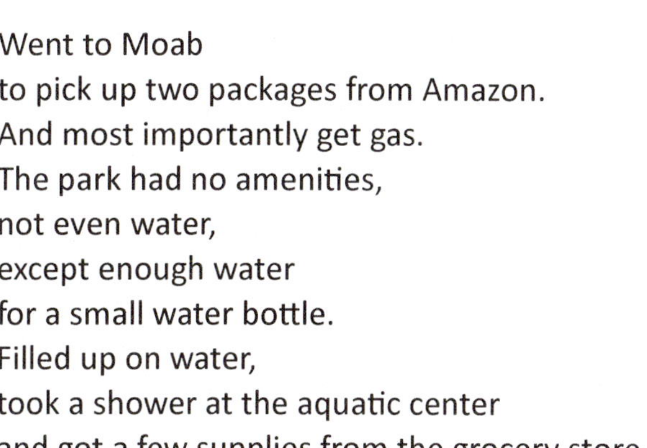

Went to Moab
to pick up two packages from Amazon.
And most importantly get gas.
The park had no amenities,
not even water,
except enough water
for a small water bottle.
Filled up on water,
took a shower at the aquatic center
and got a few supplies from the grocery store.

Talked to Ben with the 4x4 off-road vehicle
at the gas station.
Mentioned I went down Shafer Canyon
in my minivan.
He didn't say anything,
but the look on his face was priceless.

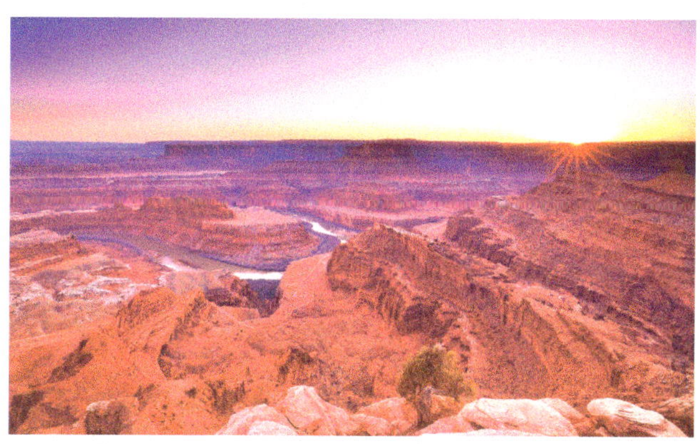

Spent the rest of the day
at Dead Horse Point State Park
waiting for sunset.
Gorgeous.
And a beautiful picture.

DAY 33 / MARCH 22

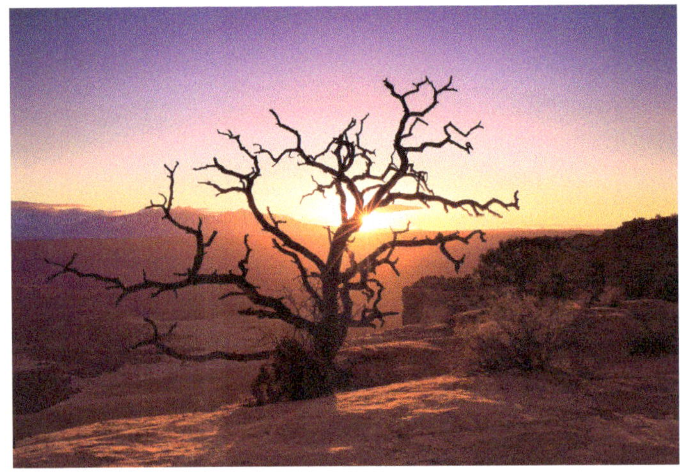

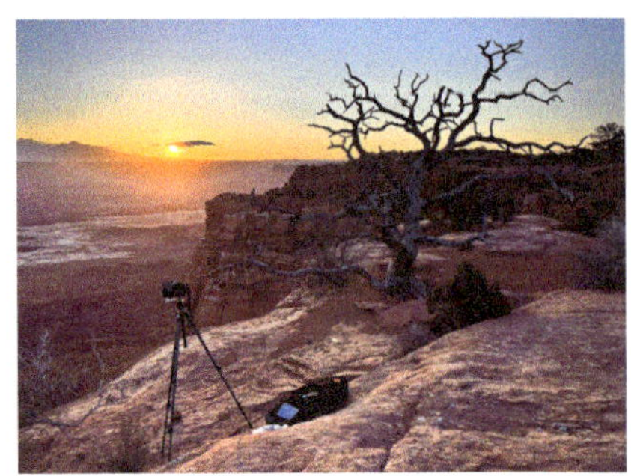

Got out of bed for sunrise,
and how worthwhile it was!
A picture of my favorite tree in Canyonlands.

Spent the rest of the day
cooking in windy conditions.
I moved over to the vacant site opposite me.
The handicapped site was cement mostly,
with very few options
to stake down the privacy tent.

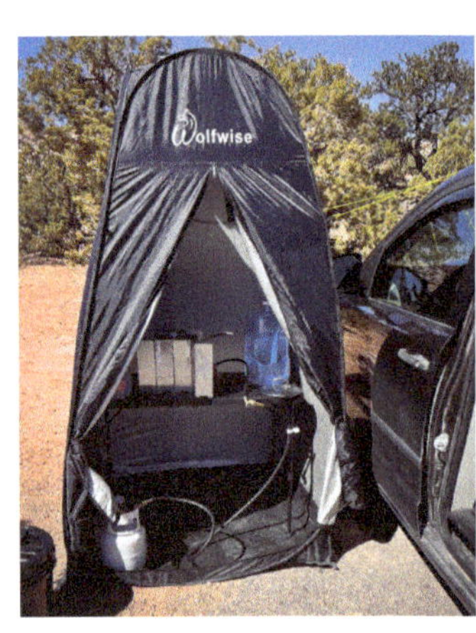

The shower privacy tent
had become a very valuable asset.
Wasn't used much for the initial intent.
And I had no clue how big a role the wind would play
during outdoor cooking.

The magnets on the roof where
the awning attached to the van,
had become versatile as well.

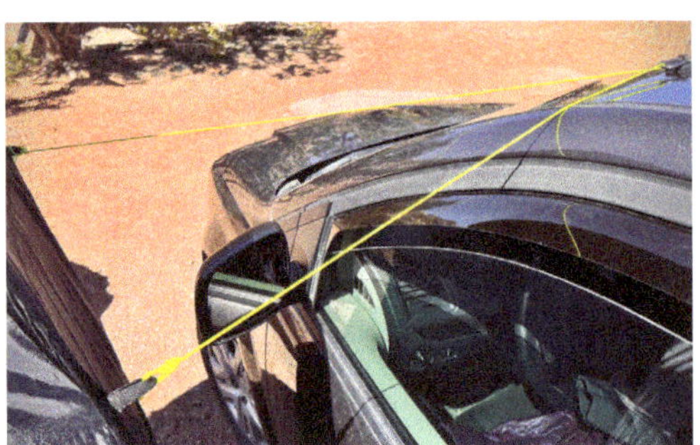

Used the 3-gallon water container
to weigh the lightweight table down.
I was afraid the gusting wind
against the tent
could knock the propane stove over
and start a fire next to the van.

Don't worry,
there was a fire extinguisher in the van.

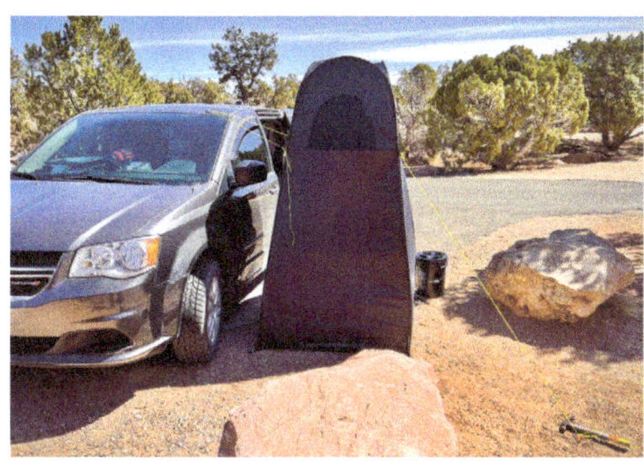

I made curry coconut cream chicken,
enough for at least a week of dinners.
The 400-watt Ninja chopper
worked excellently
off the 500-watt Jackery battery pack.
Good for making smoothies
and chopping onions and carrots.

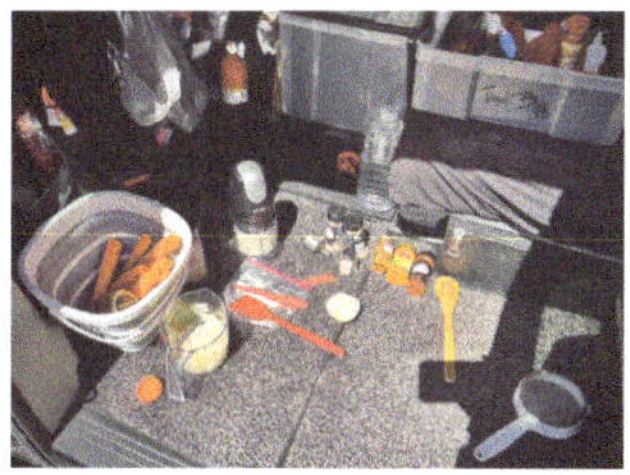

My cooking production was close
to the pay station in the campground.
Somehow,
I became "information booth" for the day.
A doctor from Germany
needed information
about camping
and how the first-come first-serve setup worked.

Two travel nurses showed up
and the campground was full.
I offered to move back to the handicapped site
and they could have my site.
One of the nurses was on his way to an assignment
in Spokane, Washington.

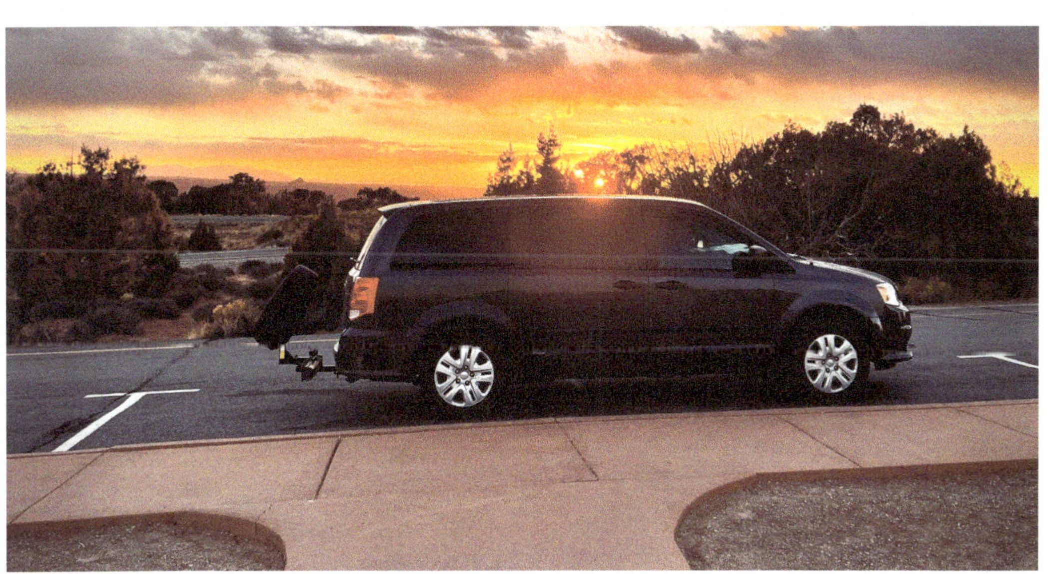

DAY 34 / MARCH 23

Left Canyonlands National Park.
Drove down the Colorado River,
checking out the campgrounds,
which were all full.
Very scenic and worth
investigating for future camping.

I found a few handwarmers I forgot I had.
They were fantastic!
Put one in the sleeping bag and slept with warm feet.

Stayed at Willow Creek BLM overnight.
The road in was very rough and bumpy,
but it's off-roading.

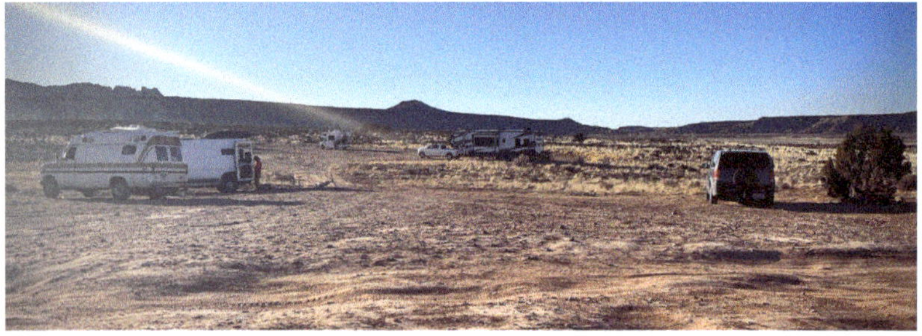

Beautiful view of the mountains.

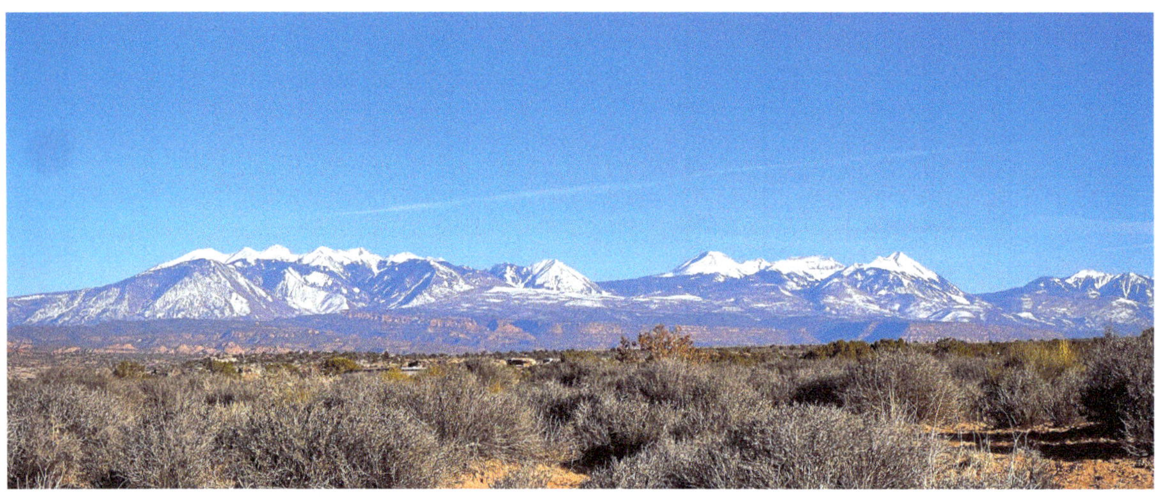

DAY 35 / MARCH 24

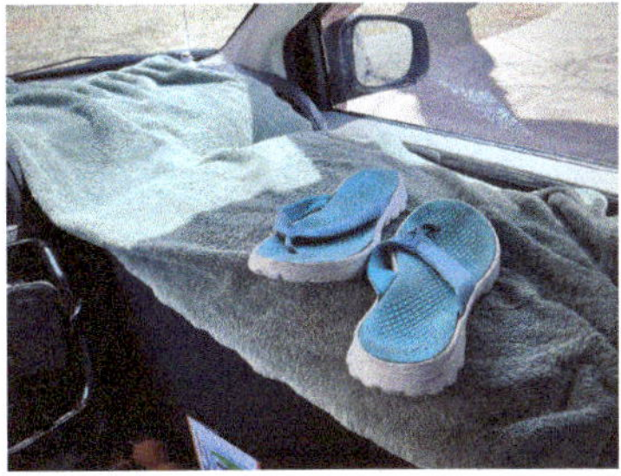

Showered at the aquatic center in Moab.
When I washed socks and underwear
in the shower,
had to dry them afterwards.
At home it's easy.
Putting them on the dashboard took care of the problem.

The flip-flops and towel dried well on
the black refrigerator.

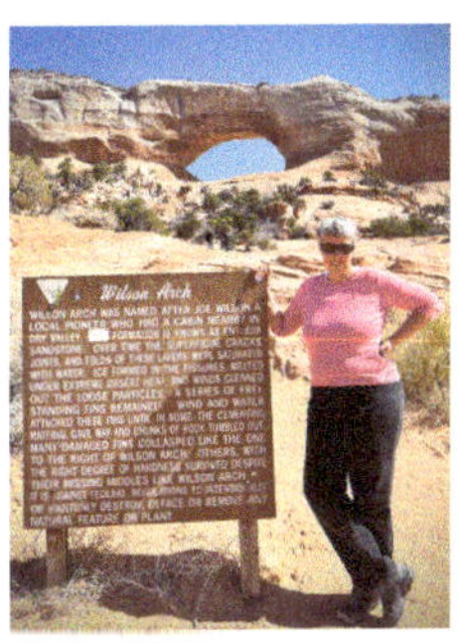

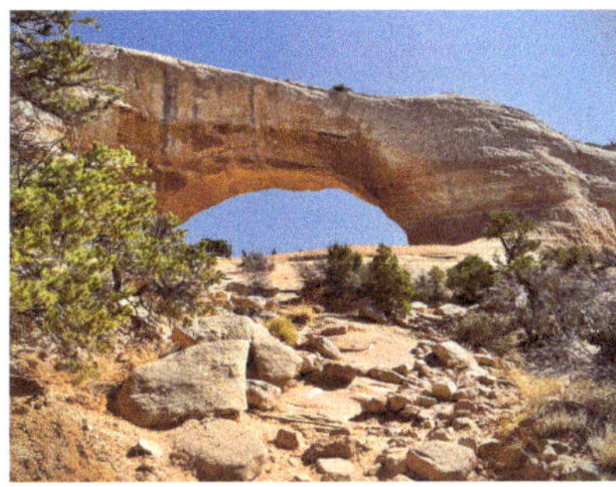

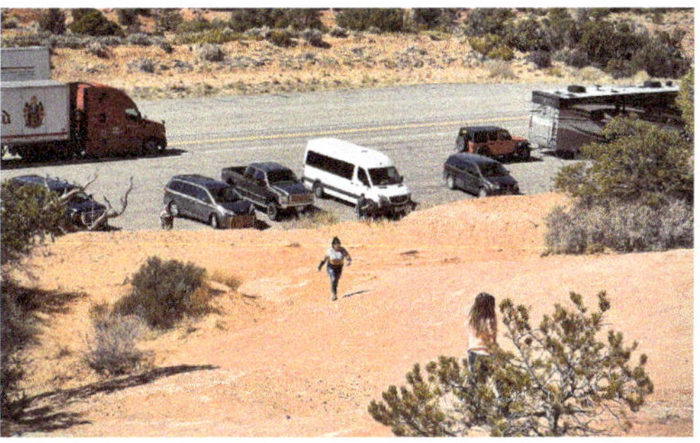

Headed south and stopped at Wilson's Arch.
Grand Central Station,
and amazed how many people
stopped to climb up to the arch.
I made it halfway
before better judgment kicked in.

Met a truck driver, Doug from El Paso.
We talked for at least 30 minutes
about the life of a truck driver.

His regular route was to Washington state
and back to El Paso weekly.
His other route was
4,500 miles to New York state
and back to El Paso.
Very tiring.

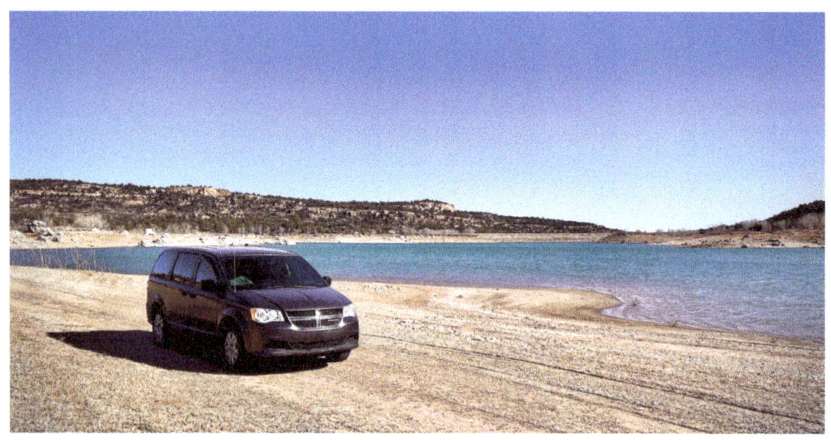

Considered staying at the reservoir,
but it was very windy.
And I did not feel comfortable
with how long it would take to get out
and back to the highway in case of trouble.
So, it was a pass.

Stayed at a gas station in Branding
with their permission.
The cashier said there was a campground
next to the gas station.
I mentioned my road trip
and my limited budget.

The gas station was not on the iOverlander app,
but I asked for permission,
and it was granted.
Got some gas and dinner
to support the business.

DAY 36 / MARCH 25

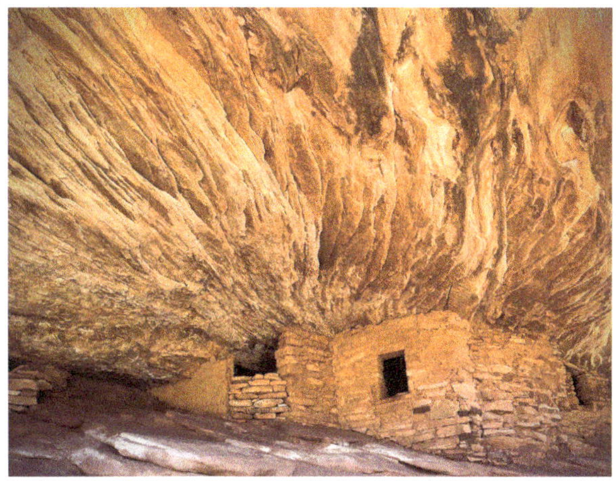

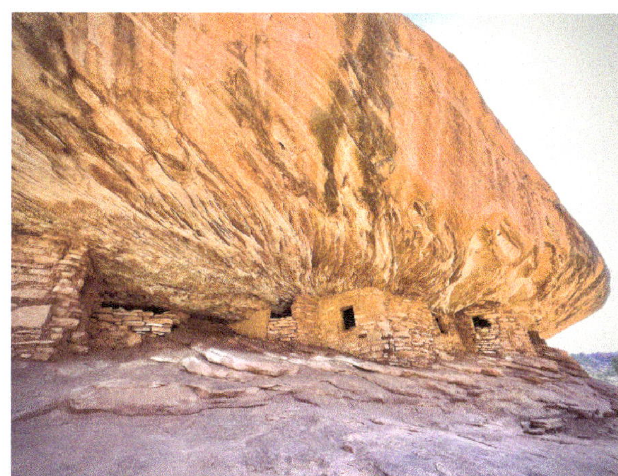

From Blanding, Utah headed to "House on Fire."
It was very hard to find.
Good thing I downloaded directions
Google Maps was not helpful.
There was no signage coming from the east,
but when I turned around to backtrack,
a sign indicated the turn off the highway.

Finding the trailhead
was equally hard,
and if I didn't see people
disappearing into a ditch,
I would have been none the wiser.

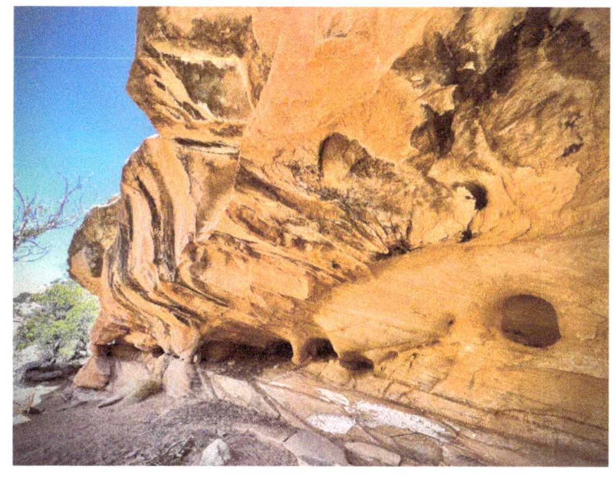

I was running late, the optimal time
to see it was between 10 and 11 am.
Did a quick trot up the 1-mile trail.
Never done a mile
in less than 20 minutes
on uneven terrain.

Met many awesome people from
Canada and Sedona
including Winter, a small dog,
who wanted me to pet her
and sit on my lap.
The trail had many outstanding rock formations
and I took many pictures.

About 30 miles up the road
was Natural Bridges National Monument.
I was fortunate and found a spot
in the campground.
I had a backup plan for BLM spots
along the highway.
The park had three huge bridges,
carved by wind and water over time.
Unbelievable scenery.
Some of the trails to the bridges
included climbing down metal ladders.
Not for me.

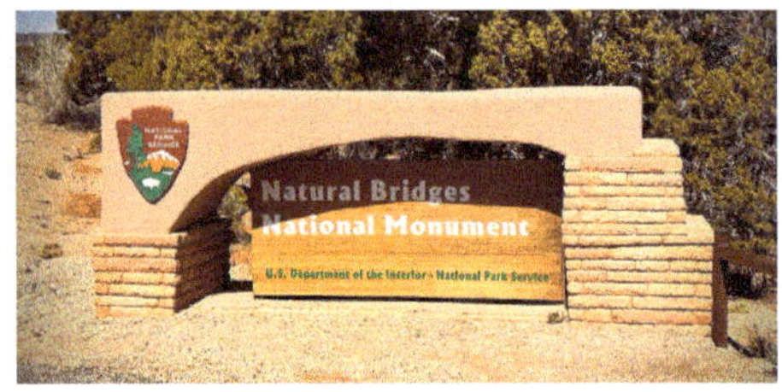

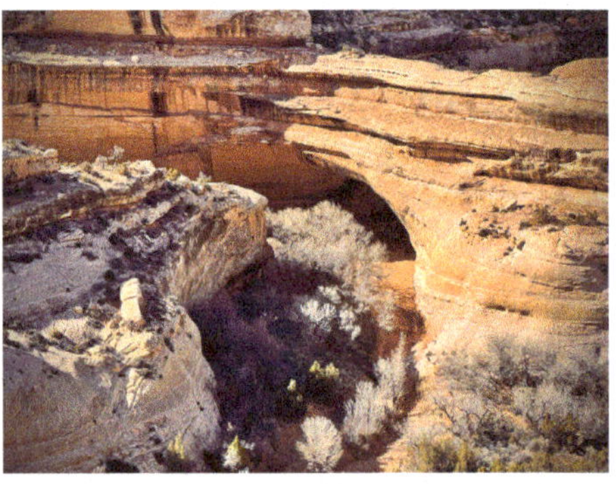

Met Ken and Valerie from Massachusetts
who traveled in a 38 foot RV.
Talked at length about RVs and they gave me
a tour of their RV.
Wonderful to be able to stand up in it.
They requested a tour of the van,
and I noticed afterwards
the urinal was in plain sight.
Insert eye roll here.

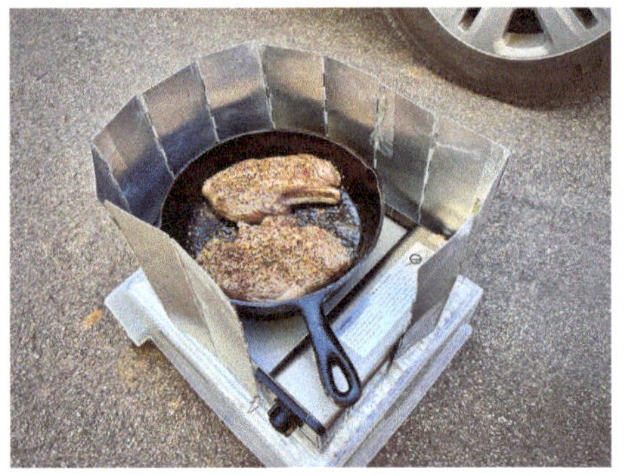

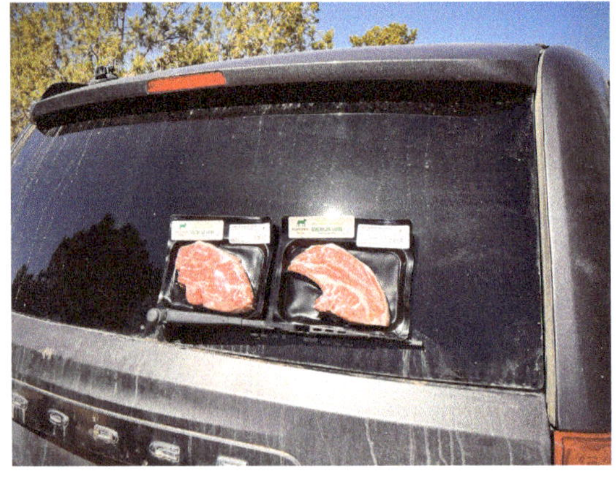

Lamb chops for dinner.
Easiest way to defrost the meat,
put it on a black surface facing the sun.
Didn't take very long to defrost.

DAY 37 / MARCH 26 / 3,484 MILES

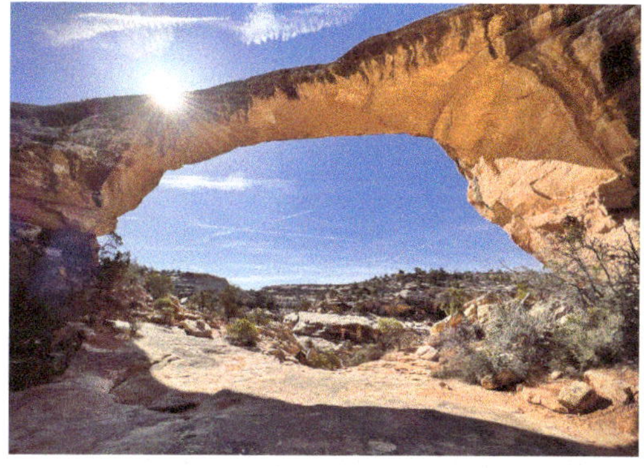

Hiked the easiest trail
to the Owachomo Bridge.
Majestic.
Unbelievable.
And huge.

Climbed,
crawled
and scooted
down a steep incline
to get a good shot of the bridge.
Sometimes you are in more trouble
than you thought you would be in.
But I made it back out in one unharmed piece.

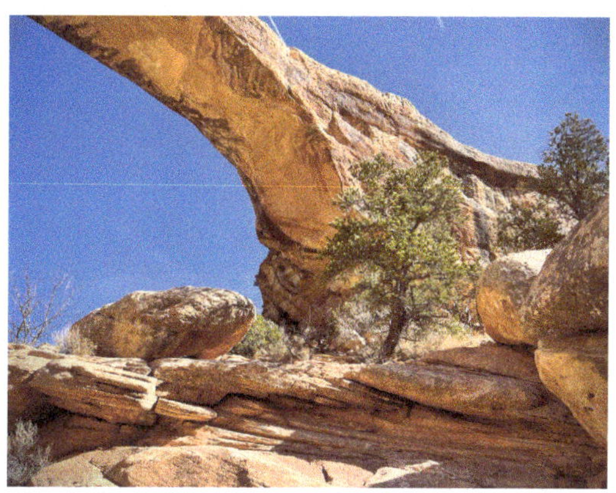

Not to lose the van keys,
put it in my bra.
The shorts and T-shirt didn't have any pockets.
After the hike I was standing next to the van
feeling for the keys.
Not a thing.
My heart about fell out.
I had a spare key under the van,
but it was better not to lose the keys.
I debated whether I should backtrack
and go look for the keys.
Checked the hiding place in the bra again
and thank God hallelujah,
they were down further in the valley than I thought.

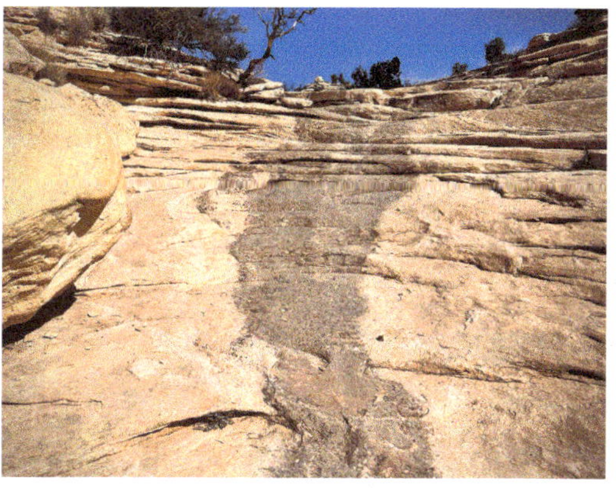

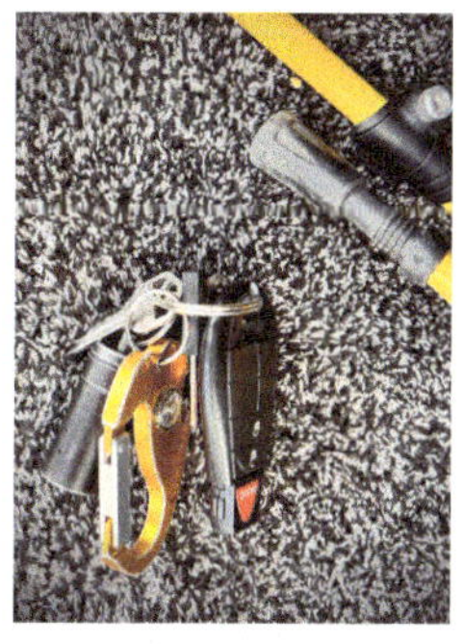

Headed south
to the top of the Moki Dugway
where a dirt road turned to the right
for about 5 miles to Muley Point.

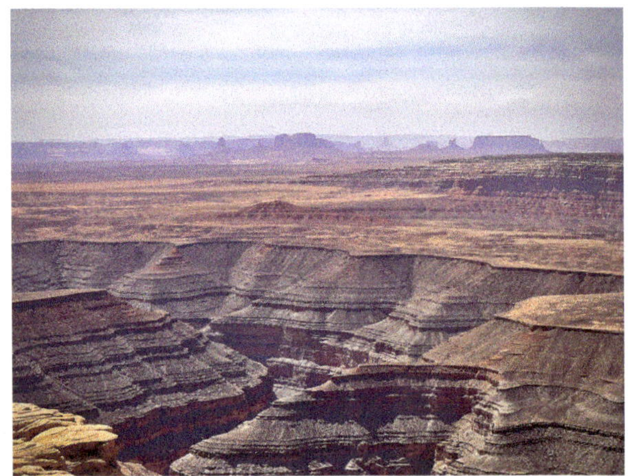

Saw it on a YouTube channel
and put it on my bucket list.
The most incredible views over canyons.

Monument Valley off on the horizon.

And boondocking spots
along the edge of the canyon.

Saw two kids getting engaged.
No one was taking photos.
I texted them the few I got,
when I realized what was happening.

I slept about 12 feet from the edge of the canyon.

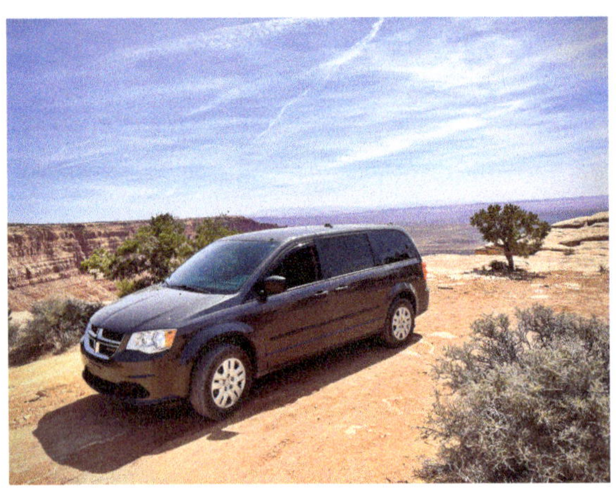

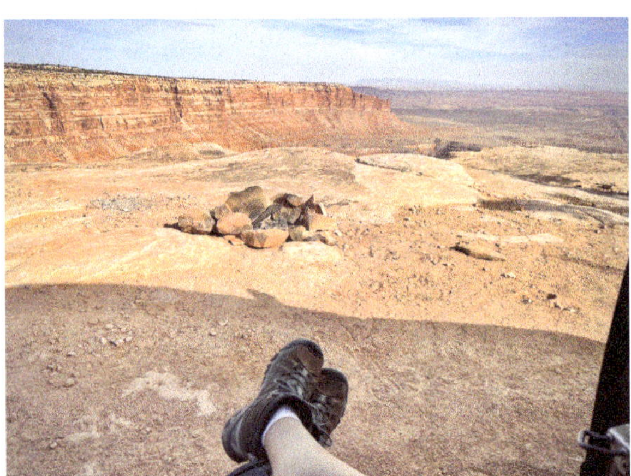

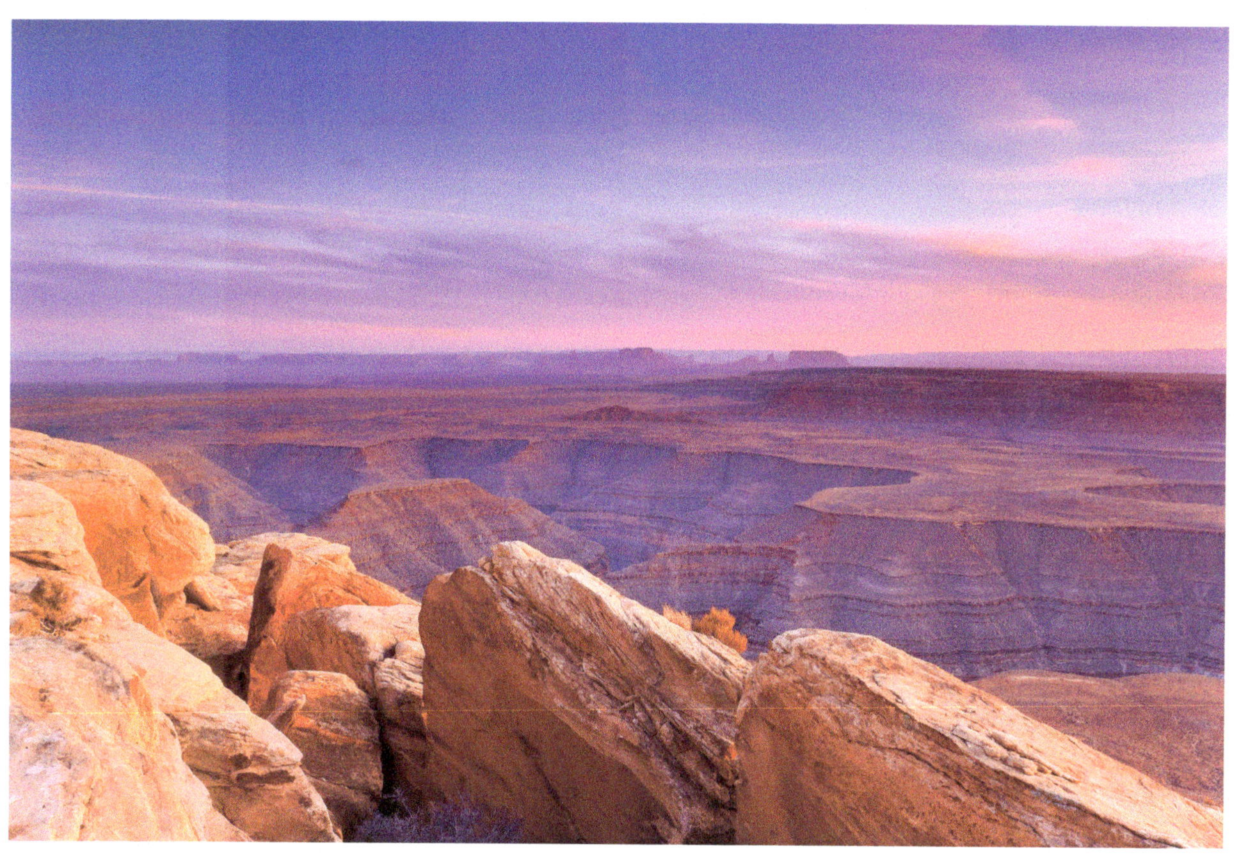

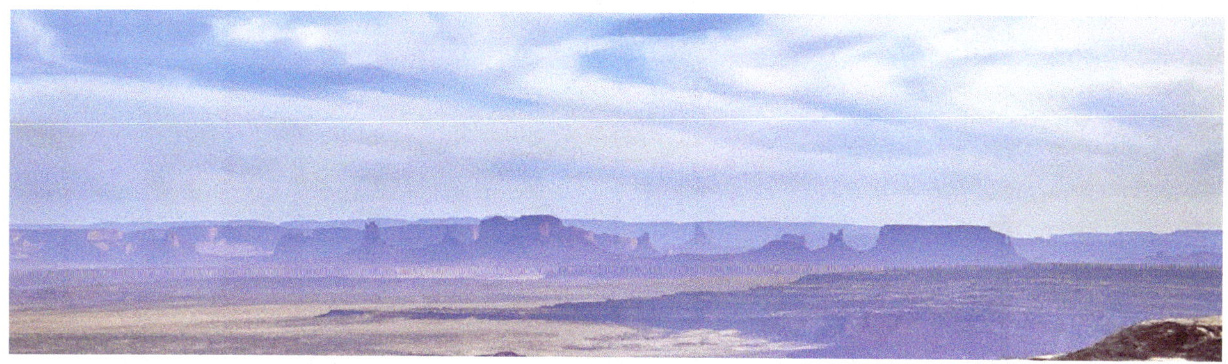

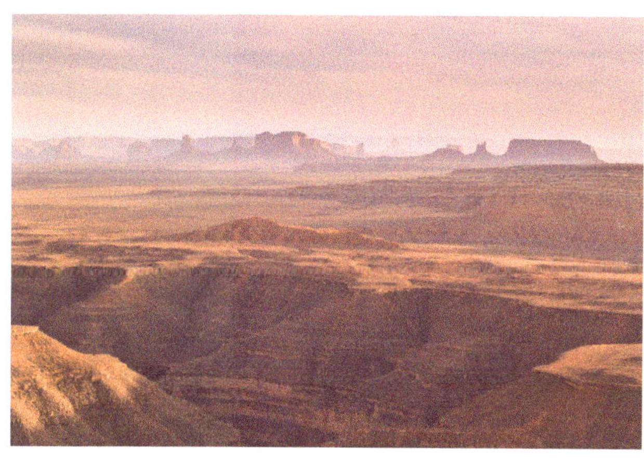

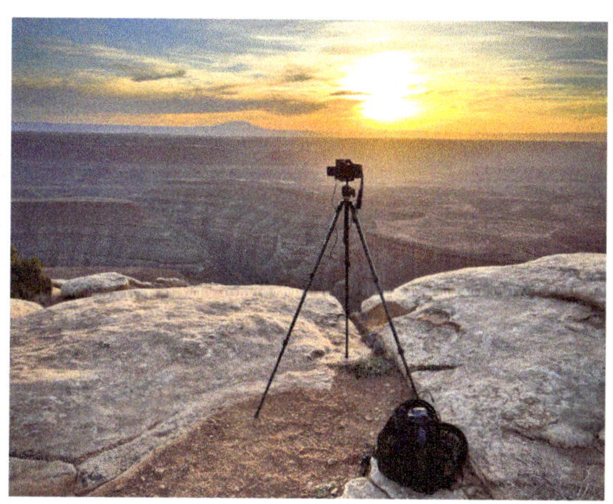

DAY 38 / MARCH 27

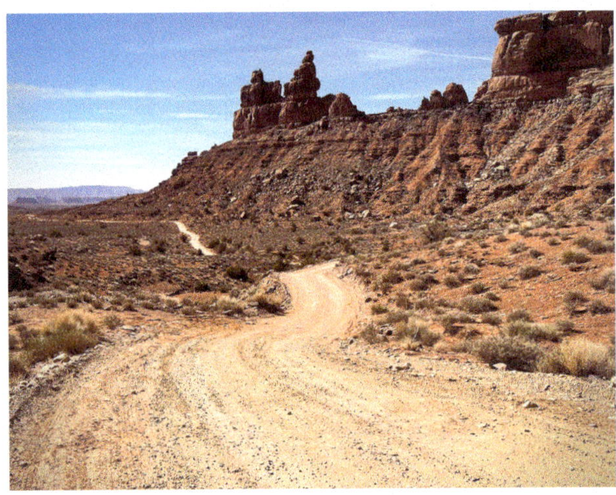

Passed on sunrise pictures
and slept in until 8am.
Drove down the Moki Dugway,
a dirt road carved out of
the wall of the canyon.
Pretty hairy driving it in a RV.

At the bottom of the Moki Dugway
was Valley of the Gods.
A 15-mile road of amazing rock formations.
The van got a new name after making
it up a 14% incline on the second try.
Badass.
I could have better driving skills
on dirt roads.

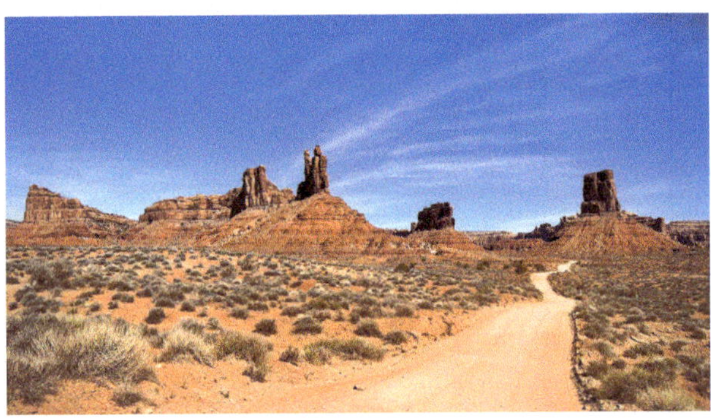

I would love to have seen
how those zig-zag patterns
were formed over time on Raplee Ridge.

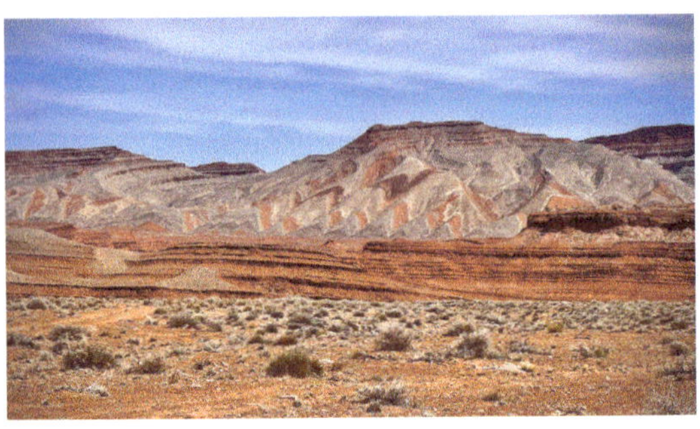

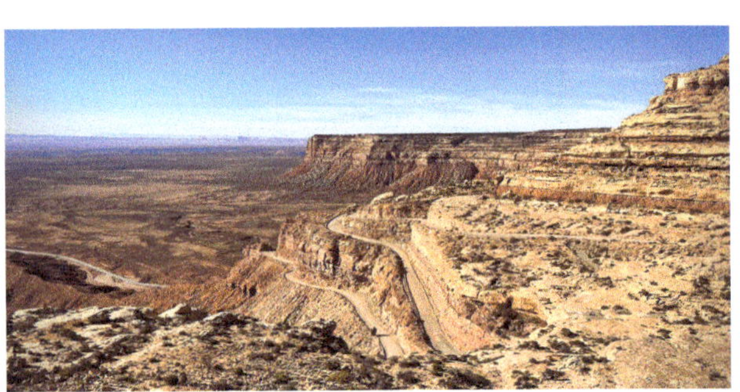

The next spot on the bucket list,
Goosenecks State Park.
Very primitive with no amenities.
Not even water.
Well-maintained toilets.
I should start a toilet Google review service.

One of the most unbelievable
and incredible views on the trip.
It was difficult to fit the two horseshoes
into a wide-angle picture.
And the wind blew like crazy.

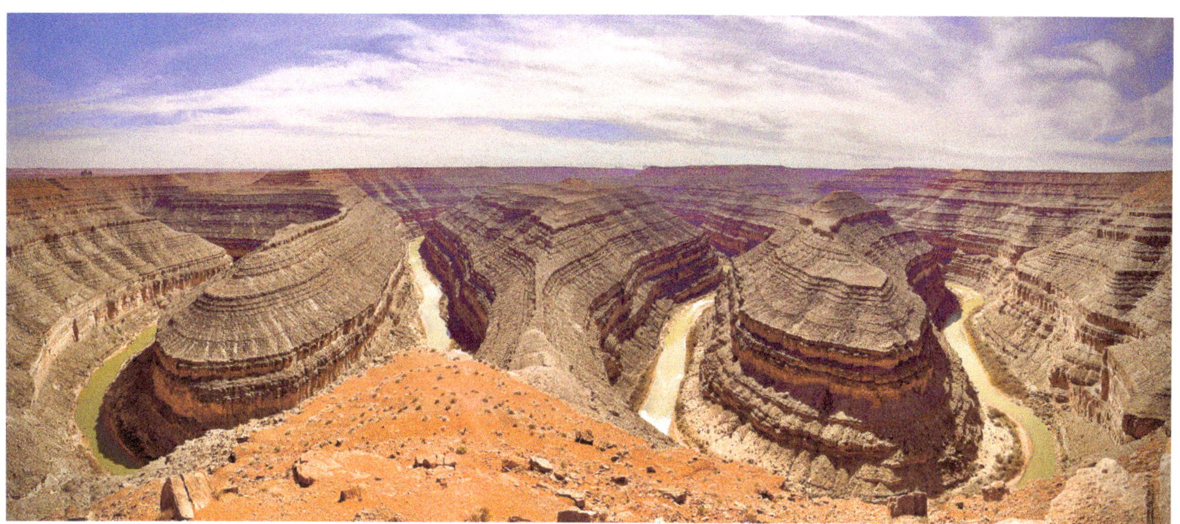

Andrew was speechless
when he saw the suspension lift on the van.
Didn't know minivans could have suspension lifts.
I didn't either until I saw it on Facebook.

I met Mike and his family
from Salt Lake City at the overlook.
He was impressed with the van modifications
and my road trip.
He told me about Diane Thomas, in her 70s,
who did a road trip to Alaska.

Where are you from?
Shitville.
Washington state.
What do you do?
I'm a photographer.
Sounds better than disabled with a brain injury.
Starting to sound more acceptable.

Two levels to choose from.
Both had value
when I decided where and how to overnight park.
Level back to front
and level side to side.
Being level side to side would be more comfortable.
Level back to front was more forgiving
if my feet were on the downhill side.
I didn't use blocks to level the van.
Too much work.

See the toilet paper moving in the wind?
The door was closed,
and the wind was coming in
through the toilet.
The speed and temperature of the wind
outside the latrine was what you would feel
on your butt when sitting on the toilet.
The colder outside,
the more unpleasant the experience.

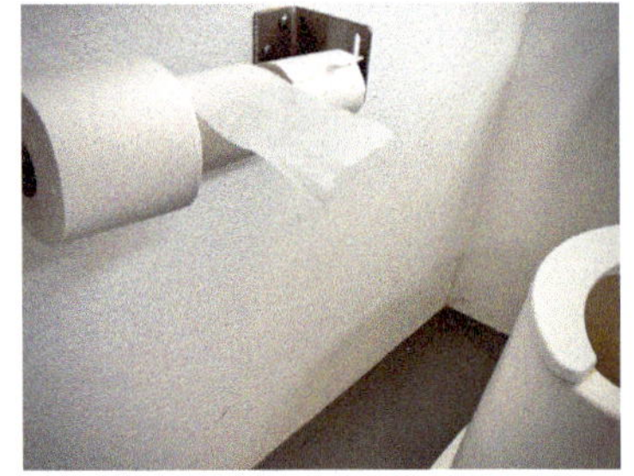

Slept in another night of heavy winds.
People from Seattle
camped in the site next to me in a tent.
Winds didn't blow them into the canyon overnight.

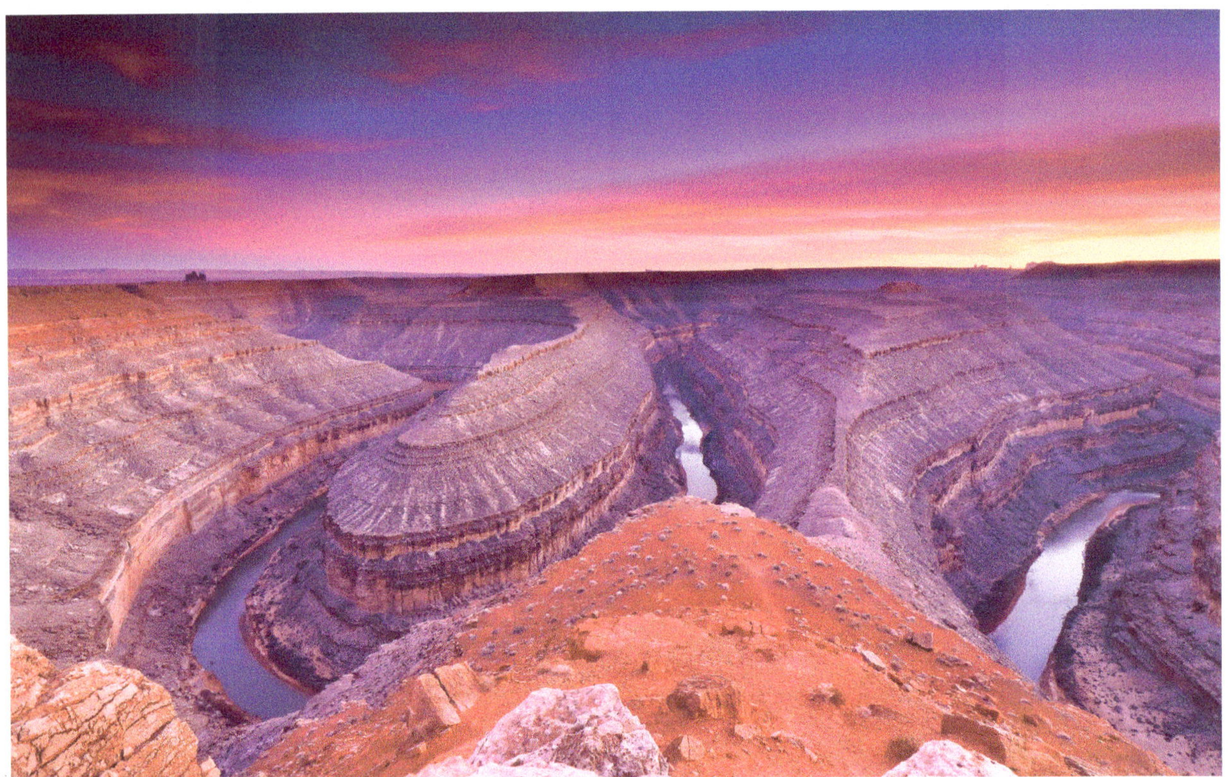

DAY 39 / MARCH 28

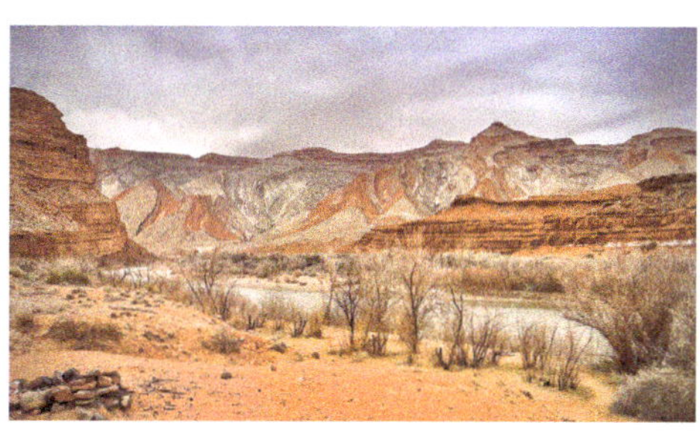

Took off from Goosenecks State Park
and stopped at Mexican Hat Rock.
Drove down to the river spot
I marked on Google Maps
and researched on Google Earth.

Bundu-bashed through the bushes,
scratched up my arms,
but got a good shot of the river.

The colored up and down red rock pattern
on the side of the mountain
was nothing I'd seen before.

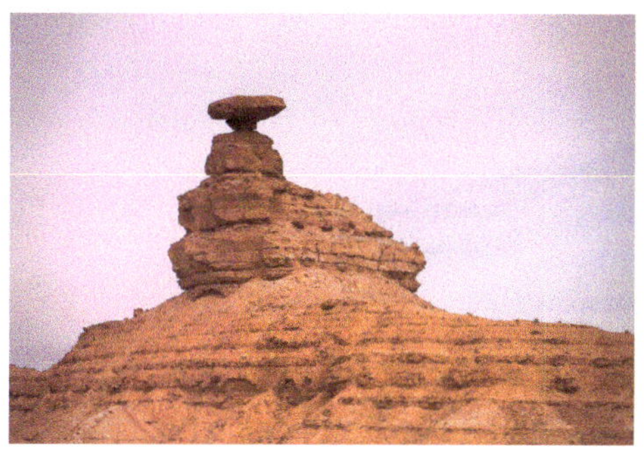

The rough ride back uphill to the highway
reminded me to secure the drawers of the
kitchen cabinet with a bungee cord
before taking off
unless I wanted to retrieve the contents
all over the van floor.

Stopped at the Forrest Gump spot on the highway.
Lots of traffic.
Went to Monument Valley.
My father-in-law John Ready
had pictures of the rock formations
on the wall in their living room.

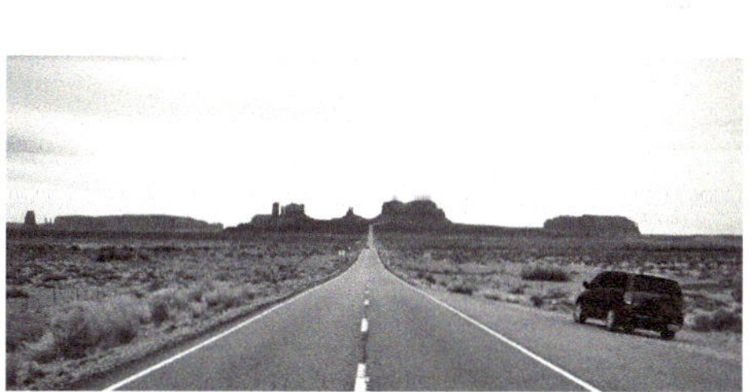

The park-mandated 2-hour limit to drive the loop
put a damper on the enjoyment.
I set the alarm to not be late leaving.
The wind escalated fast into a full-blown storm,
taking pictures outside the van was impossible.

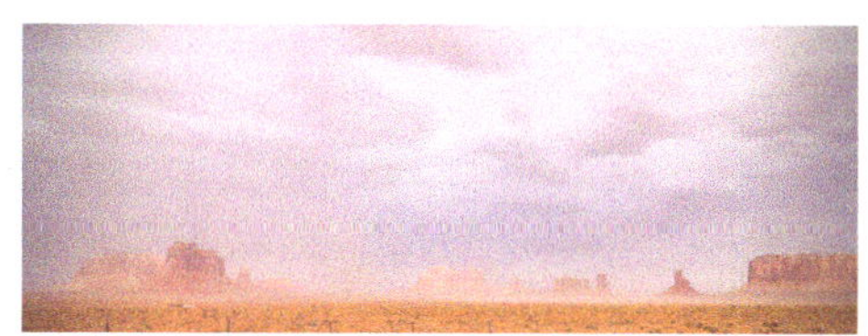

Took a rest break at the Navajo Welcome Center,
hoping the wind would calm down,
and started south towards Kayenta, Arizona.

Many scenic locations on the side of the road.
A beautiful solitary rock with horses in a meadow
got my attention and I pulled off the road,
parking next to two other vehicles.
I was tired
and didn't want to get the camera gear out.
Snapped a few shots with the phone,
ready to leave.

I saw a man in the driver-side mirror
coming around the back
walking very close to the van.
Instinctively started rolling up the window.
A native man in his early 20s said quietly

"What did you just take a picture of?"

I looked down to the phone without answering.

"No, don't do that."

I looked up and saw the pistol in his hand
aimed at my head.

Stepped on the gas hard.
The van, still in drive,
shot forward.
I heard the crunching noise of the pistol
caught between the top of the window
and the rain guard
as the window continued to roll up.

I didn't look back to see what was happening.
Joined the highway without traffic
and the engine whined
as I tore down the road.
My heart was beating hard in my chest
and my legs shook.
The rain guard got displaced by the pistol
and flapped in the wind.
I held onto it until I was sure
no one was following me.
Pulled off the road
to push the rain guard back into position.

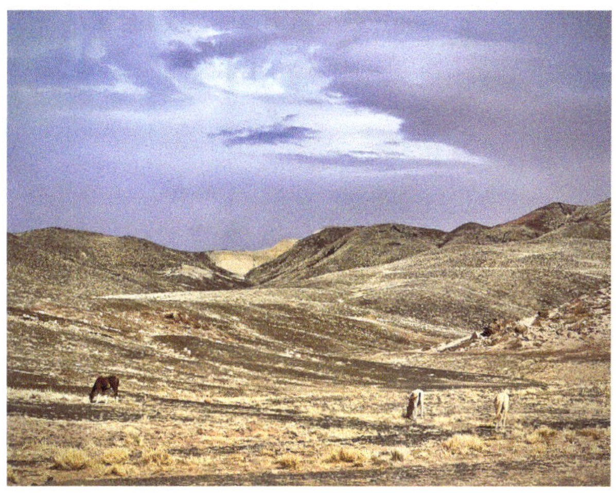

I wanted to call the police,
but no cell service.
I kept driving and looked
for the police station in Kayenta.
Somehow,
I had doubts
and changed my mind
about reporting the incident.

I stopped at MacDonald's for WiFi,
the van idling while looking at maps.
How much further was it
to get off the reservation?
About 2 hours of driving.

I was exhausted
and it would be dark soon.
Burger King allowed overnight parking
for cars and semi-trucks.

Backed into a parking spot behind the building.
The spare tire would be out of sight
and not make the van identifiable.
It would be easier to take off
without having to back out of a parking spot.

I slept in my day clothes,
the driver seat in the driving position,
the back of seat down.
I could step onto the driver seat from inside the van.
Keys next to me,
and the pepper spray
and taser.

Thought about going back home to safety.
I was too naïve about the world.

DAY 40 / MARCH 29 / 3,648 MILES

Got gas the next morning.

Drove back to the location of the incident.

No *private property*
or *no trespassing* signs.

"Fuck you, boy,
you don't dictate how I live my life."

"And you got your ass kicked
by a middle-aged woman with gray hair."

Took off to Farmington, New Mexico.

Once in Farmington,
settled in at Walmart with their permission.
There was no way
I could tell Mark on the phone
about what happened.
It had to be a face-to-face conversation.
He would see I was safe
and unharmed.
It had to wait until we met
in Corpus Christi Texas on April 11.

I called Daniel,
my photography friend from Seattle,
who grew up in New Mexico
for advice and information.

It was a huge relief to talk to someone
who understood the area.
And who understood
that I couldn't talk to Mark about it.

We talked about photography spots
and his upcoming photography road trip.

Planned on meeting
where our routes intersected for a photo shoot.
Preferably at Bisti Badlands
with no formal hiking trails.
Since I was directionally hopelessly confused,
it would be a good idea to go with someone
who would get me back to my vehicle.

Cooked a nice dinner
with leftovers for the next day.
I invented a new way of cooling off the pan
without burning the carpet.
Balanced it on the upside-down lid.

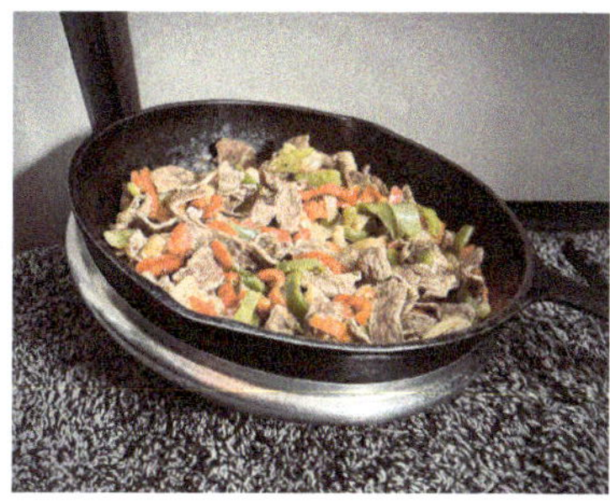

I was very vigilant parked at Walmart,
ready to take off at a moment's notice.
Regarded everyone with suspicion.

I knew I wouldn't always have cell service
on the trip.
Emergency calls without a signal
were possible on an iPhone.

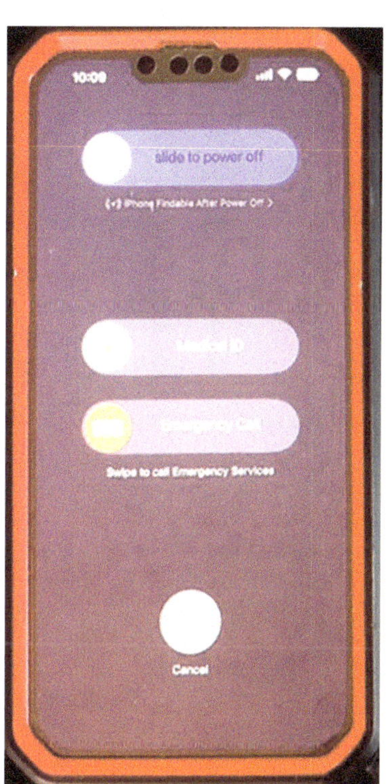

I forgot how to do it.

I forgot that it was even possible.

Googled it.

Hold the volume up and the power buttons

down simultaneously.

The option for an emergency call
will appear on the screen.

DAY 41 / MARCH 30

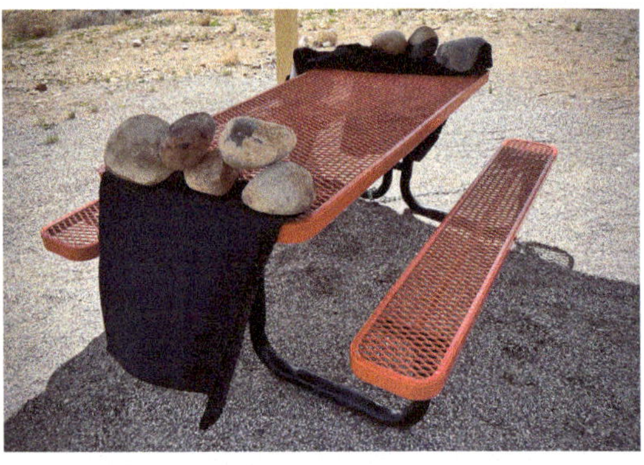

Went to Lake Farmington.
The campground did not have a good vibe.
Met a lady and her dog who shared the impression.

Well, shit.
I didn't tighten the lid on the water bottle
and the mats were soaked.
Dried them on the picnic table in the wind.

Downloaded Gaia GPS maps for Bisti Badlands.

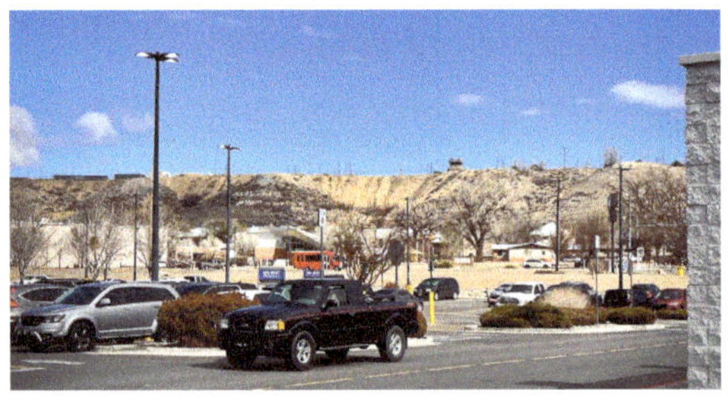

Got a permit for a local campground
from the BLM office.

The last 3 miles to the campground was dirt road
with a sign "*Impassible when wet.*"
The weather report said no chance of rain.
The clouds in the sky said something different.
Bailed on the campground.
Didn't want to get stuck in mud.

Distilled water had been in short supply
due to the pandemic.
Target had a few gallons available.
$5.35 per gallon.
How badly do you want it?
Checked out at $1.39 per gallon.
I had serious visual and reading issues.

Filled up with gas and fresh water.

Broke one of my rules
"No turning left across traffic without a traffic light."
Saw nothing coming and stepped on the gas.

Out of nowhere a pickup truck right in front of me.
Slammed on the brakes hard.
Stuff hit my seat from behind.

Oh jeez.
That was INCREDIBLY STUPID.

Timed how long it took
to roll up the van window,
from pushing the button
to where the top of window was level
with the rain guard:

3.28 seconds.

From where I saw the asshole
coming around the back of the van,
to stepping on the gas,
hearing the gun crushed
between the top of the window and the rain guard:

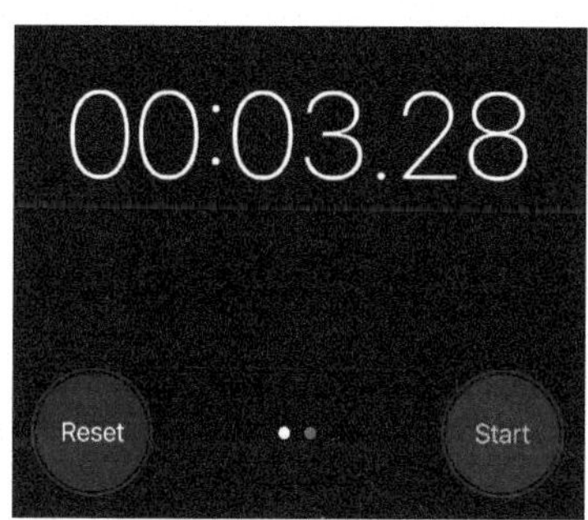

3.28 seconds.

He intended to point the gun at my head
when he approached the van.

DAY 42 / MARCH 31

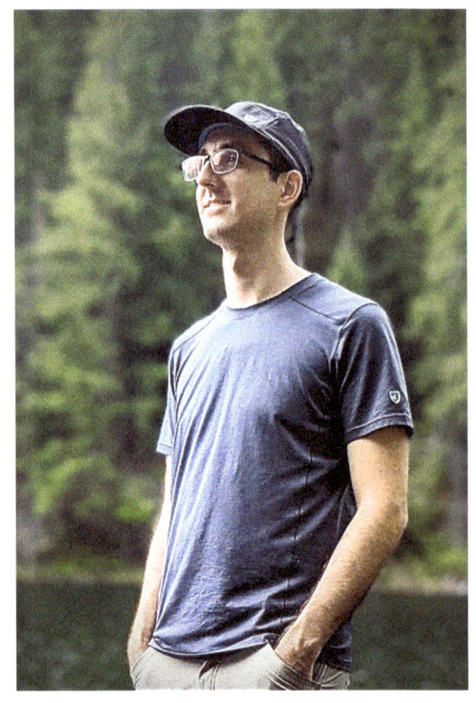

Headed towards Albuquerque.
Passed on Bisti Badlands.
It was about 1,000 miles to Corpus Christi, Texas.

Daniel left Seattle on March 30 for
Zion NP, The Wave, Monument Valley, Shiprock,
Bisti Badlands, Goblin Valley, and Antelope Island.
All in 2 weeks.

I had to start driving to Corpus Christi on April 1.
No meetup in the cards.
Hopefully later in the year in Washington state.

We met in a photography class
on the Olympic Peninsula in June 2020.
We were both immigrants,
he was born in Spain and spoke 3 languages.

Met with Daniel and Ying (his wife) at Lake Wenatchee
last year for a few days of photography.
He encouraged and gently pushed me
to resume photography.

As an occupational therapist I knew
people lost their drive and motivation
after brain injuries.

I had no clue how debilitating it was.
To do nothing for days and months
and not care.

Lost the desire to participate
in my life and meaningful activities.
I was obsessed with photography
before the injury.

Photography was erased from my life.
Like my job.
My existence.

Looked up pictures of pistols.

The man aimed a Glock at my head.

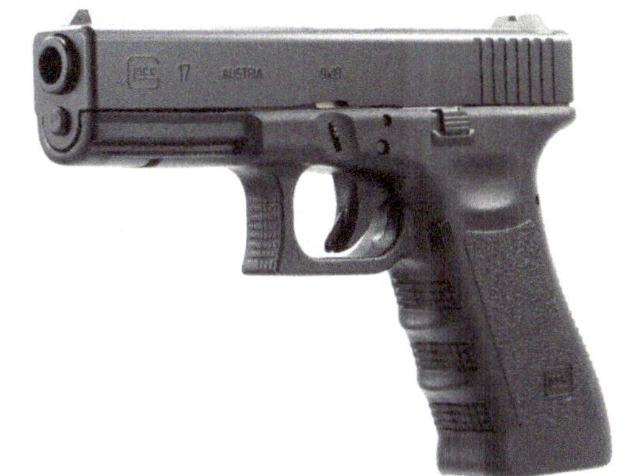

The dashboard became multifunctional.
Dried the carpet on the dashboard.
Convenient.

And for God's sake,
don't drown the mats again.

They took forever to dry out.

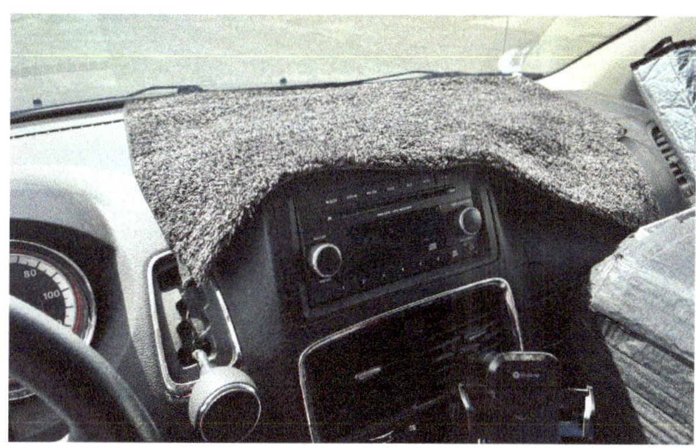

Eating crunchy and noisy foods
while driving
helped me to stay focused
and not space out.

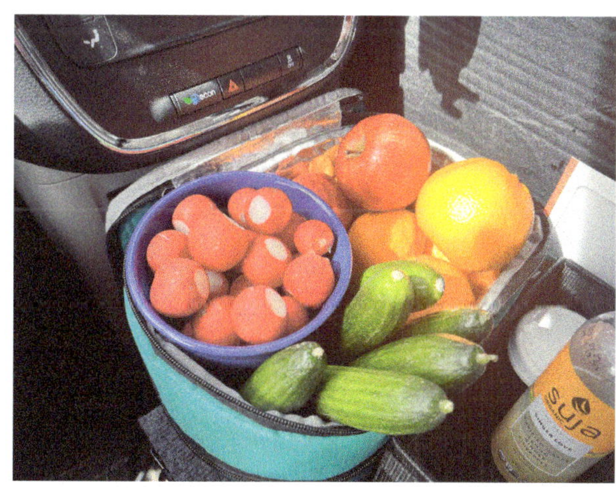

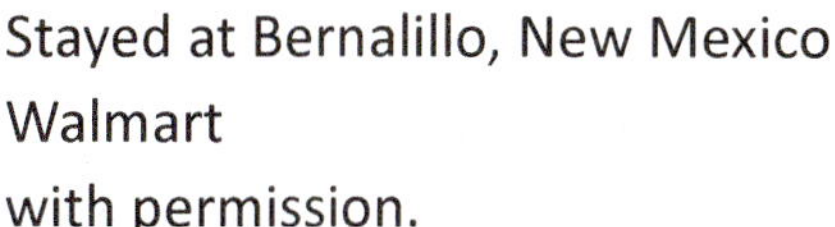
Stayed at Bernalillo, New Mexico
Walmart
with permission.

DAY 43 / APRIL 1

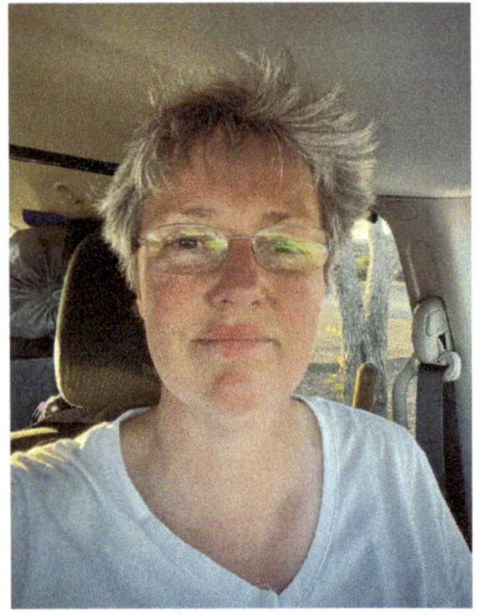

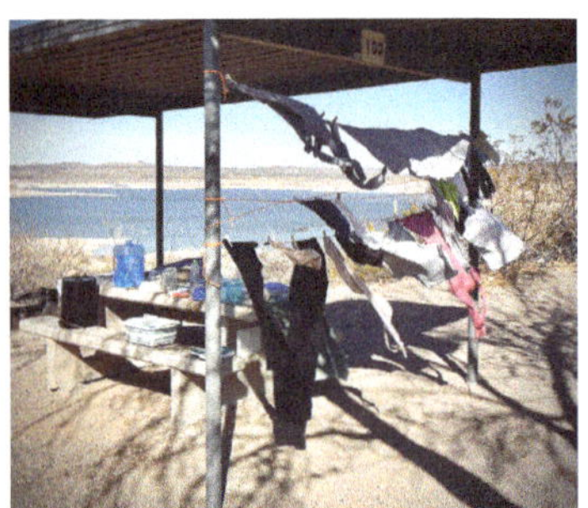

Drove from Bernalillo, New Mexico
to Elephant Butte State Park.

I paid for parking by the water.
It looked very sandy.
And the lady at the park entrance
warned about getting stuck.

Took a shower and washed my clothes
in the bucket while showering.
Hung it on a makeshift clothesline.
It was windy and my hair dried quickly,
standing in all directions.
Only took an hour to dry my jeans.
Passed on the camp spot by the water.
Moved to Truth and Consequences, New Mexico Walmart.
The parking lot was in the shade
of a lot of solar panels.

Daniel sent a picture of
Black Magic Canyon in Idaho.
Saved the spot on my map.

Spent a peaceful and quiet evening
with the other overnight guests.

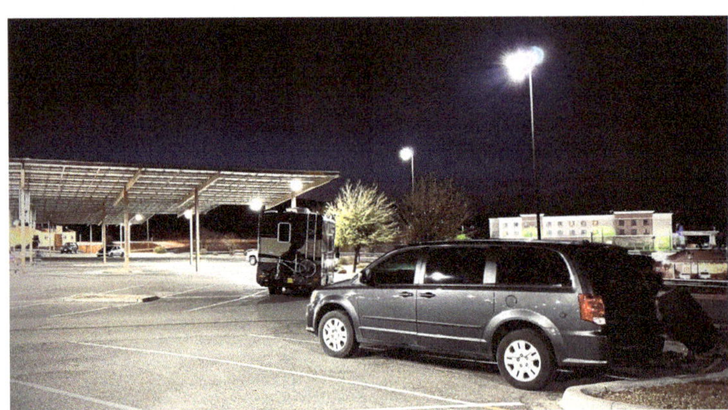

DAY 44 / APRIL 2

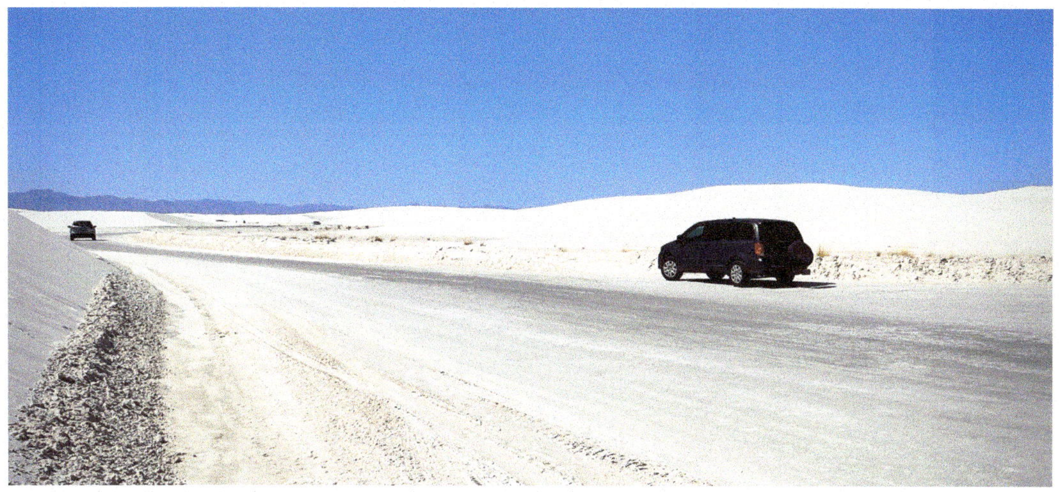

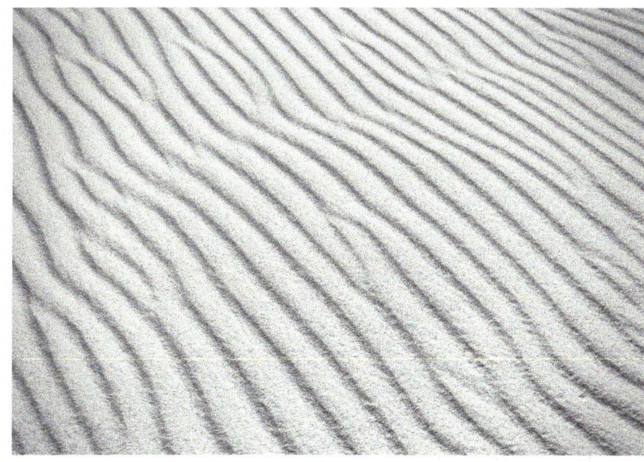

Drove from Truth and Consequences, New Mexico
to White Sands National Park.
A long straight downhill and very windy trip
down the Organ Mountain.
A great view into tomorrow.

The park was very busy
with lots of tracks on the dunes.
Not photogenic.

Early in the morning would be a better time.
Took video to show Mark.

Checked in at Walmart in Alamogordo, New Mexico.

DAY 45 / APRIL 3

Headed for Carlsbad.
Drove through Cloudcroft, Daniel's high-school town.
A wonderful ski-resort town vibe.

Stopped in Hope, New Mexico.

Felt like Sunday afternoons
on my grandmother's farm.
Warm, dry.
The sound of wind.
Deserted.
Nobody.

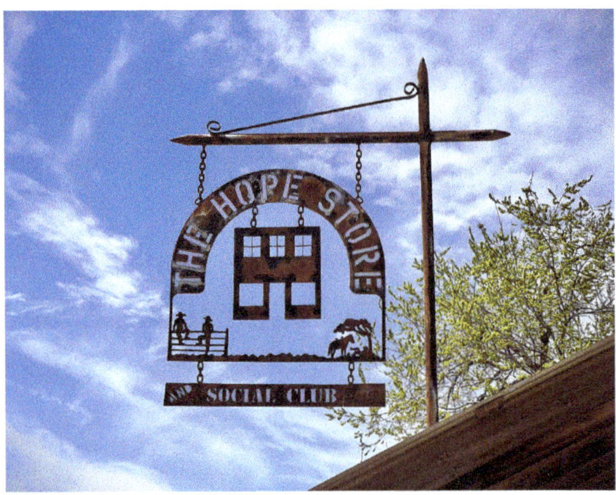

The Hope Store – Social Club.
Hope?
Hope of what?

Getting my life back?

Being normal again?

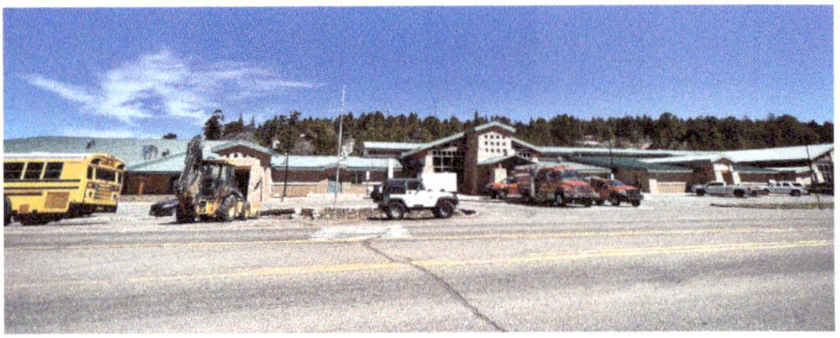

Able to read books?

Going to work every day?

Stuck in Groundhog Day.

You don't get the day off
from having a brain injury.

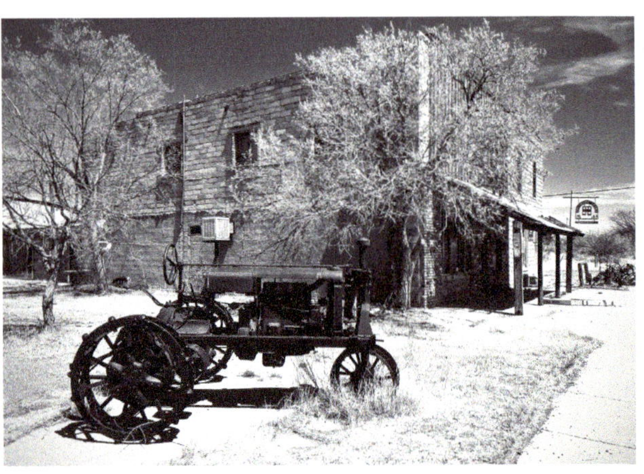

You have it every day.
It starts over every morning.
I could tell from how many times
I lost my balance
walking to the bathroom in the morning
what kind of day it was going to be.
How bad my reading would be that day.

Shitville Social Club for one.

Stayed at Carlsbad, New Mexico Walmart with permission.

Went to the buffet in town
and the waitress kept coming back
to talk to me about my road trip.

Called Orli, a fellow South African friend
since 1997, to catch up on my travels.

She invited me to visit.
Memphis was "close" to Corpus Christi.
I would think about it.
Called Mark, he said I should do it.
I had to make a reservation for
Carlsbad Caverns National Park for the next day.
Had to time it
to have enough time to get there,
do the tour and make it
to the next overnight spot before dark.

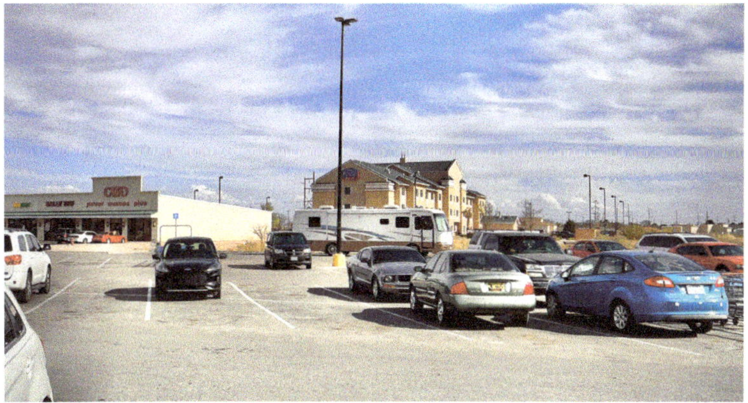

DAY 46 / APRIL 4

Didn't sleep well.
I didn't like where I was.
And I wasn't talking about geography.
How much did the gun episode
affect my thinking and state of mind?

I had to leave by 10am
to be on time for my reserved timed entry.

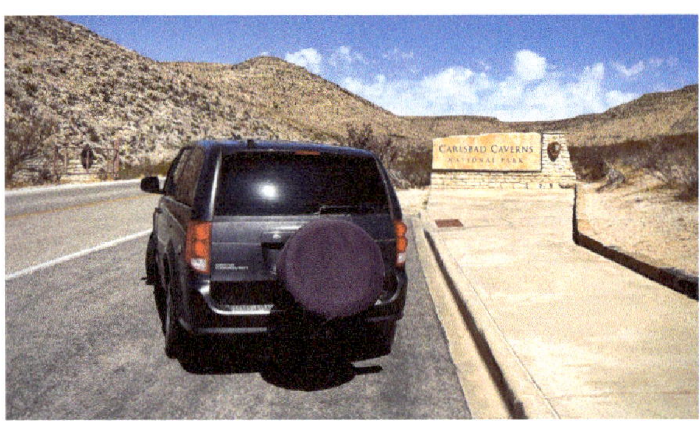

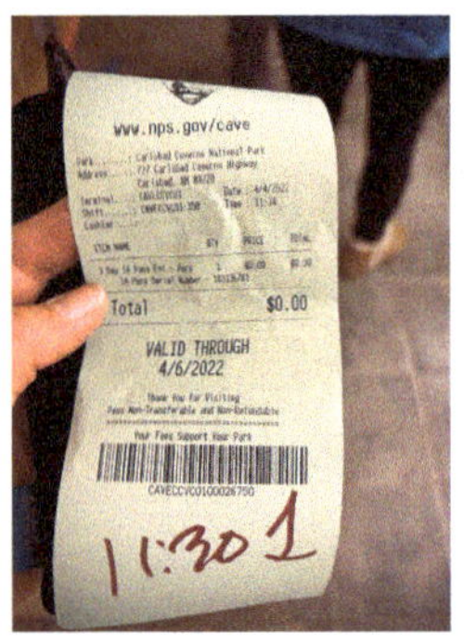

I stood in line at the visitor center for a half hour
listening to people talk and announcements.
Earplugs, sunglasses and a hat
to block out the incoming sensory stimulation.

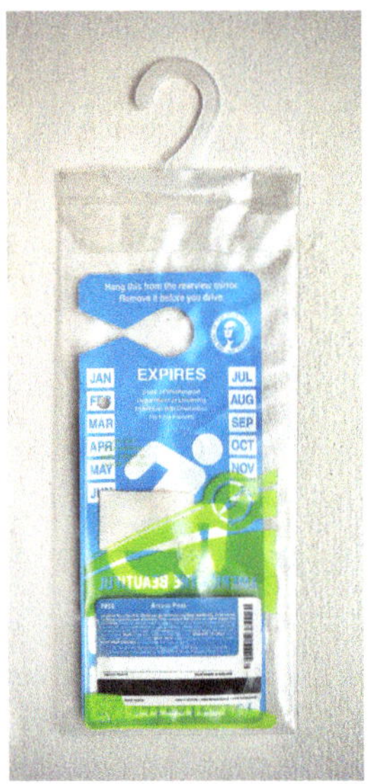

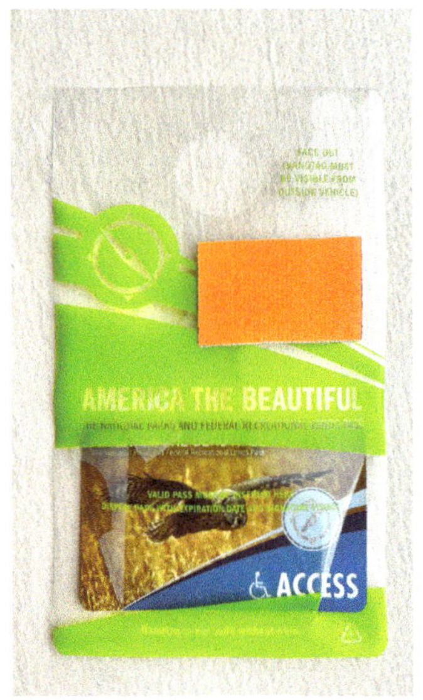

"You can't have the Access Pass taped to the holder."
The irritation in his voice cut through my soul.
I didn't understand what he wanted.

He took it out of the clear plastic envelope
I kept it in with the blue disability parking placard,
so I wouldn't lose it.

Ripped the card out of the plastic green holder,
scanned it
and threw the green holder in the garbage can.

I had a piece of orange tape on it so I could "see" it.
Also, to remind me where it was.

He put the access pass in another green holder
and gave it back to me.

I asked for the one in the garbage can.
Which he gave back to me.

He handed me my ticket.

I tried to put the pass back in the plastic envelope
but couldn't get it open.
Felt rushed by his impatience
and the line of people.

"I can't get it open" and handed it to him.
He opened it and I put everything back in.

I walked back to the van to put the placard in the window
before I forgot what I did with it.

I wanted to hide in the van.

I've been to many national parks,
no one ever scanned my card
or wanted it out of the plastic envelope.
They verified the name on the pass and driver's license.
And they were a whole lot nicer.

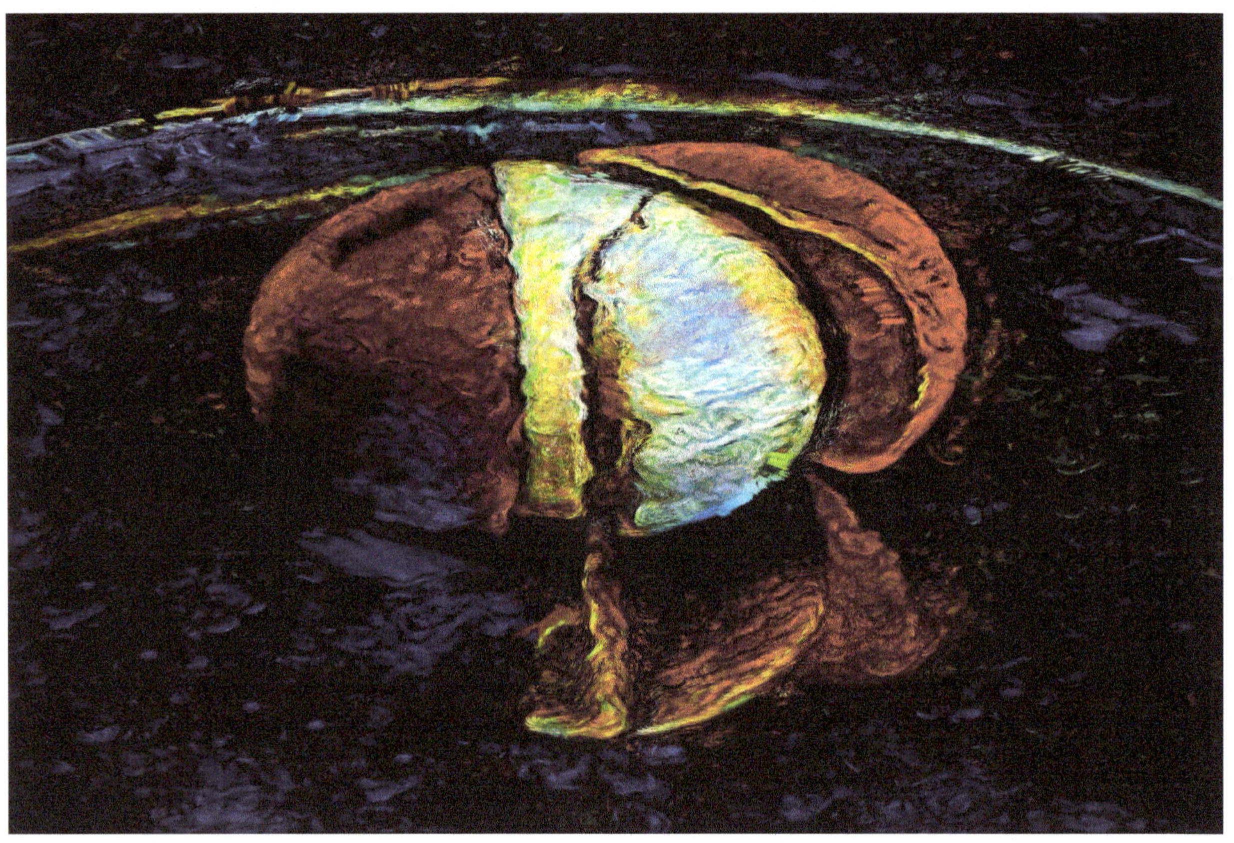

Not everyone with a disability is in a wheelchair,
or walks with a cane or crutches.
He failed miserably, rude and impatient.
Because I looked normal.

I completed the trail through the Carlsbad Cavern.
It was dark mostly and I had to use the rail
to keep my balance.
I didn't enjoy the experience,
wouldn't have missed much by leaving.
Got done and got out.

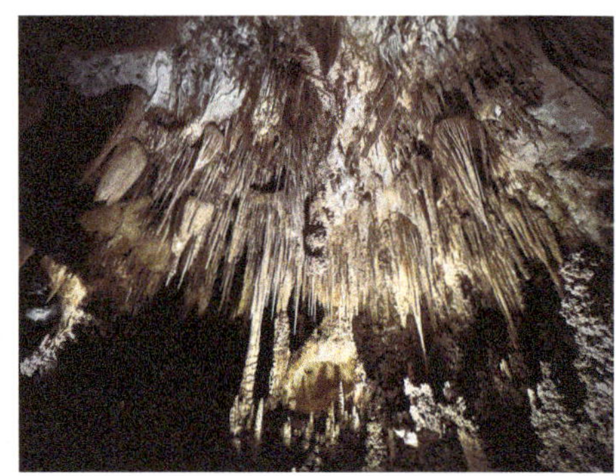

WELCOME TO TEXAS

Made it as far as Pecos.
Had permission for overnight parking at three businesses.
Couldn't get settled in.
It was 5:45 pm already and would be dark soon.
Called Mark to let him know
I'm heading for the next town.

Continued to Fort Stockton, Texas.
The Walmart had a great vibe
with many other overnight campers.

Met Hailey from Florida.
Had a very educational visit about traveling.
She gave me a piece of Velcro, very handy.
I used it to fix the back window cover.

I researched the distance and time
to possibly make it to Big Bend National Park in Texas.
Wanted to see Boquillas Border Crossing to Mexico.
Saw a YouTube video of a man with a small boat
rowing people across the river
to shop and have lunch/dinner
and take them back to the crossing.
How cool was that.
Too bad I didn't have my passport.

Daniel sent pictures of Goblin Valley
and Factory Butte Utah.
It stormed when I was in the area.
I'll have to try again.

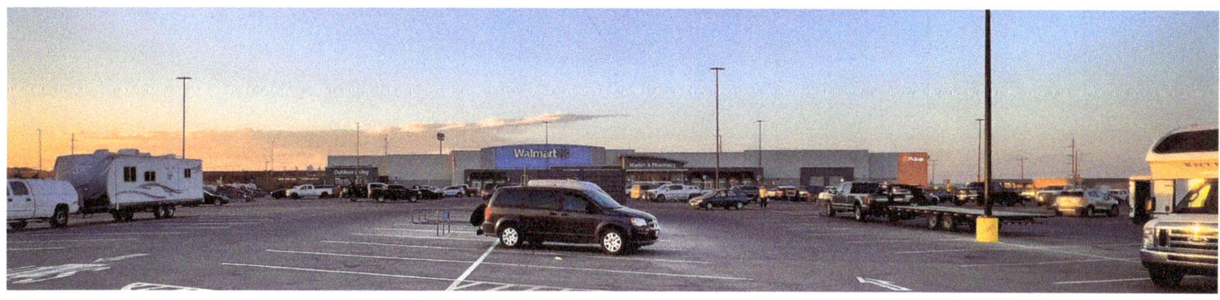

DAY 47 / APRIL 5

A long day of driving.
And it was hot, 97F (36C).
The rest-area picnic tables had covers.

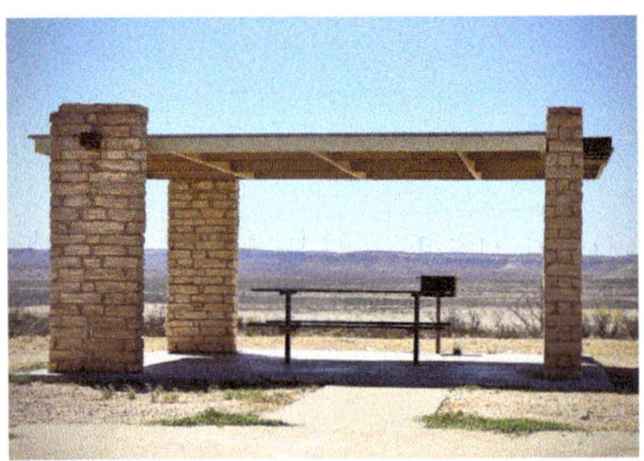

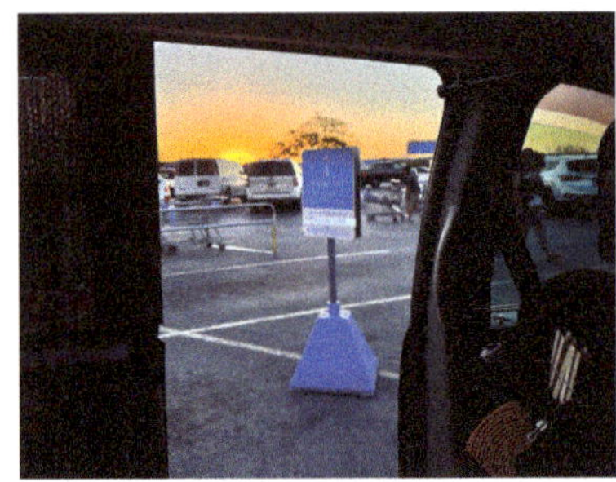

Stopped at the visitor center at Ozona, Texas
for lunch and bathroom break.
The very nice lady helped me
plan my route to Corpus Christi,
to bypass the San Antonio traffic.

Orli called and invited me
to give a motivational talk
to occupational therapy faculty
and students where she worked.
I would think about it.

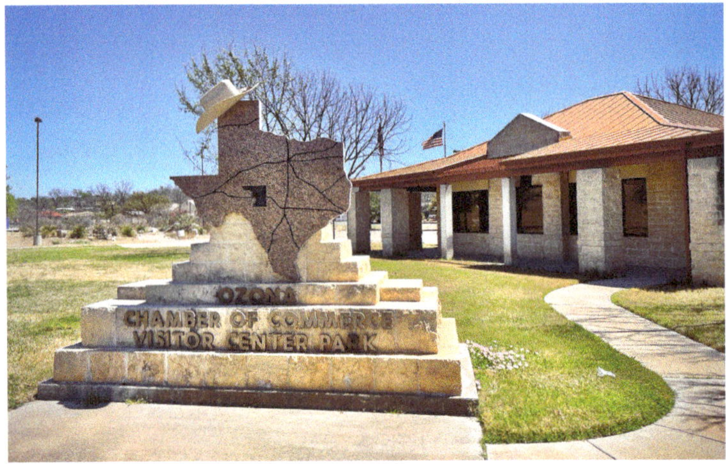

Decided against going to Big Bend National Park.
It would be a lot of driving
and too much.

DAY 48 / APRIL 6

Stayed at the Walmart in Kerrville, Texas.

The battery level was 50%
when I took off from Kerrville.
Checked again at noon,
not charging,
the breaker under the hood was flipped.
Reset it.
Charging as usual.

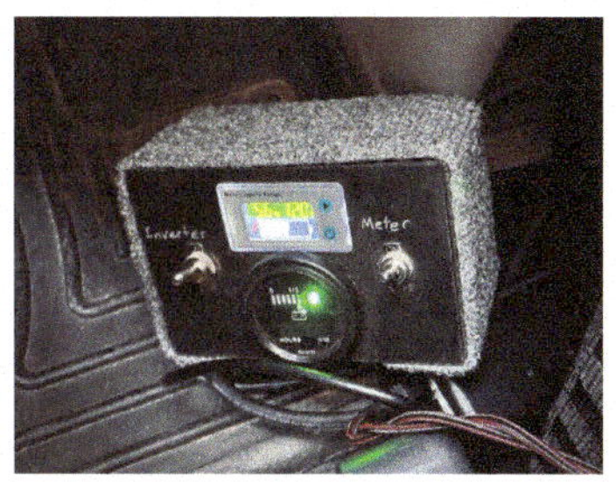

Made reservations
at Lake Corpus Christi State Park
to use the electric hookup
to charge the batteries.

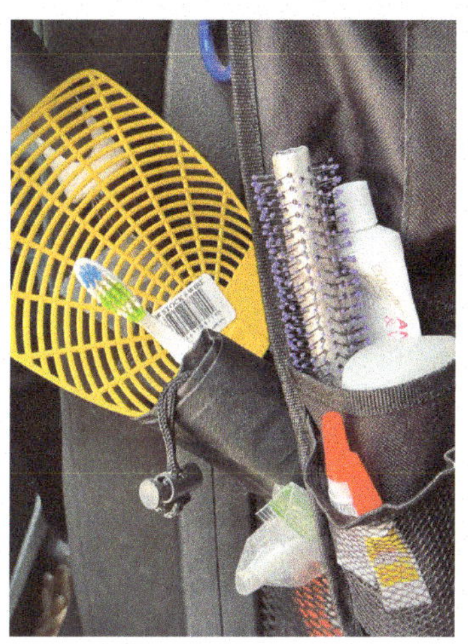

I found my toothbrush.

I put it away while talking
on the phone two weeks ago
and stuck it in with the fly swatter.

Since it was supposed to be
with toothpaste and hairbrush,
my brain couldn't see it
and therefore "lost" it.

I had a backup toothbrush in the shower bag.

I accepted Orli's invitation to talk
about living with a brain injury.
I had to start thinking
like an occupational therapist again.

I took pictures of
the compensatory strategies I used
to deal with visual dysfunction in the van.

Colored tape on the tag
of the spare key in the glove box.
Also on the tire gauge.
Reminders to "see" it.

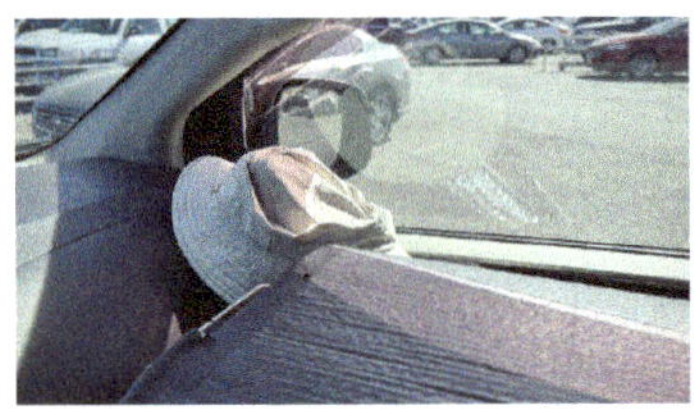

Light sensitivity
was a huge pain in the ass.
Had to deal with
light reflections in the van.
All. The. Time.

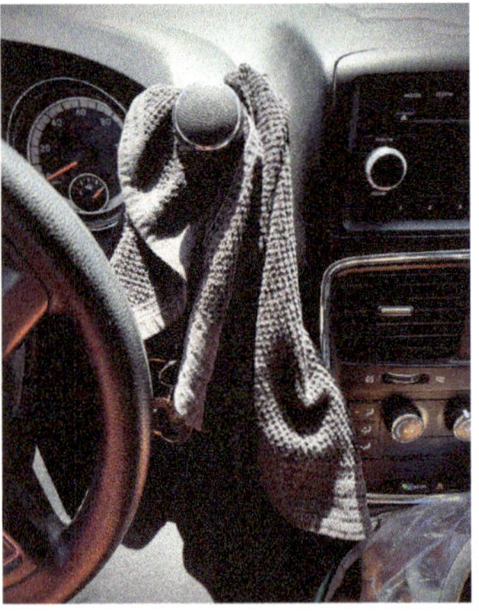

Put my hat on the
reflectix window shade
reflecting in the window,
blinding and distracting.

Put a black dish towel
around the gear lever
to block the sun
reflecting on the silver trim.

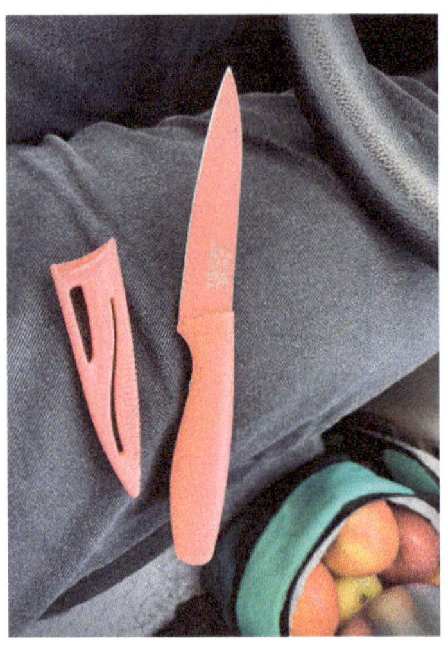

I used black items against the black interior to
limit visual fatigue and overload.

Used a brightly colored knife my brain could see
with a cover to prevent injuries.
My hands no longer had good sensation
or a sense of manipulating smooth objects.

The electricity was off when I checked
into Lake Corpus Christi State Park.
It would have been nice to know.
It would have saved me the time and energy
trying to figure if other sites
were without electricity too,
or just my site.
Learned that when the electricity was off,
the bathrooms would be locked.

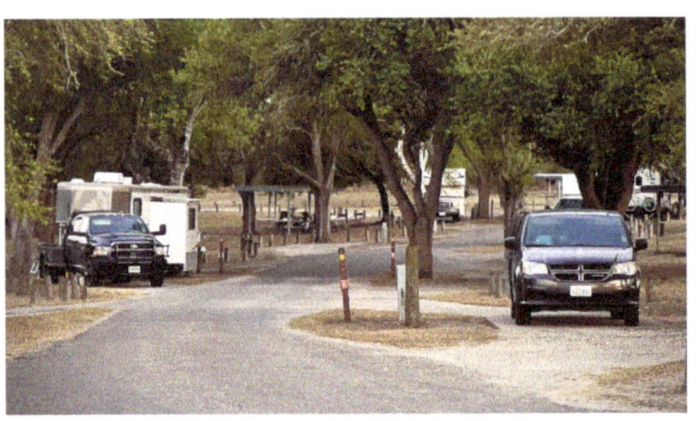

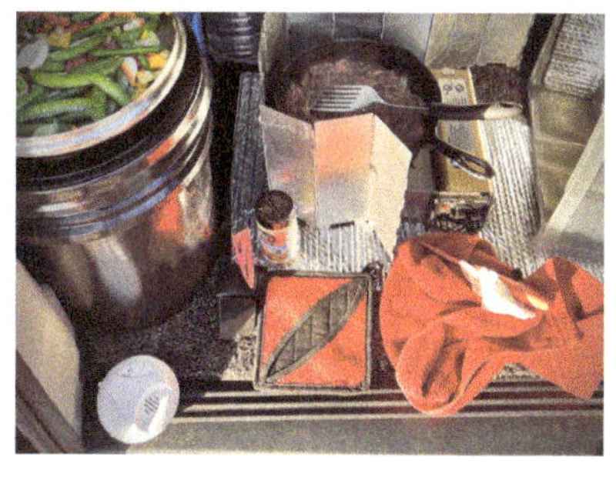

Later checked on the showers
and talked to Ken the camp host.
He and his wife lived in their RV full time.
He enlightened me that the toilets
needed electricity for the pumps.

My neighbors were young people from Cuba.
He was a truck driver
and they lived in a RV for 2 years
before buying a house 2.5 hours from the lake.

Enjoyed the luxury of using my electric kettle
instead of the butane stove.
Cooked in the van,
the wind was blowing.
Front row seat to sunset.

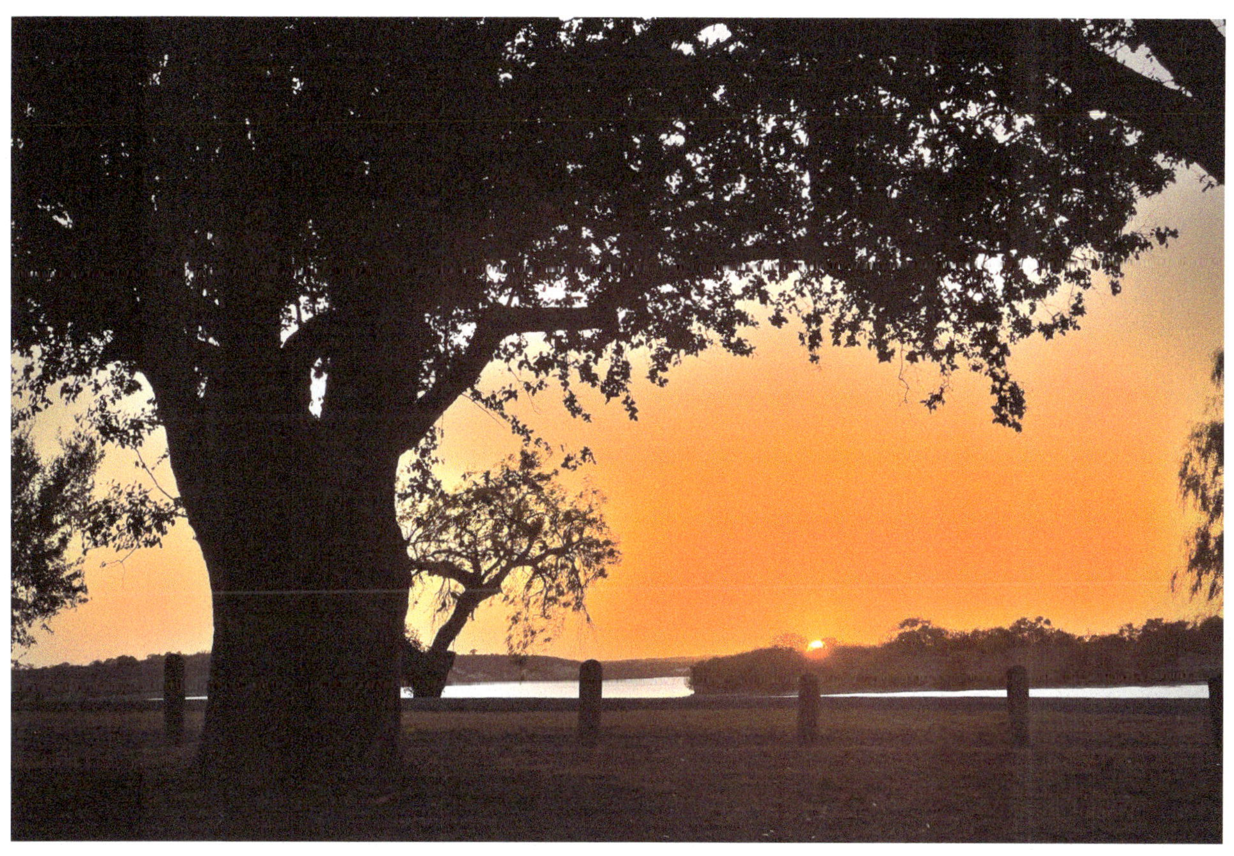

DAY 49 / APRIL 7 / 5,167 MILES

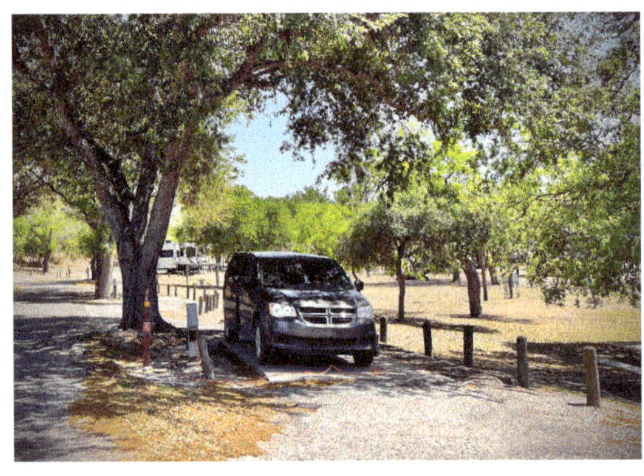

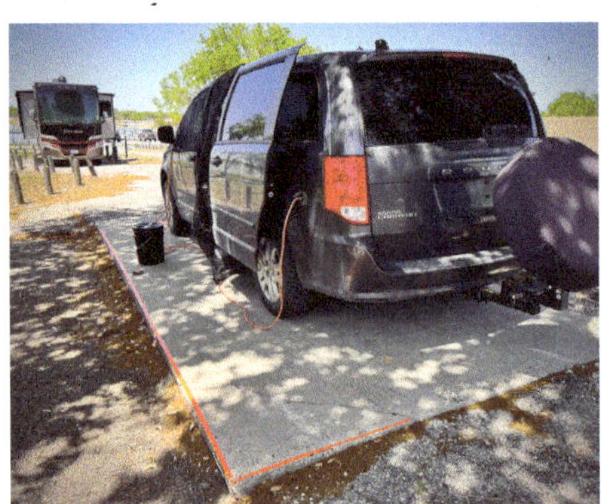

Slept until 9:45 am to my surprise.

I drove 1,324 miles in 7 days
since taking off from Farmington, New Mexico.

Moved to my reserved site for the day.

Put orange tape
on the edge of the parking pad.
I knew that if I didn't pay attention,
I would forget about the drop off and fall.
Ripped the tape lengthwise
to cover most of the edge.
Added to the shopping list.

I downloaded an app on my phone
to measure noise level.
Flushing toilets
and hand air dryers everywhere
were so loud
and hurt my ears.
And yes, they are all loud.

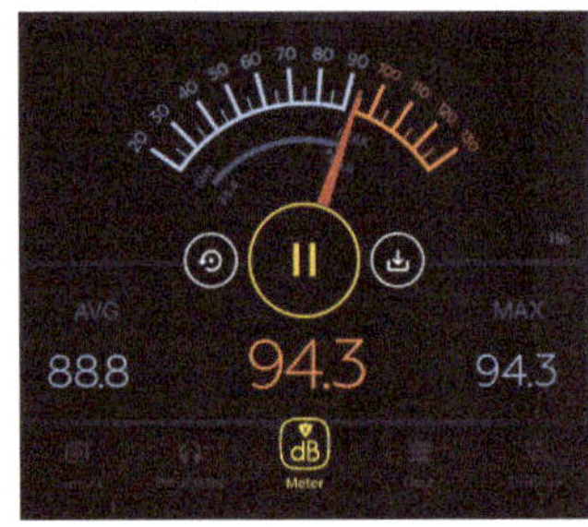

I put red film (for brake-light repairs)
over the lights and flashlights
to cope with light sensitivity.

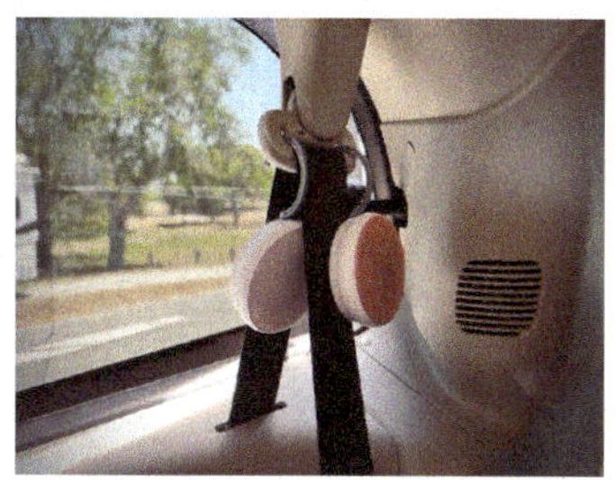

The stainless-steel water container
held 10 gallons of distilled water.
I could try and keep track mentally,
but it could be disastrous.
I made 1-gallon marks on a skinny stick.
Checked the water level periodically.

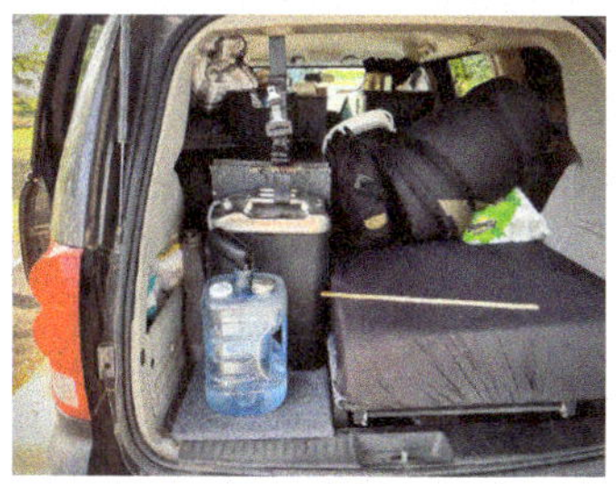

It was very easy to wash and rinse clothes
with a constant supply of water at the site.
Always took advantage of the wind
to do laundry.

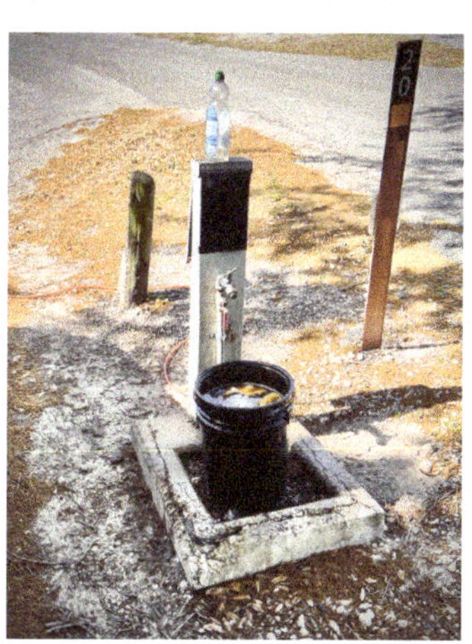

Put up a clothesline
between the picnic table and tree.
Many clothespins were a good idea.

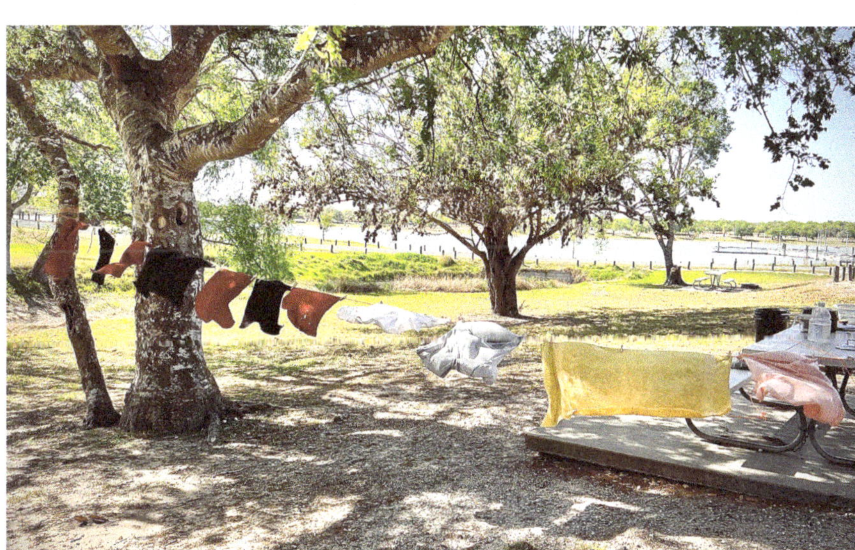

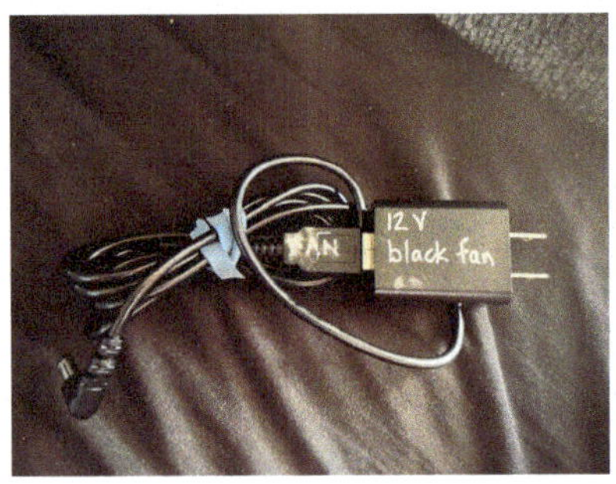

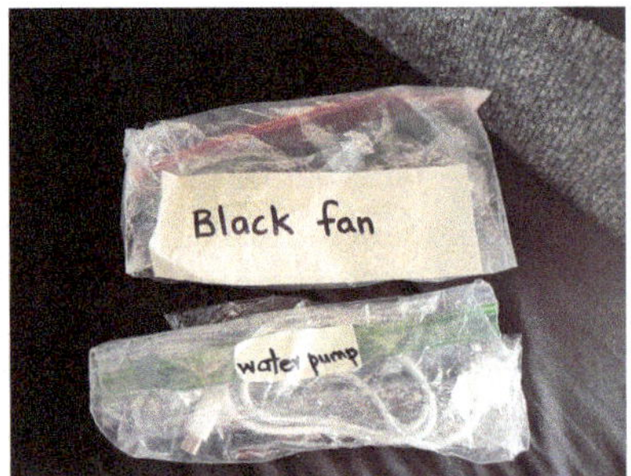

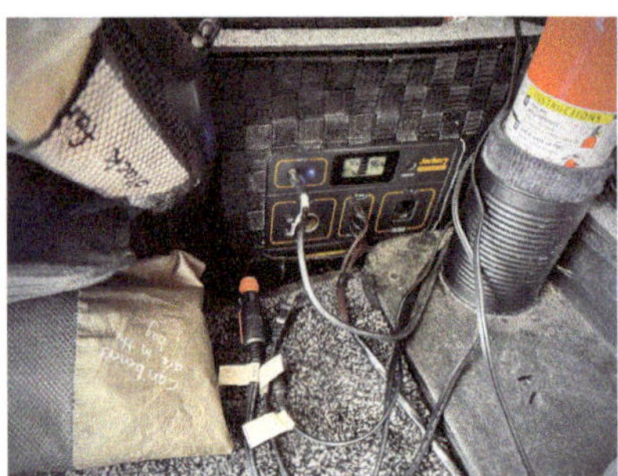

Every cord was marked at both ends
with masking tape and black ink.
The Ziplock bags
with charging cords were also marked.
Just because I knew on a certain day
what and where it was,
didn't mean I would remember
the next day or next week.

The fridge and Jackery battery pack
had a 12-volt (battery power)
and a 110-volt (wall electricity)
charging cord each.

The fridge plugged either into the inverter 110-volt
or the Jackery 12-volt/van cigarette-lighter outlet.

The Jackery plugged into the power strip (shore power 110-volt)
or the cigarette-lighter outlet 12-volt.

Which one I used also depended if I was driving, parked,
or in a campground with electricity.

Figuring how those two items should be plugged in,
was like failing an IQ test daily.

If I didn't run the van battery dead,
all was good.

If I did, I had an electronic battery jump starter
and jumper cables.
Long ones.

It’s very hard to focus on small print
and exhausting to read.
I received these magnifiers with lights,
just the right brightness,
from the Lilac Foundation
in Spokane, Washington.
They assisted people
with visual dysfunction.

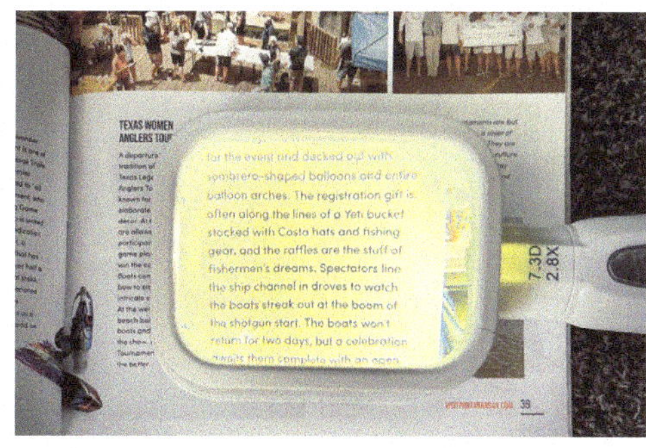

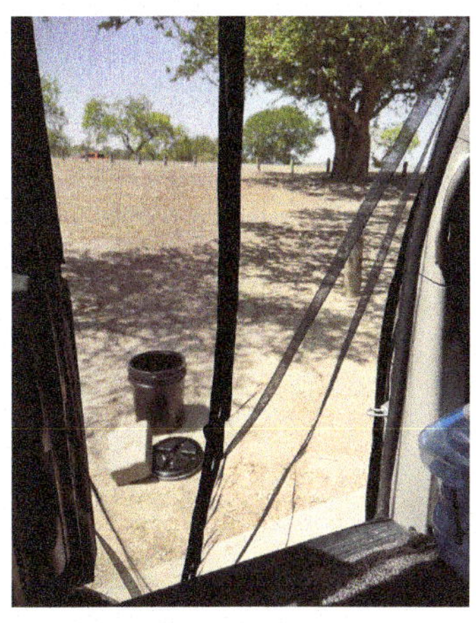

Bug screens were a must.
Got these off Amazon.
They were attached to the van with magnets.
Essential to cut down on the bug annoyance factor
and help with ventilation.

Talked to Ronald fishing at the lake.
Learned that you didn’t need
a fishing license for catfishing in the park.
Good to know.

Met Bev and Katie the dog from Wyoming.
They were camping in a horse trailer RV
and her husband brought
his Harley Davidson motorcycle.
The motorcycle rode in the back of the horse trailer.

Heard from Daniel.
He was at Bisti Badlands
and it was so cold at night during the star shoot,
“The pee froze as it hit the ground.”

DAY 50 / APRIL 8

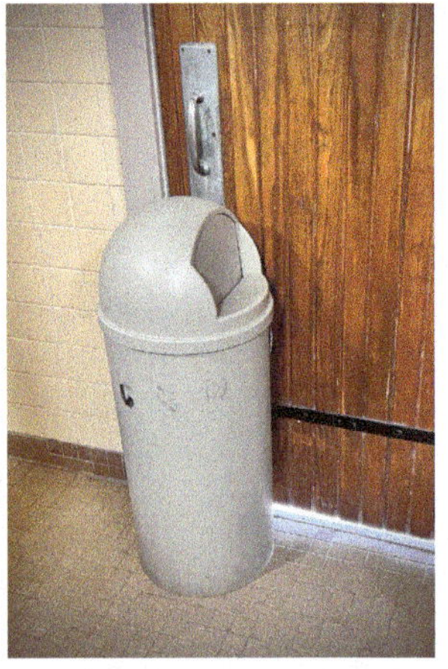

Started the day taking a shower.
The door to the building
couldn't lock from the inside
and the shower stalls
had shower curtains.
No doors that could lock anywhere.

The building site next door
had at least six workers.
Anyone from the campground
could walk in anytime.
I put the garbage can in front of the door,
and my fish fillet knife
in the soap dish.
Hoping I would hear
someone opening the door.

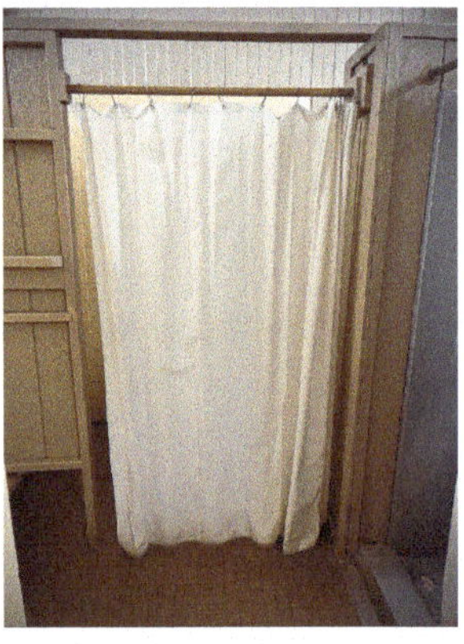

Anyone coming through the curtain
would connect with the knife.
And I meant business.

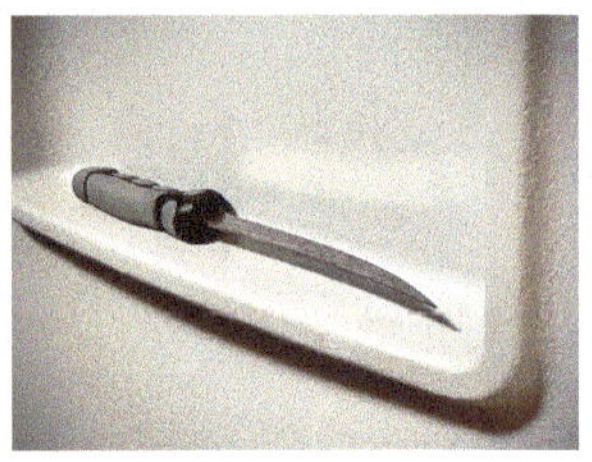

Drove to Padre Island.
Stopped on the pavement
and walked onto the sand
to check out the beach.
There were several vehicles
including a minivan on the beach.

A man fishing on the beach approached me.
"What's wrong with your van?"

"Nothing. Just checking where to drive
so I don't get stuck in the sand."

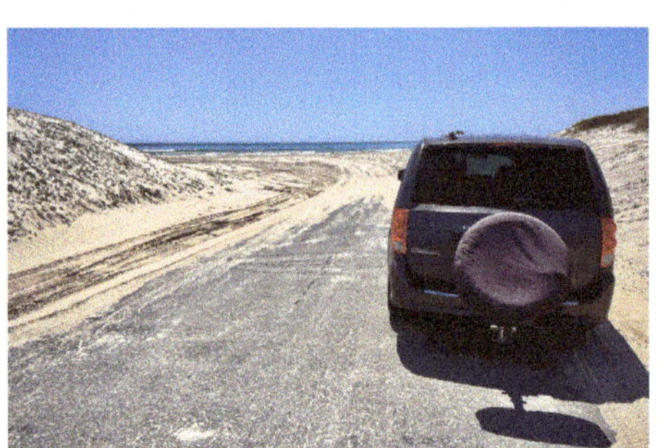

"You'll be fine.
If you get stuck,
I'll pull you out."

Good to know.

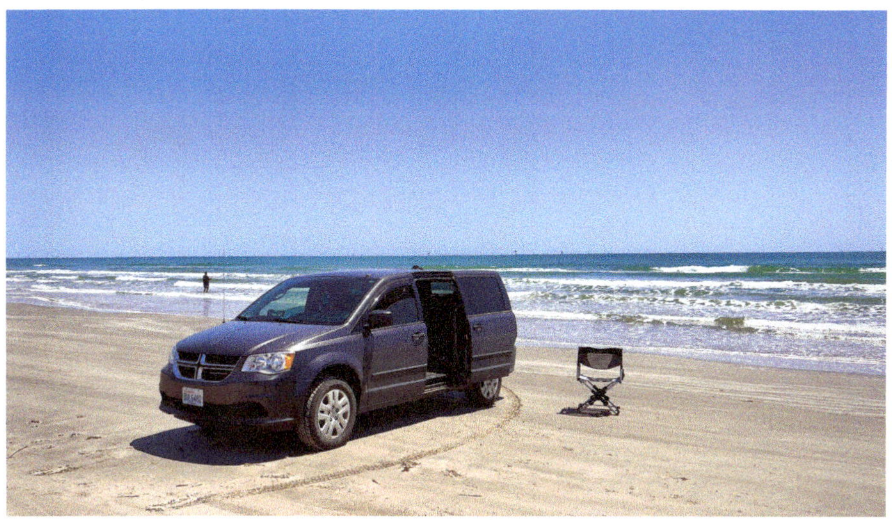

Drove onto the beach
and parked.
I made it to the Gulf of Mexico!
Number 1 item on my bucket list:
drive on the beach
to see the Gulf of Mexico.

Just got situated,
and Anthony fisherman walked over.
People were stuck in the dry sand.
"I could pull them out with my jeep,
but I don't have a tow strap."
No kidding.
He was going to pull me out
if I got stuck.
With what?

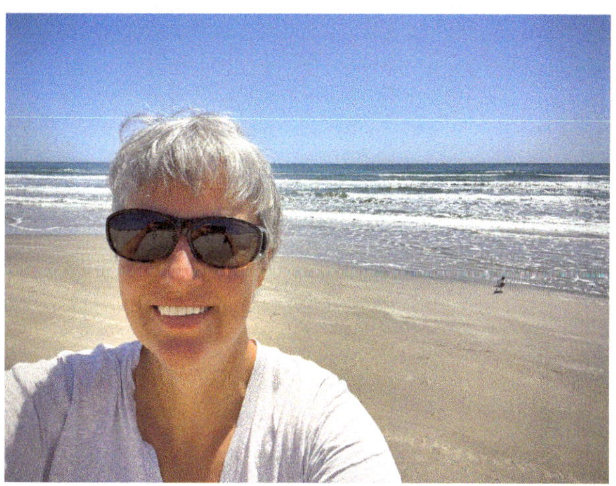

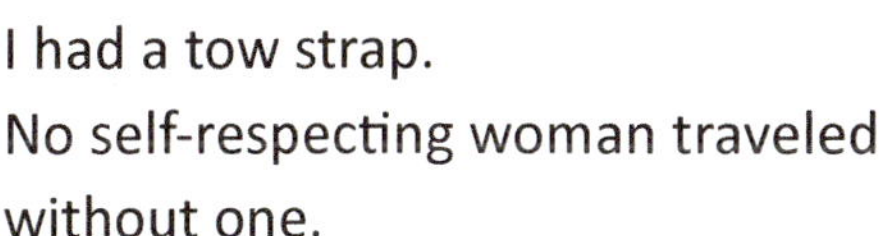

I had a tow strap.
No self-respecting woman traveled
without one.

We walked over and he pulled out
two stuck vehicles.
People were driving onto the beach
taking shortcuts through the dry sand.
Even I knew better.

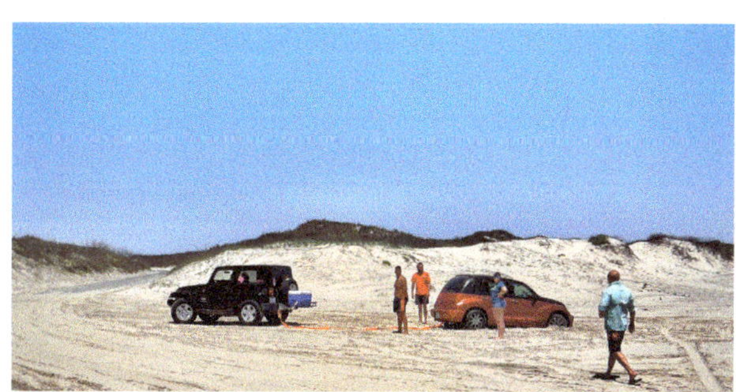

The drive back to
Lake Corpus Christi State Park was hectic.
Lots of traffic
and the speed limit was 70 mph.
And lots of tailgating.
Super exhausting.

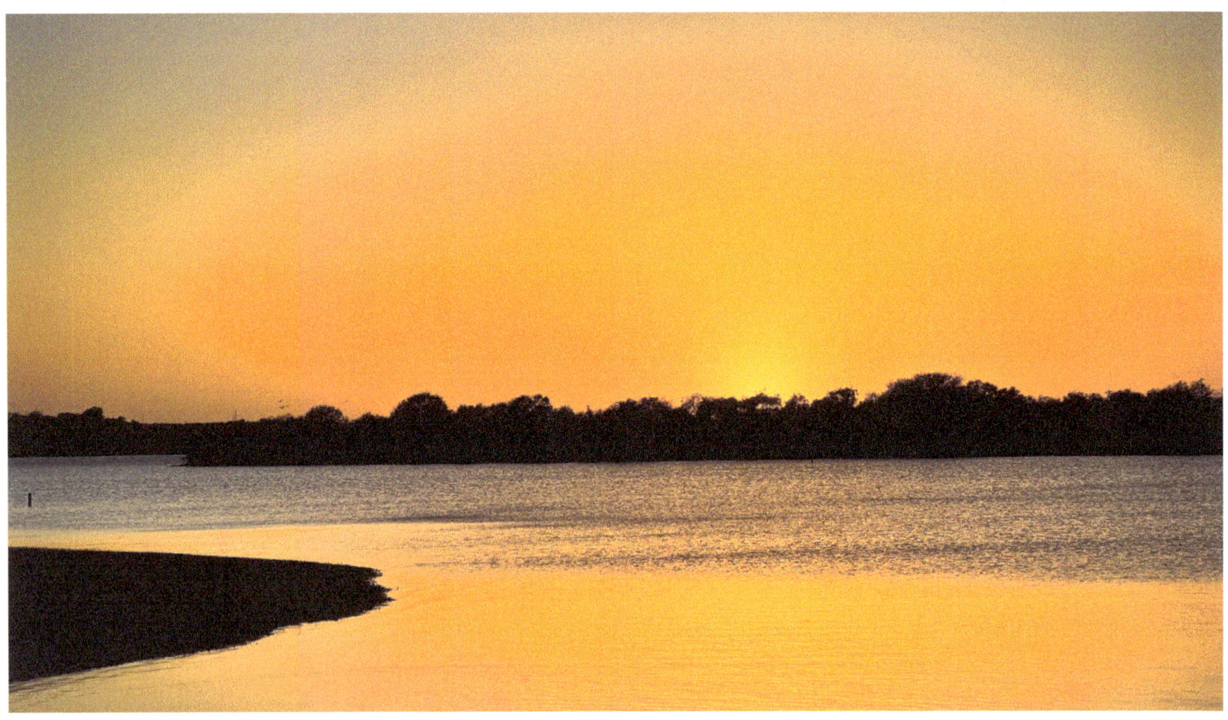

Dave and Bev walked by during the sunset picture shoot.
Great conversation.
Shared I was born and raised in South Africa.
Dave commented that's why I wasn't afraid of traveling alone.
Bev invited me to visit the next day.

DAY 51 / APRIL 9

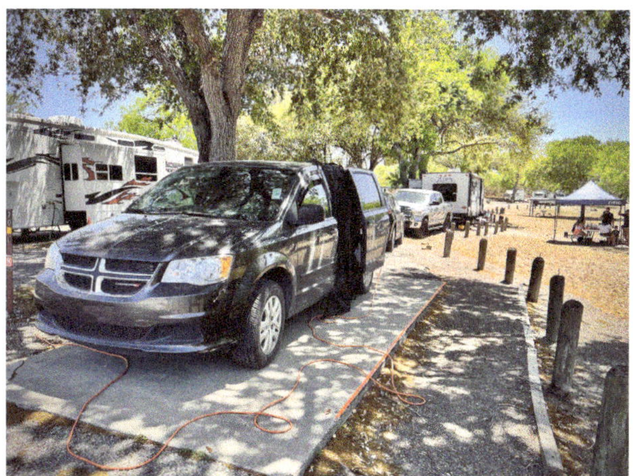

Bev came by and invited me to breakfast.

Wow, never seen a horse trailer
that looked like a luxury RV inside.
They had the work custom done.

Gave Dave and Bev a tour of the van.
I was supposed to camp
on the beach on Padre Island
and therefore,
didn't have a reservation for the night in the park.

I was very tired and felt disconnected
after the drive the day before.
Driving to Padre Island was a bad idea.
The park was full,
and I couldn't get a reservation for that night.

I planned to stay at the truck stop.
Bev offered that I park behind them in their site.
The best people are from Wyoming.

Heard from Daniel briefly,
he was OK out in the cold.
Traveling like crazy to make it through his destination list.

DAY 52 / APRIL 10

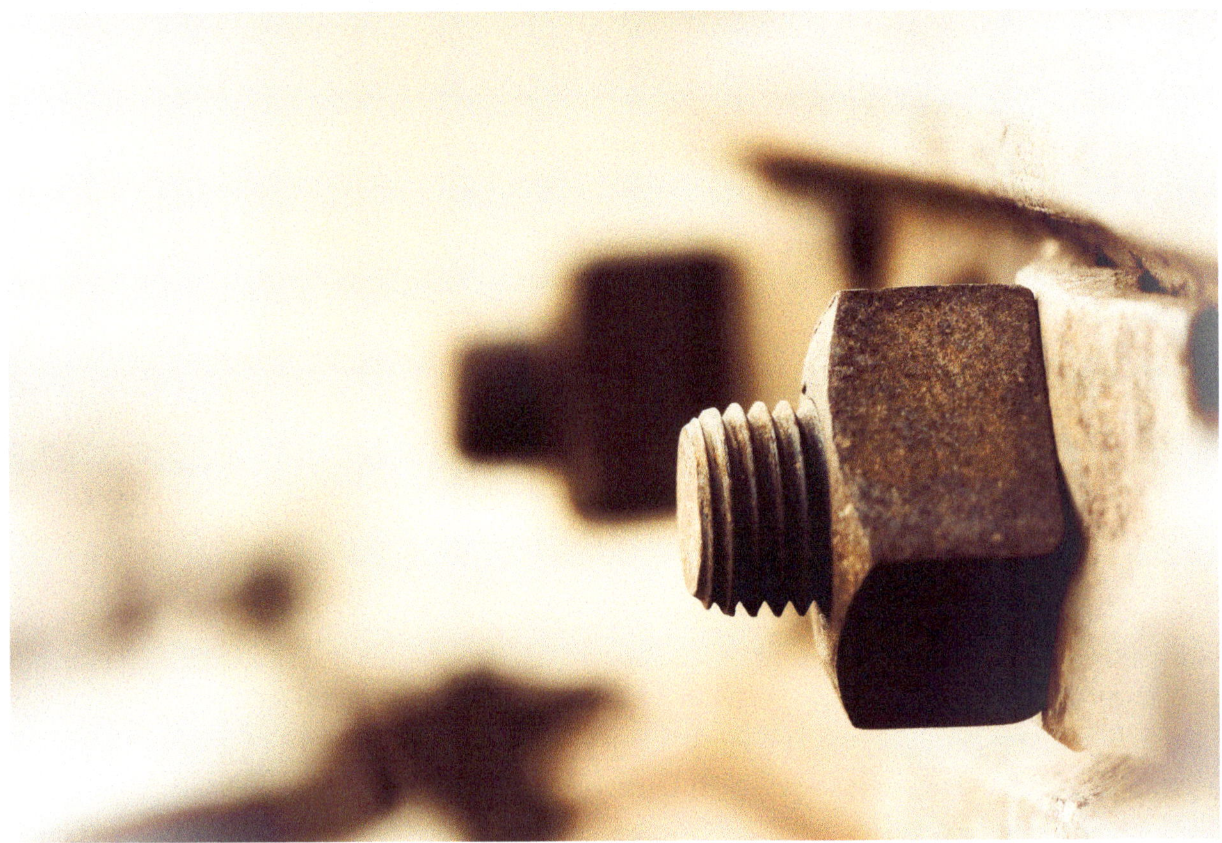

Today was our 11th year wedding anniversary.

Mark was a great husband
and a saint for letting me go on this trip.

The bolt and nut that kept the shit-show together.

And he could fix anything.

And he let me have 5 dogs.

Still a little spaced out from the driving two days ago,
went to the store in Mathis, Tesax to get distilled water.
I probably stood at the counter for 5 minutes
before I saw the sign to ring the bell for assistance.

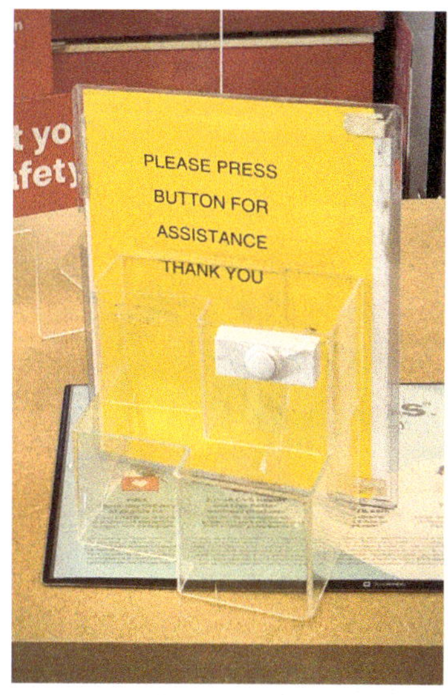

Did laundry and washed the sheet and mattress cover.
It was super windy
and I had to watch the laundry
in case the wind blew it into the lake.

Took a few lamb-chop bones to Katie the dog.
It would be a shame to put them in the garbage
if a nice dog could enjoy them.

Met Dave and Bev at the lake during the sunset shoot.
I was taking off the next day to meet Mark in Corpus Christi.
I asked if I could take their picture.

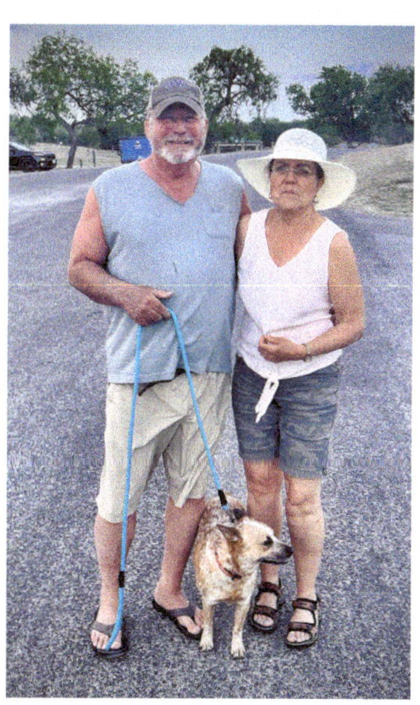

Bev: "I'm not wearing a bra."
Me: "I'm not wearing a bra either. It's too hot."
Dave: "I'm not wearing a bra."
Time to say goodbye.
I would send Bev flower prints when I got home
to thank them for their kindness and providing me a safe spot
to park in overnight.

DAY 53 / APRIL 11

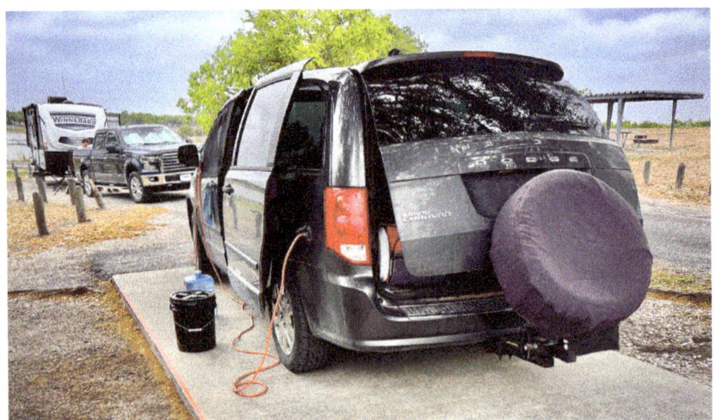

Time to take off.
My brain cells were very puffy.
It was cloudy.
Thank God I didn't have too far to go today.
I could check into the hotel at 2pm
and wait for Mark to arrive.

Holy shit.
Got a message from Daniel.
He was back home.
His wife was visiting family in China
and announced she was leaving him.
What do I say?
That was awful.
I would call him once I got to Corpus Christi.

I wound the extension cord
around the side mirror when setting up.
To be sure not to drive off while still plugged in.
The orange cord helped with seeing it.
Walked around the van a few times
not to forget something.

Mark had an old-school flip phone
and printed the map and directions
from San Antonio airport
to the hotel in Corpus Christi before leaving home.

The plane landed at 2:50 pm
and I was expecting him at the hotel around 5:30 pm.

I was getting worried and stood by the door
to check when he pulled into the hotel parking.
He called to let me know he was on his way,
and I could help somewhat with directions.
It was a relief to see him again after 53 days.

Called Daniel while I was waiting for Mark.
He was devastated.
All I could do was listen.

Mark arrived and we went to dinner.
Alex, Mark's daughter, came by to visit later
after she got done working.

I was debating when I would tell
Mark about the gun episode.
I would wait until the next day
when he was rested.

DAY 54 / APRIL 12

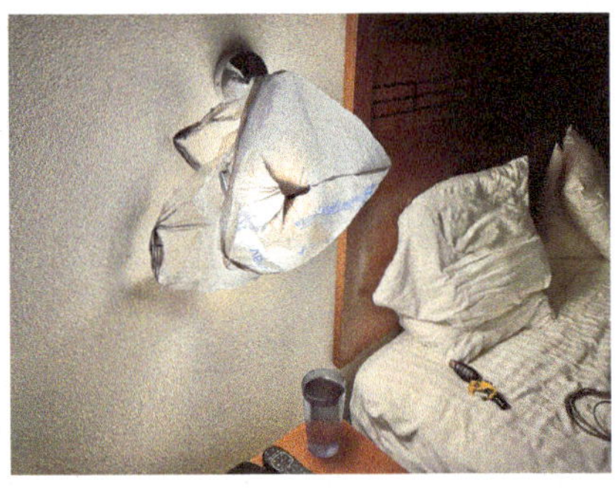

After we had our morning coffee,
I asked Mark to sit on the couch.
I had something to tell him.
I told him the details of the gun episode,
and that I didn't want to share the news over the phone.
My husband, who seldom looked angry,
was very disturbed by the incident.
But he could see that I was fine
and in good health.
He was proud of me for how I handled it
and said I should continue with the trip.

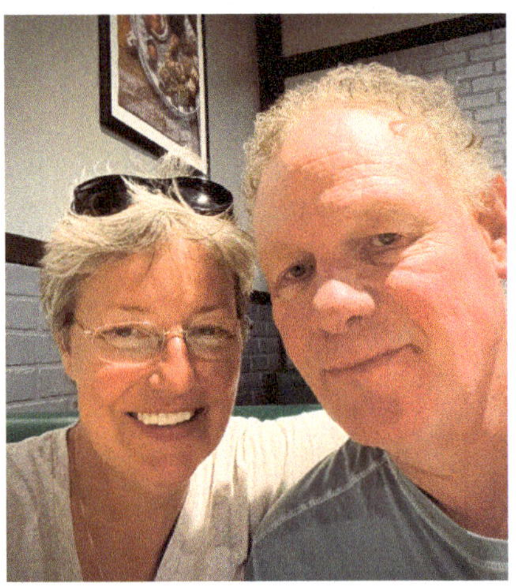

The lights by the bed were very bright.
Pulled a Walmart bag over them which
helped a lot to diffuse the light.

We went to dinner with Alex
to celebrate our wedding anniversary.
Delicious meal.

Later in the evening:
This is an excellent example of how differently
my brain worked after the injury.

Words have lost their meaning
and the pictures are the only thing I "see."
When I saw the picture on the right,
I thought there was something wrong with the oven
and it got burnt.

HE IS RISEN!
HE IS NOT!
HAPPY EASTER!
HAPPY PASSOVER!

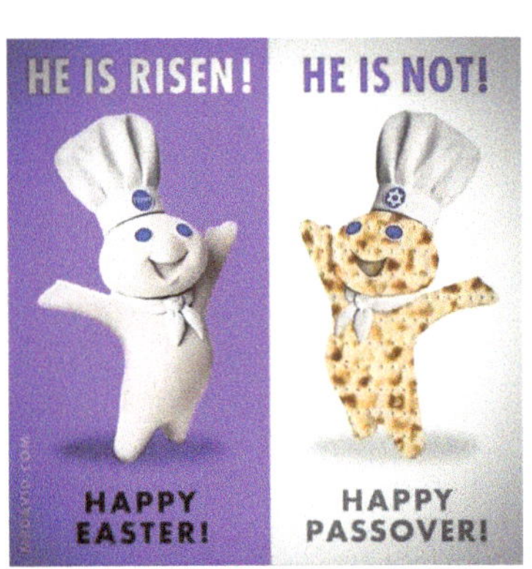

DAY 55 - 57 / APRIL 13 - 15

We visited in Corpus Christi and stayed at the Best Western hotel.
Alex visited as much as she could and gave Mark a tour of the area
while I took the van for an oil change.

I shopped for supplies, distilled water,
cleaned up the van, did some minor repairs
to the window covers
and reorganized the van.
Bought engine coolant to fill up the reservoir
and kept the rest in the van.
Mark helped me shop for a product to un-squeak
the sliding door and rain guards.
Downloaded audio books and offline maps.

I had a double page reserved in my notebook
where I planned my shopping list, to-do items, checked them off as I went.
I took notes in pencil, and erased items as they got done.
Repeat items such as food, water and gas stayed on the list.

We were supposed to swim in the Gulf of Mexico.
But the wind was too unpleasant all week.

Ordered a decal with the new van name BAD-ASS.
Travel Bug was way too wimpy.
Bought supplies and spices for crackers
and "biltong" South African jerky I would make at Orli's house.
Amazon delivered stainless-steel extra-large baking sheets for making crackers.
They wouldn't take much room in the van,
and I would take them home with me.

Planned the trip to Memphis, checking overnight parking options.
Mark made tomato soup for the trip to Memphis at Alex's apartment
while I was fixing the window covers.

And so, time went by, and we would take off the next day.
Mark for San Antonio and I for Memphis.
It was great to see Mark and spend time with him.
I was thankful for the time Mark could spend with Alex.
We only saw her once a year when she came home for Xmas.

DAY 58 / APRIL 16

Took off from Corpus Christi around noon.
800 miles and 4 days to get to Memphis.
I was tired and not in the mood for driving.
Did only about 100 miles
and overnighted at Walmart in Victoria, Texas.
Called ahead on impulse and a nice girl directed me
to the other Walmart in town which allowed overnight parking.

Called Mark, he was home safely.
Called Orli, Jennie and Daniel to catch up.

DAY 59 / APRIL 17

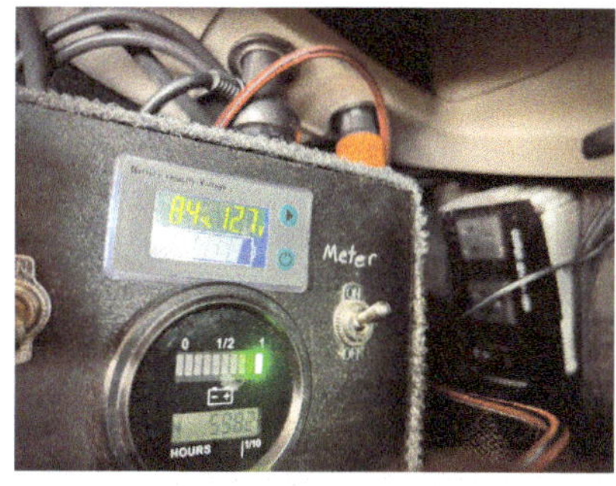

It looked like the DC-DC charger was inconsistent
with charging the deep-cycle batteries.
229 miles of driving for the day.
Speed limit in Texas was 70 mph, even on back roads,
most of the time.
Took more energy to keep up the driving tempo.
Made it to Crockett, Texas.
A really hot day and even hotter in the van.
The little fan did help some,
but a bigger more effective fan
was on the shopping list.
Talked to Mark about DIY AC.
Bought a bag of ice
and jerry-rigged the fan
positioned by my boot
to cool things down.

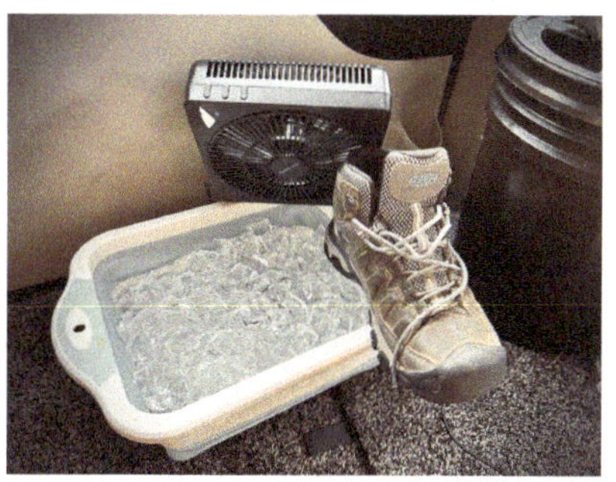

Maybe by 3 degrees while raising
the humidity from 25% to 65%.
I didn't think it helped much.
A bigger fan was a better idea.

Texas had nice sunsets.

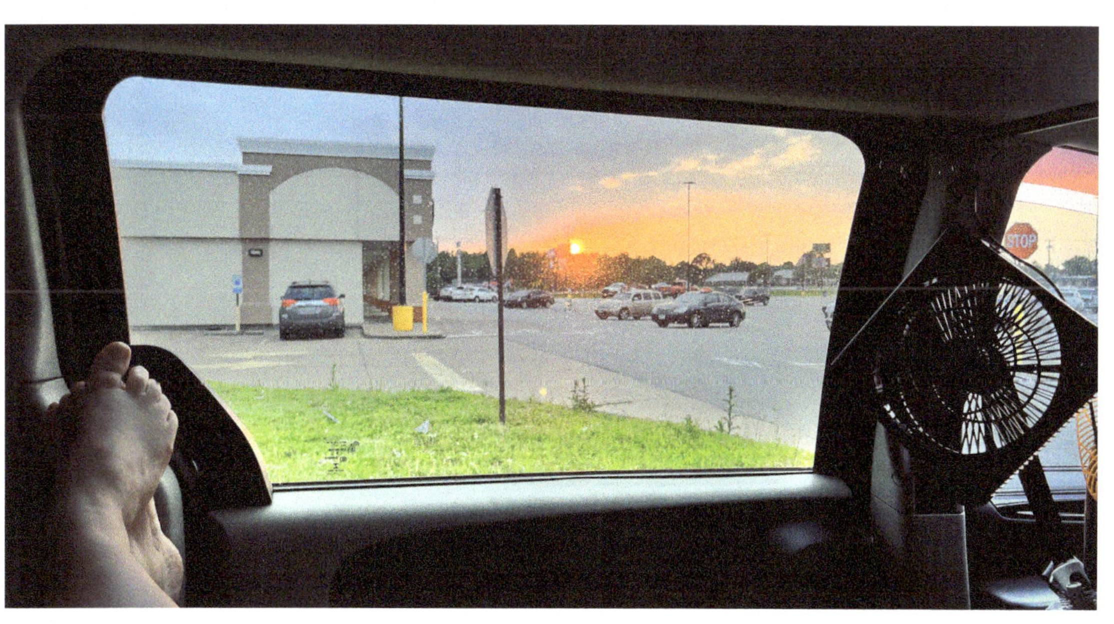

DAY 60 / APRIL 18 / 5,779 MILES

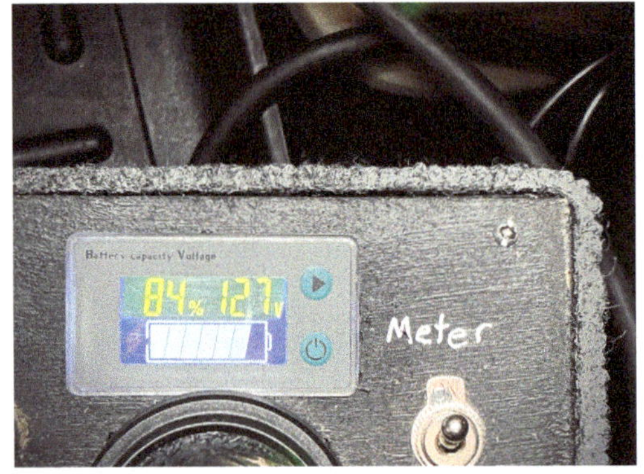

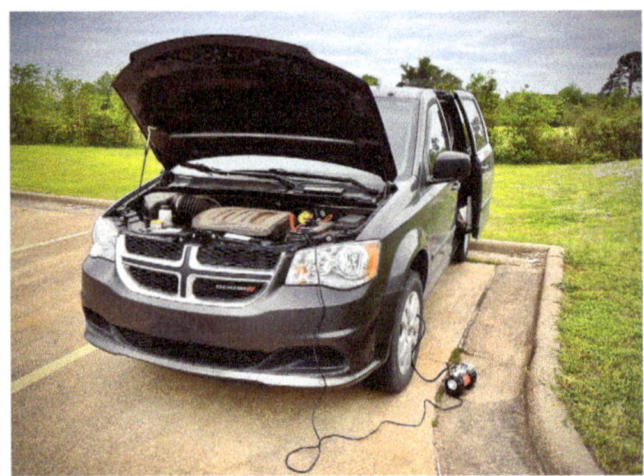

OK, I knew for sure
the batteries were not charging.
First thing I checked every morning.
Plugged the fridge and Jackery into van 12-volt outlets.
I completed a pre-takeoff checklist every morning:

checked the oil and coolant before starting the engine,

no puddles under the van indicating something was leaking,

filled the window washer water and add a few drops of soap,

eyeballed the tire pressure,

checked the temperature settings for the fridge and freezer,

made sure the swing-away hitch was locked in position,

all the doors closed properly, and the back window closed.

Nothing more annoying than to stop after getting started
to close the window (road noise) or the 'open door' light was on.

Also, took thyroid pill, used eye drops
and brushed my teeth.
I needed a reminder to brush my teeth.
Just didn't occur to me.

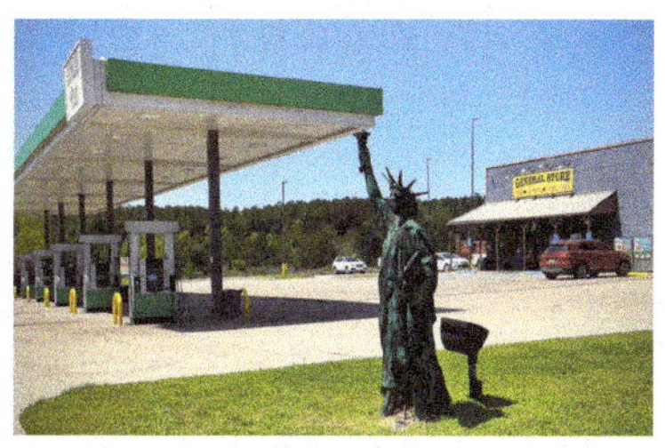

Crossed into Louisiana, a state I've not been in.

Stopped at the Walmart in Minden
and called Mark about the battery problem.
He recommended buying a multimeter
to check the electrical components once I got to Memphis.

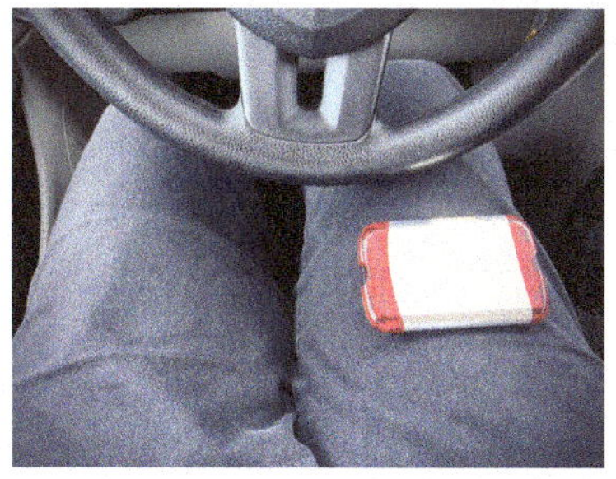

Looked for my wallet before going into the store.
I only took the wallet out of the van
when I needed it for shopping or getting gas.

It was gone.

Not in its usual spot next to the driver's seat.

Not in my bra where I kept it when my clothes didn't have any pockets.
A sick feeling to my stomach.

Bloody hell.

What happened to it?

Maybe I dropped it when I was shopping at the convenience store?

I could call them and ask if it got handed in?
It's not that far, I could go back and look for it?

I had cash in the van, but I didn't have an extra driver's license.

Then the "brain" light came on.

I have been wearing shorts and t-shirts for the last month
and got in the habit of putting my little metal wallet in my bra.
The shorts didn't have any pockets.
I forgot I was wearing jeans that day.
With pockets.

I had put my wallet in my pocket.
And left it there.

Jesus, you really got to get with it.
Your thinking will give you a heart attack.

WELCOME TO ARKANSAS

I lived in Arkansas briefly in 2003/2004
and haven't been there since.

Stayed at Pine Bluff Walmart
after driving 376 miles.
It was a lot of driving for one day.
I wanted to get as close to Memphis as I could.
I didn't want to arrive in Memphis during 5pm rush hour traffic.

And the flushing toilets and air hand dryers were loud.
Wore earplugs everywhere.

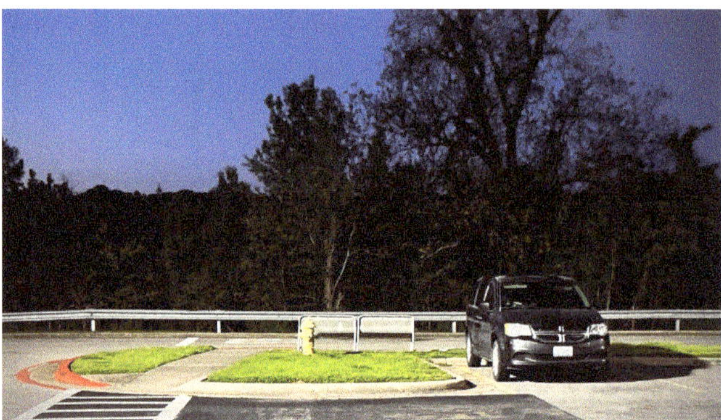

Beautiful sunset as usual.

Found a nice quiet parking spot against the curb.
The green space protected me from people
speeding through the parking lot.

I bought reflective yellow tape
to sew onto the spare tire cover to make it more visible.

By backing into the parking,
I could take off easily in a hurry if needed,
and the curb behind the van protected the spare tire.

DAY 61 / APRIL 19

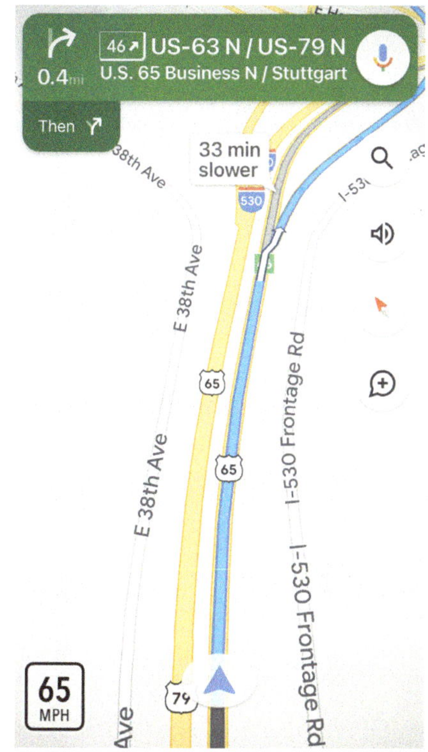

My absolute favorite thing to do:
Listen to Google Maps' verbal directions.
The more words the MERRIER!
And then she repeated it a few times!

In 0.4 miles take exit 46, US-63 N, US-79 N

That's 19 words to listen to.
I lost her after exit 46, the words came at me too fast.
The words didn't stick in my brain.
I tried to replay the words,
while she continued to talk,
while scanning the road signs
for what she possibly said.
For God's sake, just SHUT UP.
By the time I figured out the words,
I missed the exit.
I turned the sound off
and looked at the picture
of what to do.

I stayed on back roads as much as I could
and pulled over for a rest break
before joining the I-40.

Orli had great timing and called during my break
to check on my ETA.

Steve and the dogs would be home to welcome me.

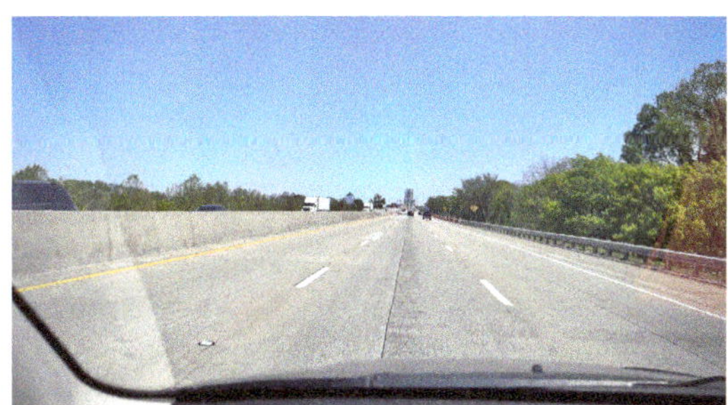

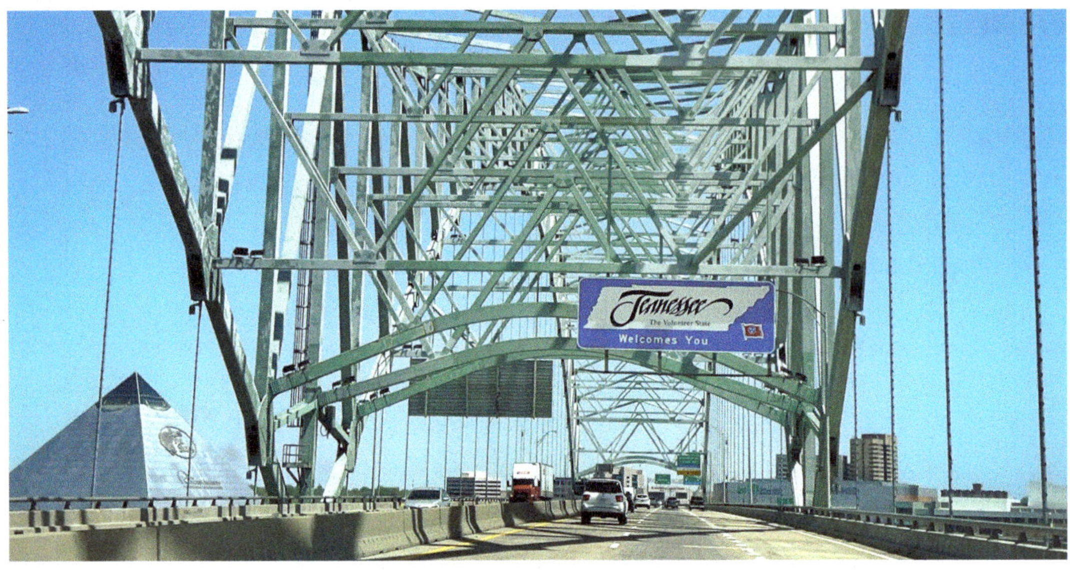

WELCOME TO TENNESSEE!

The last time we were in Memphis
was in December 2013
to watch Orli run a half marathon
and my 50th birthday.
Memphis had a huge ice storm
and the race got cancelled.

Steve welcomed me, helped offloading
necessary items from the van.
We went to Costco to buy meat
for the great biltong making
event of the year when Orli got home.

Biltong is a South African culture you didn't want to miss out on.
Jerky for the American version.
I only shared biltong with a privileged few.

Steve was my first American friend
after arriving in the country in 1997.
He even speaks a few words of Afrikaans.

It was great to see Orli again!
We both arrived in the U.S. in 1997 and worked for the same company.
She was born in South Africa and grew up in Israel.
Teaching Occupational Therapy and a great artist.

DAY 62 / APRIL 20

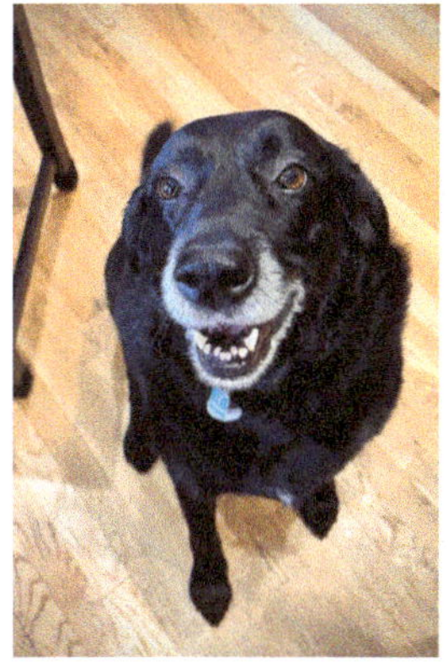
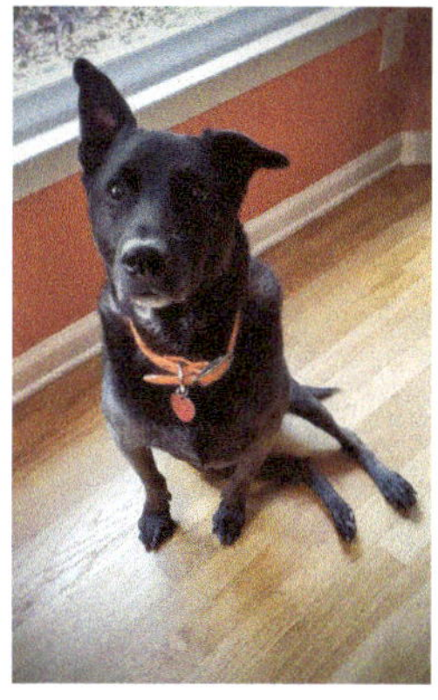
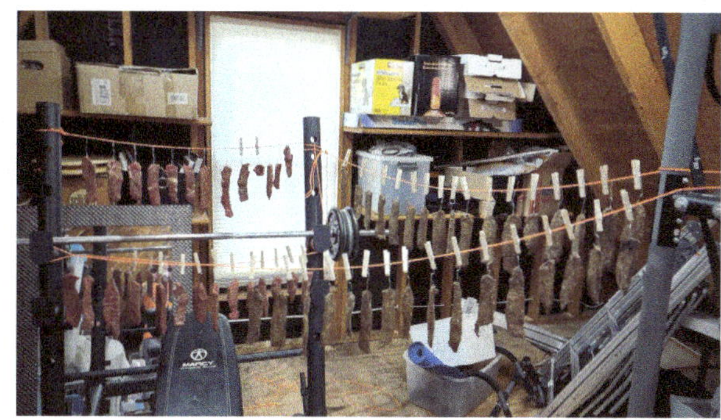

Mira and Nicki were great company,
especially since I haven't seen
our 4 wiener dogs in 62 days.

And a real washing machine!
A great pleasure to use after 2 months
of hand-washing clothes in a bucket.
Got started on making 3 batches
of flaxseed-meal crackers.
Cooked a big pot of stew
and put it in Ziplock baggies for dinners for 6 days.
Checked on the biltong in the loft.
Could start tasting soon.

I put an album of pictures together
for my motivational talk coming up.

Orli recommended doing a slide show in Google Docs.

I started working on it.

It was torturous.

Visually exhausting.

She helped me by checking for duplicate slides.

I had 4 days to get ready for the talk.

DAY 63 / APRIL 21

I took the fridge out of the van
as well as the "kitchen" set of plastic drawers.
Took the platform out that covered the electronics.
I had a clear view of it,
took a picture and sent it to Mark.

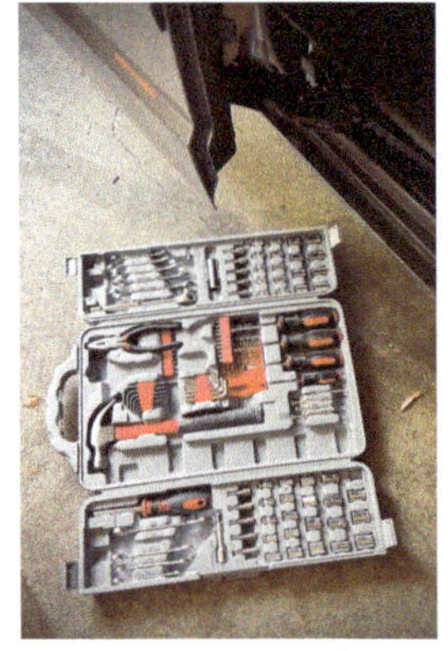

He called me for a phone troubleshooting session.
The man was very brave.
He gave verbal directions to test different circuits
to his wife with a brain injury who had trouble
following verbal directions.

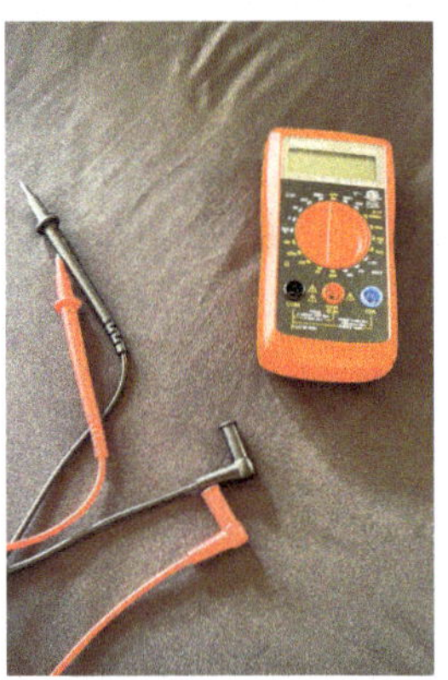

He explained how to turn on the multimeter
and the settings to use.
I couldn't get the wires connected.
They had plastic plugs covering the ends.
No one told me about it.

"Take the tape off the main wire coming through the firewall
and check the connection."

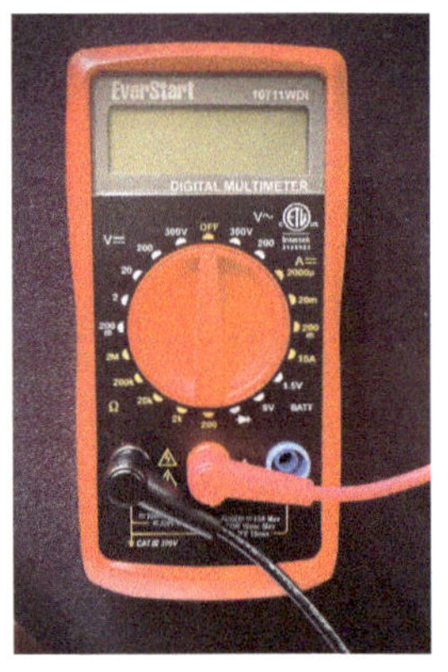

"Don't shock yourself."

"Don't start a fire."

Holy shit.

"Should I turn off the breaker under the hood?"

I was sweating like a pig.

Even more.

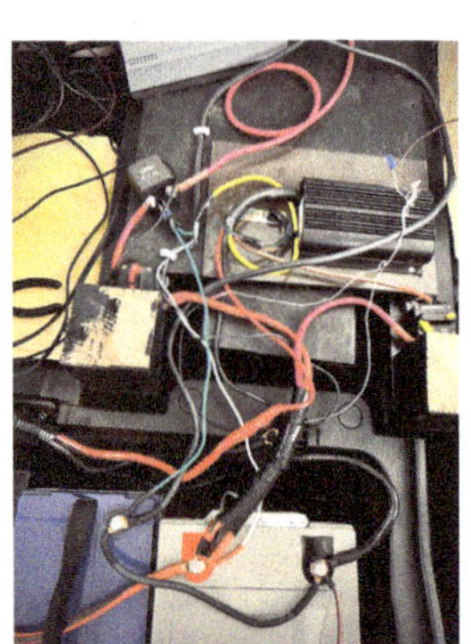

My heart was beating too fast.

Following the directions the best I could.
After taking the tape off the main wire
and finding a good connection, taped it back up.
Went to turn the breaker back on.

And the breaker was on.

I was sure I turned it off.

I was touching a live wire.

Jesus.

And I didn't get shocked.

There was no definitive answer to the problem.
The conclusion was Mark would look at it when I got home.

After I got home, Mark fixed the problem.
The breaker under the hood didn't fail outright,
it allowed 5 volts through intermittently instead of 12 volts.

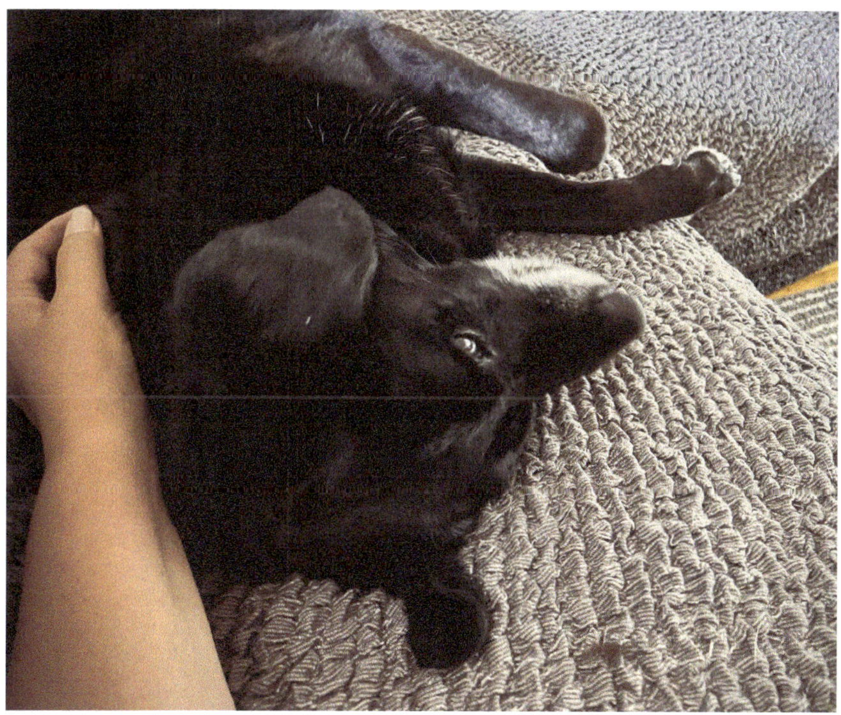

Nothing relieves stress
like sitting with
and petting a dog.

DAY 64 / APRIL 22

I worked on the slideshow in all earnest.
I realized how much work went into getting ready
for the trip and
how many occupational therapy principles I used subconsciously.

I had 5 typed pages double-spaced of things to do,
fix and reinvent
before leaving on the trip.

I had an expensive new iPhone I didn't
want to damage or break by dropping it.
I bought a metal waterproof case,
but it felt very slick,
and I could drop it without noticing.
My hands didn't register very well what they did anymore.
I saw a case with a wrist strap, but it wasn't waterproof.

I drilled two little holes in the corner of the case
and attached a wrist strap.
Solved the problem.
I just had to remember to use the strap consistently,
especially close to water and rocks.

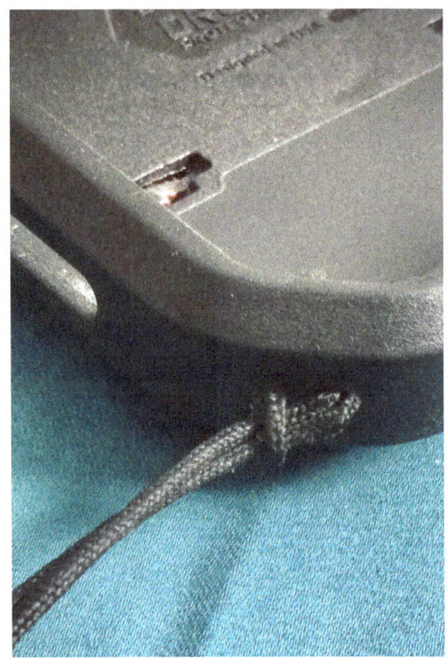

I focused heavily on energy conservation techniques
when designing the inside of the van.
Minimizing the number of steps
required to complete a task,
and having items needed stored together.

Being able to boil water in the van
without having to get out,
getting the spare tire out of the way,
opening the back door,
setting up the stove, getting the water and pot,
and boiling the water.
That was the previous setup.
Very tiring.

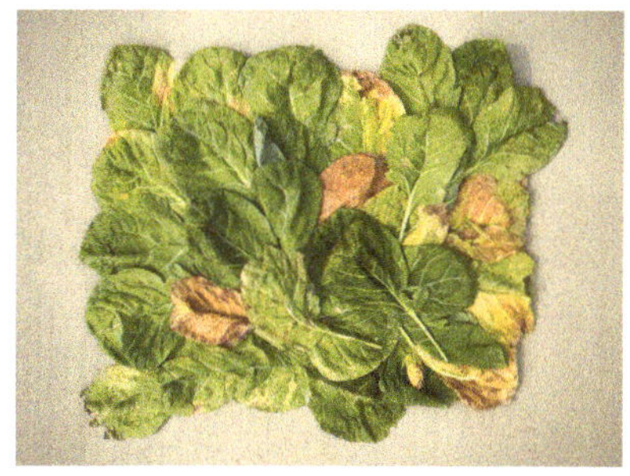
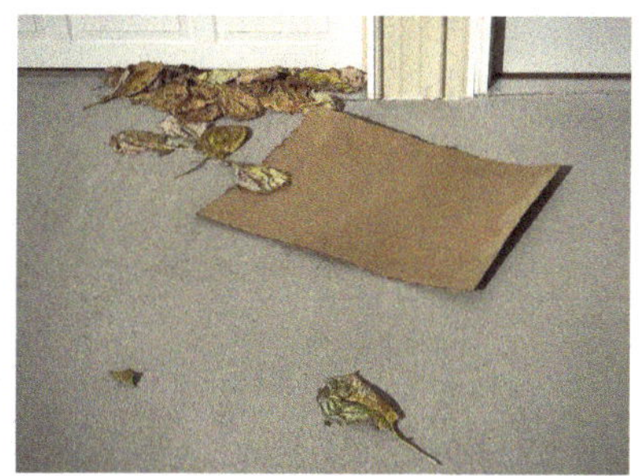
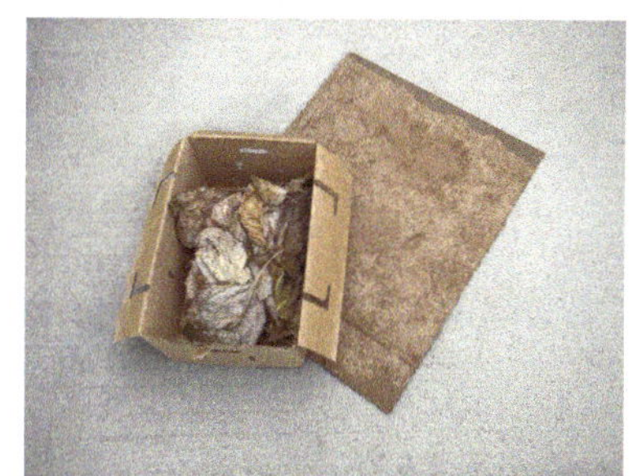

Preparing for the talk reminded me of the last almost 4 years
of going to therapies and counseling.
Struggling with the painful aftermath of the injury.
My organized normal professional life blown up.
Picked up the pieces and put them on a shelf.
Forgotten.

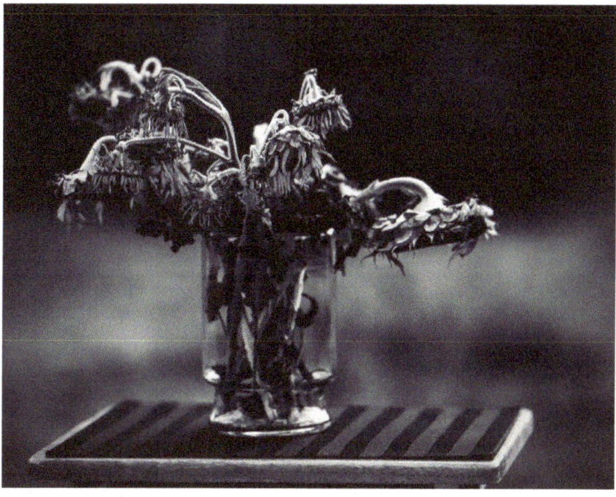

I let my occupational therapy licenses lapse
after 3 years of struggling to maintain it.
It was too hard to meet the
continued education requirements.

I was officially useless.

Without a job permanently.

Funeral flowers for my profession, my identity.

The Death no one knew about.

The funeral for one.

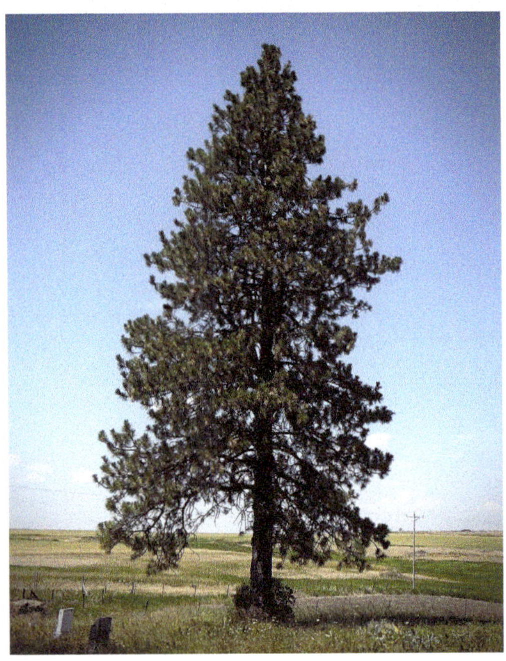

Most people who don't know me think I look normal.
Those are the people who see the healthy tree.

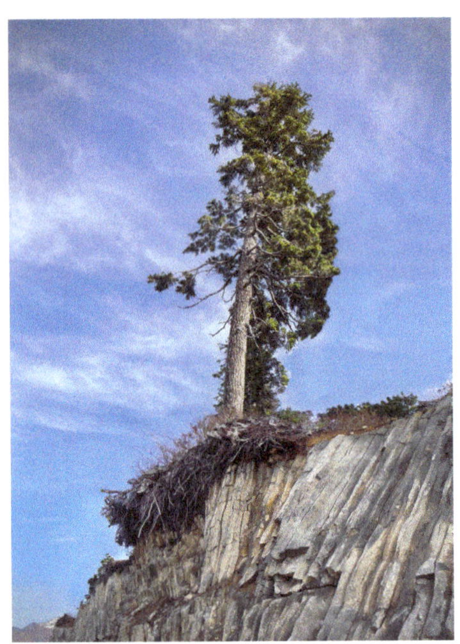

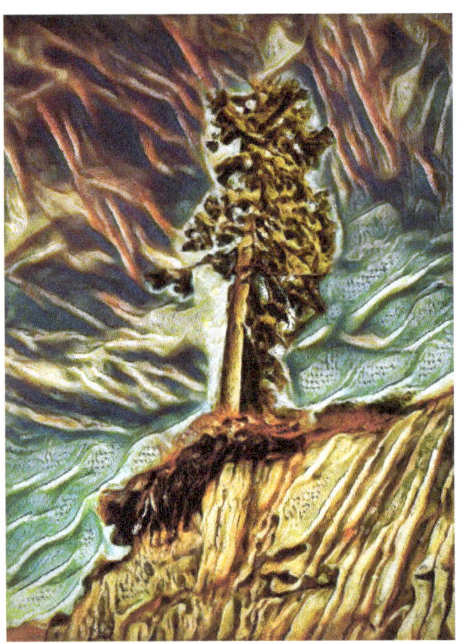

Explaining what an injured brain feels like,
having people see the tree
where half the roots are exposed, visible,
where the ground gave away and damaged the tree.
Painful explanations.
Talking about someone else,
but know it's me I'm talking about.

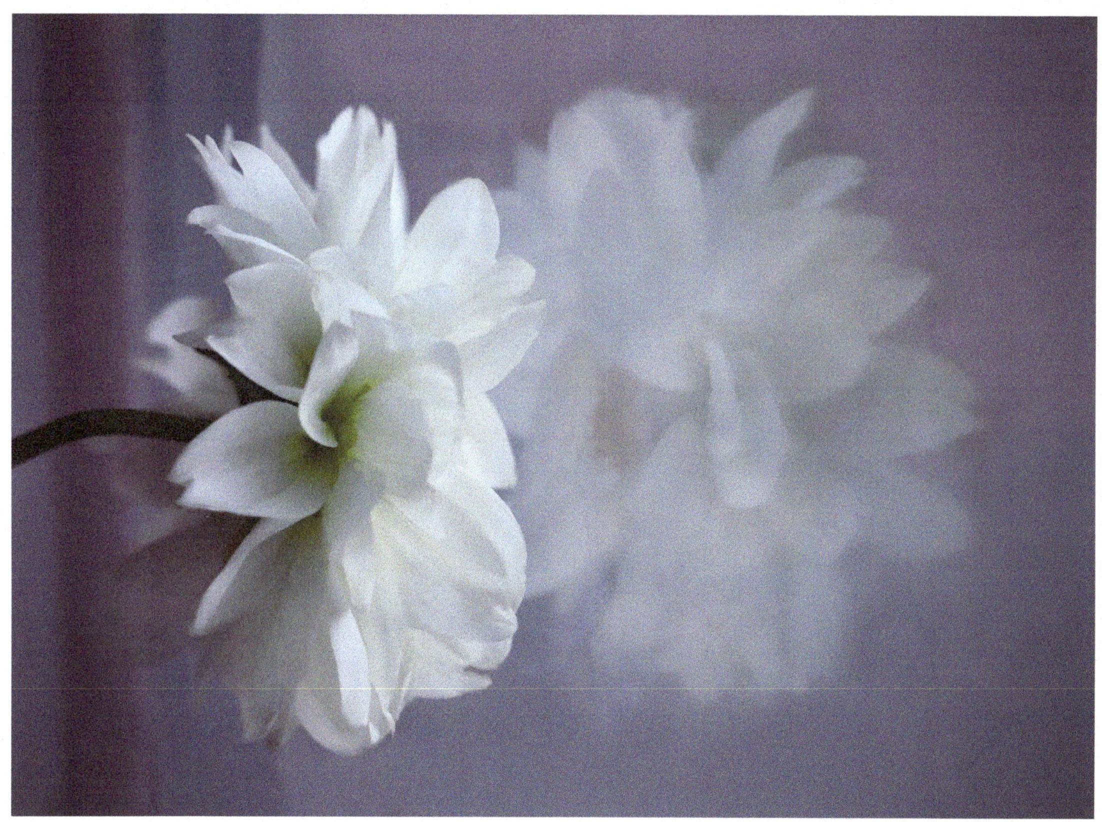

All I can see is what's left of my life.
The shadow of what I used to be.

Steve went to the car wash with me,
watching and waiting,
while I hand-washed the van
without worrying about what was happening around me.
Without worrying about my safety.

I needed two prescriptions refilled.
Albertsons/Kroger did a great job
transferring the prescriptions and filling them.

Took the van to Discount Tire, got the tires balanced and rotated.

I had to pick up a box of butane I ordered from Home Depot.
Most affordable option.
Orli took me to pick it up.
I was too tired to drive.

DAY 65 / APRIL 23

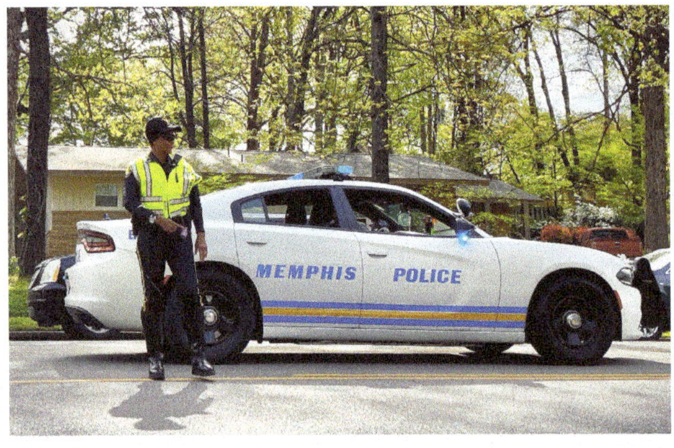

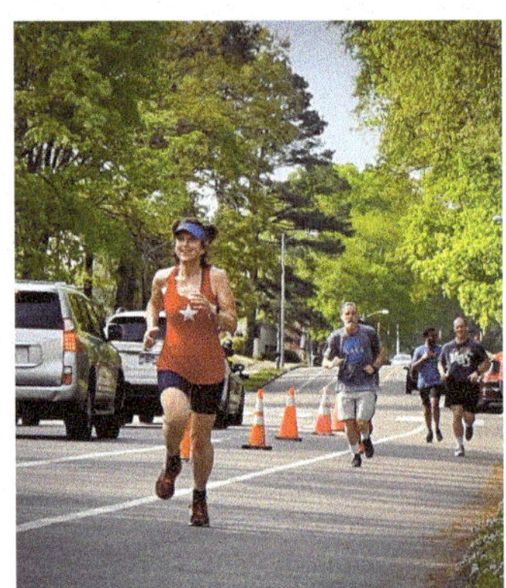

Checked off another bucket list item.
Seeing Orli run a half marathon.
The timing wasn't right for the half marathon,
but the bonus was seeing both Orli and Steve run a race.

I sat on the sidewalk watching the race.
I had a lot of time to watch the lady cop manage the traffic.
I hoped she made it through her day safely.
Dangerous job she had.
So she could go home and spend time with her family.

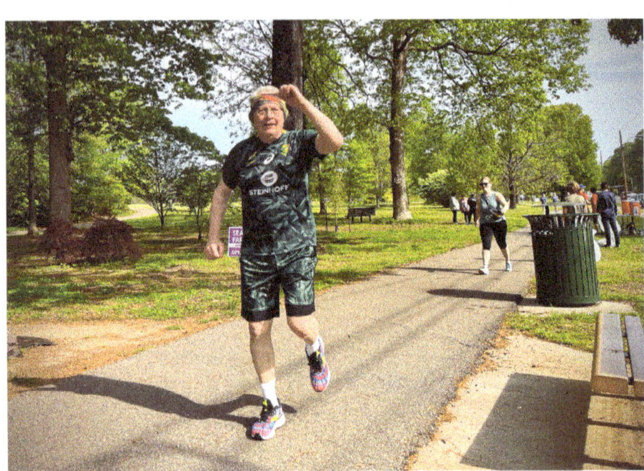

Steve walked me down the aisle when Mark and I got married.
After decorating the tables on the wedding day,
we did a practice run,
with hilarious dancing and fancy steps down the aisle,
just about rolling on the floor laughing.

While we were waiting for the music
to start at the ceremony,
Steve said, "The same as this morning?"
and I said yes.
Most memorable wedding of the year.

Steve did the same fancy dance steps
during the race when he saw me.
Got to love him.

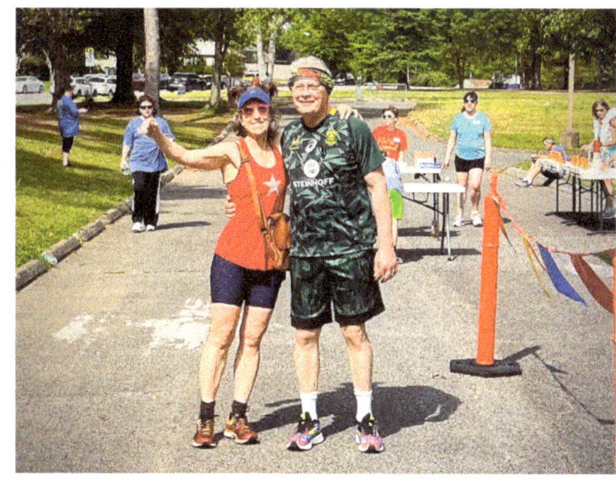

More sweating putting the slide show
together later in the day.

The thinking of an injured brain.
Not the easiest problem-solving techniques.
Herding chickens.
Or was it "herding marbles"?
Who came up with marbles in any case?
Whoever dropped the marbles
must have stood on a hill
when they scattered them.

Thinking is not in a straight line.
Distractions.
Dead ends.
Sidetracks.
Forget as you think about it.
Exhausting.
Why does it have to be so hard?

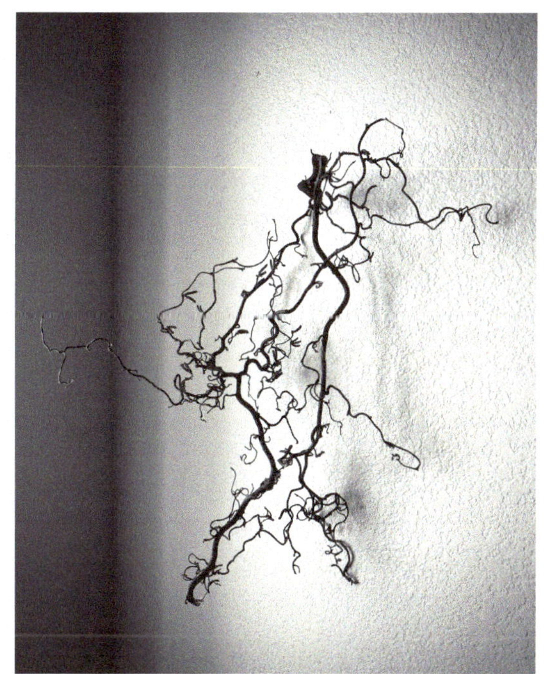

DAY 66 / APRIL 24

Orli took me to the
University of Tennessee
Health Science Center.
Showed me where I would be giving the talk and where to park.
I would call her when I arrived,
and she would accompany me into the building.

It was raining and my brain felt like it
was stuffed with cotton balls.

It was getting very real,
and I was very nervous
and felt guilty for agreeing to do it.

I didn't want to embarrass her by doing a crappy job.
I didn't want to bail.
I like to do what I said I would.

I called Mark and confessed
my doubts about my abilities.
He said do my best
and he knew I could do it well.

I also called Daniel.
He was closer to the students' age
and had a different perspective.

"You know something they don't.
Talk about it."

DAY 67 / APRIL 25 / 6,305 MILES

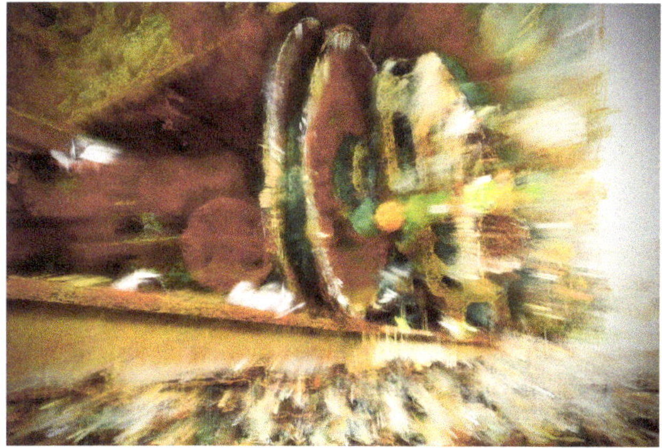

I woke up feeling like something exploded in my head.
A train ran over me last night.
It was raining and I felt very disconnected.
Orli had the slideshow, and it would all be set up when I got there.
I drove to the college avoiding the interstate.
I wanted to be there early and rest in the van to recover from the drive
in the rain with the wipers on.

Orli came and waited with me
until it was time to walk into the building.
The room was buzzing with
the students enjoying lunch.
I asked to wait in a quiet room.
Orli gave a great introduction
to faculty and students.
She showed me the remote for the projector.
I had such a deer in the headlights feeling,
I forgot to thank her
for the invitation and introduction.

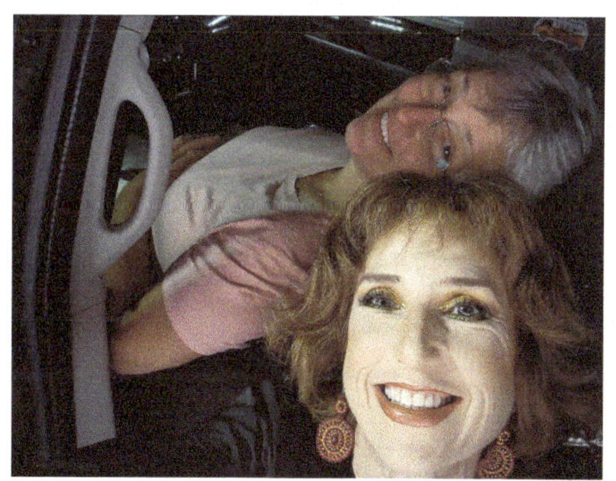

I started the timer on my phone
for 45 minutes.
I was just praying it wasn't the time
to look for words
or forget what I was going to say,
or they could tell
how hard my heart was beating.

I made it through the slideshow
with 5 minutes to spare.

Orli had a huge smile on her face,
and a big applause in the room.

She invited everyone to a van tour
in the parking garage.
I was surprised and impressed
with the questions the students asked.

Orli said the students were listening while I talked.
The best compliment to any speaker.

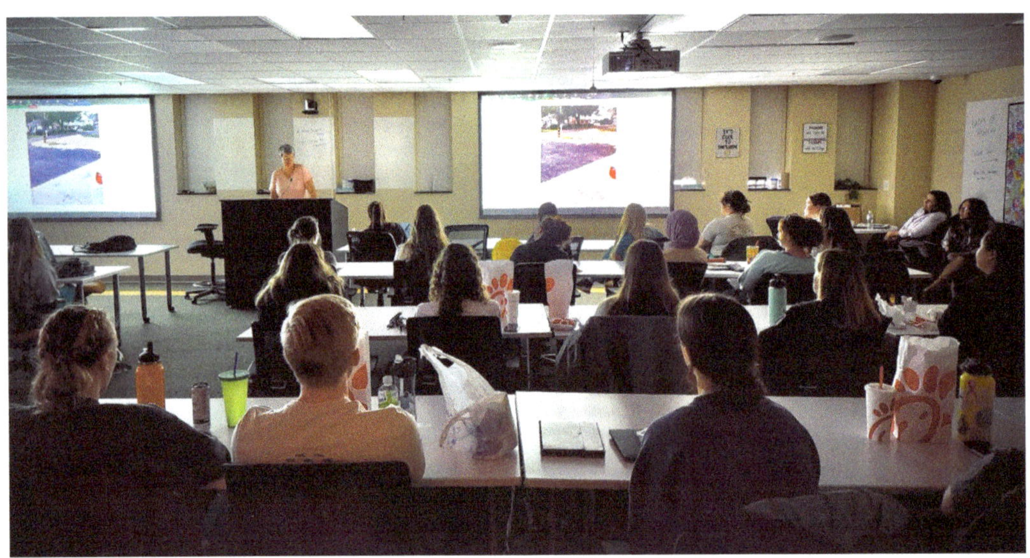

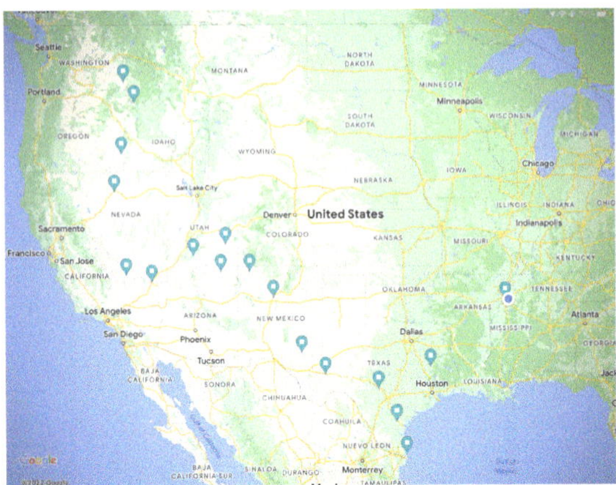

DAY 68 / APRIL 26

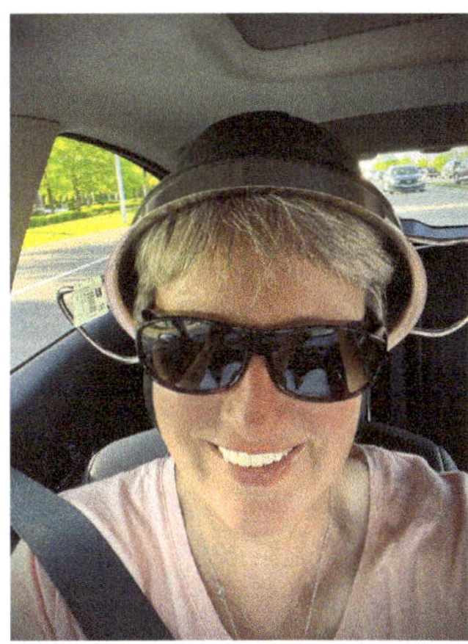

The last day of the Memphis visit with dear friends.
Steve helped me load the heavy stuff.
Daniel helped me with suggestions
for the route back to Moab, Utah.

Steve gave me a handy back scratcher.
I used it regularly to turn off the dome light
on the dashboard after I was in the back of the van already.
Orli, the true occupational therapist,
gave me bubble-wrap baggies.
I put the butane canisters in them
to stop them from rattling while driving.

We went to Ikea and
Orli gifted me a collapsible colander.
It was very handy and as usual
everything was used in multiple ways.
I had to shop for a charging cord for my Bluetooth speaker.
Those cords must have fallen off the planet,
couldn't find one anywhere.
I found a rugged speaker with good sound
I could listen to, very affordable.

Downloaded new audiobooks
and offline maps for my route to Moab.

I had a favorite author with a series of 67 audiobooks.
The same characters I was familiar with.
I couldn't remember the details of the stories
but knew the people.
I would restart at the first book
once I was done with the series.
I didn't have to pay too much attention
but would follow the story mostly.

I didn't like starting new books,
it took a lot of energy to pay attention
and I couldn't do it while driving.

The van was loaded and just a few details
to finish the next morning including making sure
I didn't forget anything.

DAY 69 / APRIL 27

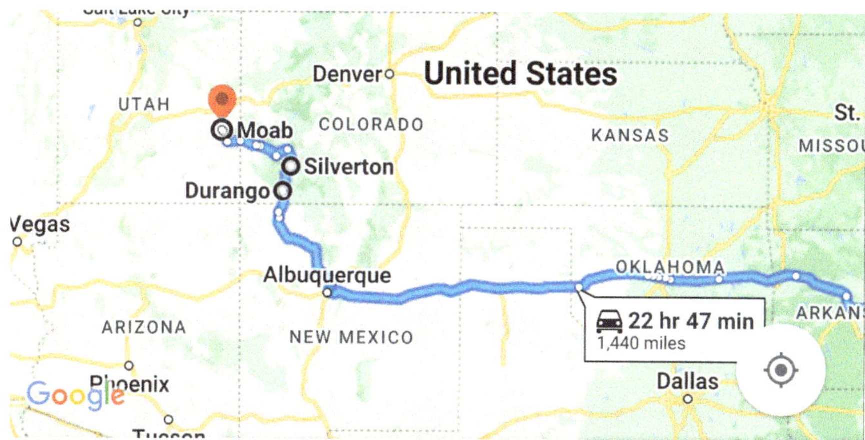

Said goodbye to Steve and the dogs.
Said goodbye to Orli last night.
A huge trip ahead of me.
Days of I-40 driving to New Mexico.

Many, many semi-trucks doing 70–80 mph.
Crosswinds.
Death grip on the steering wheel.
Pay attention, don't space out.
Follow backroad routes as much as possible.

Spent a lot of time the last week
talking and focusing on the brain injury.
Not a good feeling.

Drove across Arkansas
and made it to Fort Smith.
308 miles driving for the day.

On the border of Arkansas and Oklahoma.

Called Orli and Mark.

DAY 70 / APRIL 28 / 6,671 MILES

WELCOME TO OKLAHOMA

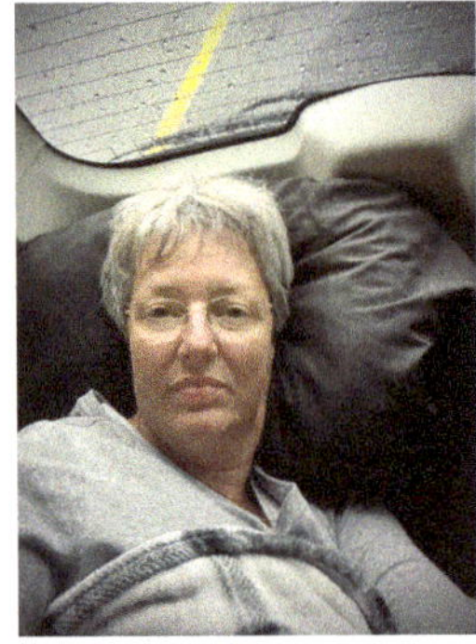

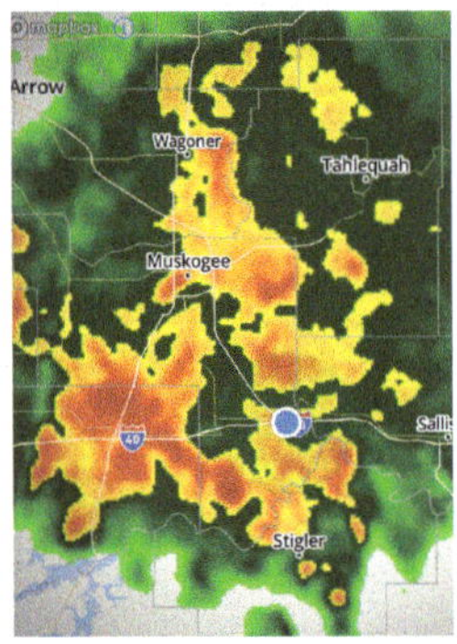

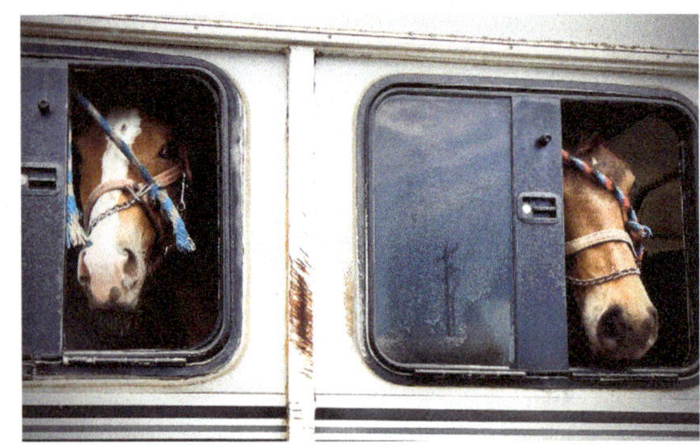

Ran into heavy rain and stopped at the Love's Truck Stop
in Webbers Falls, Oklahoma.
I didn't drive in rain, the wipers made me dizzy.
Cool neighbors of the 4-legged kind.
Stayed put and took a 2-hour nap.

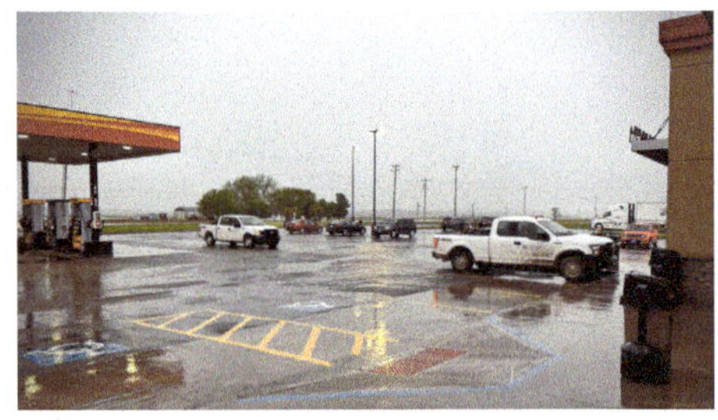

The storm subsided when I woke up.
Orli said there was a tornado in the area the next day.

I wanted to call Len, my counselor.
I did well with giving the talk,
but it dug up the pain of losing my profession.
My life.
Dead forever.
How would I make peace with it?

My Plan was looking better than ever.
I didn't want to live this painful life anymore.

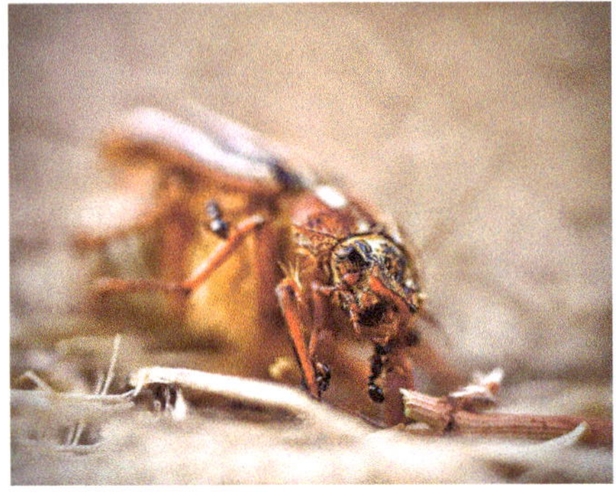

Goal for the day:
make it to El Reno, Oklahoma.
Just going through the motions.
Keep going.

And get off I-40.

Typically, the women's bathrooms at Walmart have been on the right side on the trip.
The bathroom on the right side was not the women's.
No one inside to tip me off.
And I didn't "see" the urinals.
After a few minutes saw someone leaving.
Long hair looked like a woman, until he looked at me.

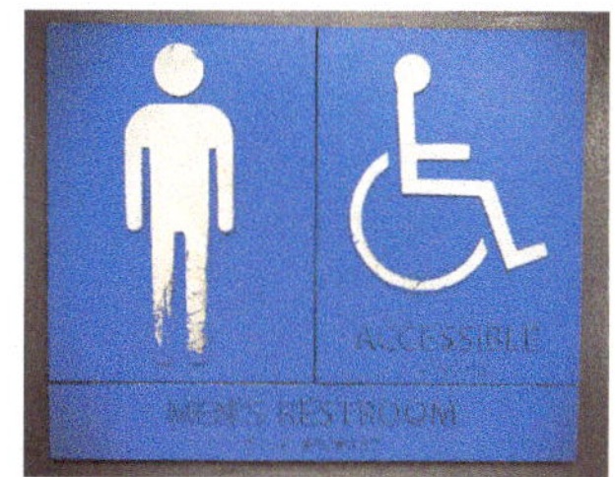

Great spot by the truckers.

Quiet and peaceful.

Called Orli to update on travel location.

249 miles for the day.

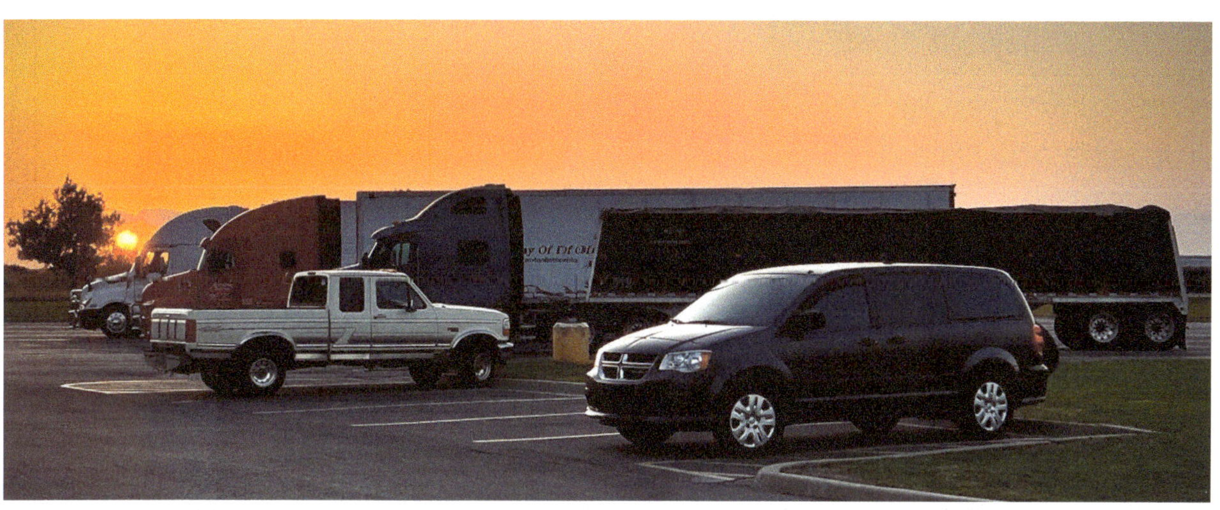

DAY 71 / APRIL 29

WELCOME TO TEXAS

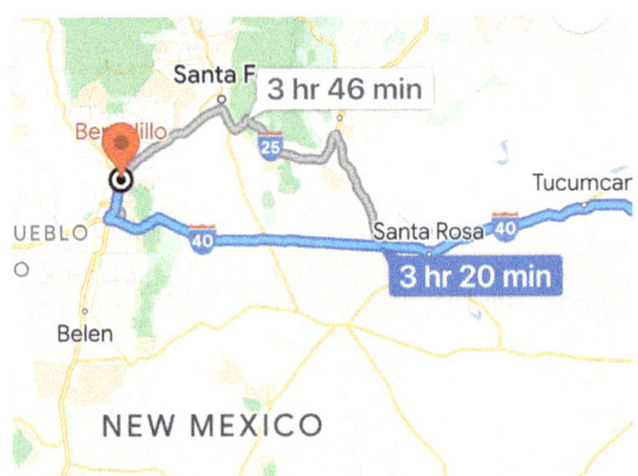

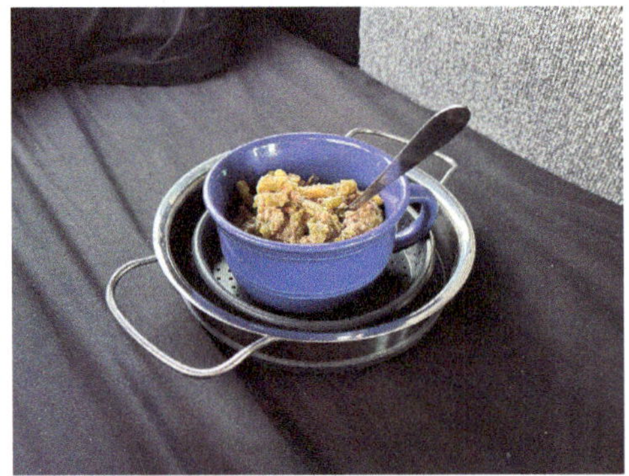

The collapsible colander was very versatile.
Especially for supporting the bowl with my lunch.

Stopped in Amarillo for gas and a break.
Super windy.
And hot.

Biltong and wine for dinner while enjoying sunset.
309 miles for the day.

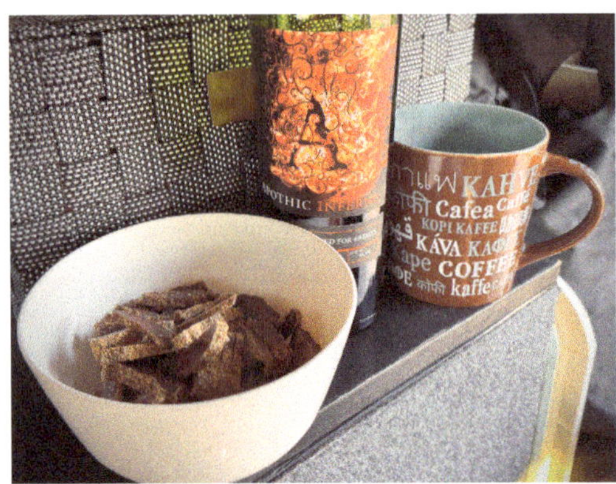

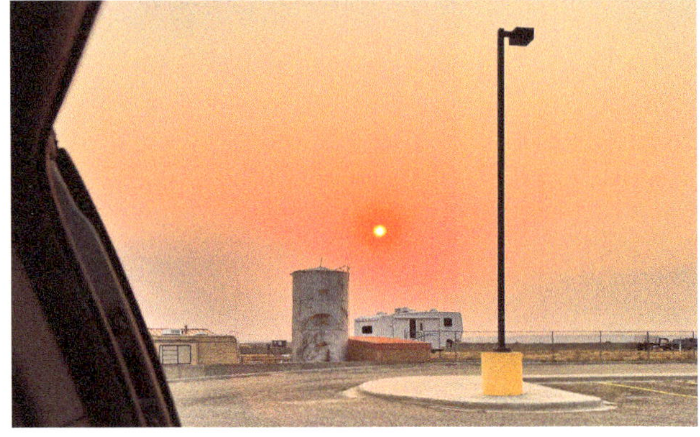

DAY 72 / APRIL 30

Left from Russell's Truck and Travel Center, Glenrio, New Mexico.
Beautiful car museum with free entry.
Needed more time in the museum.

Called Steve to say "Happy Birthday!"

Drove 275 miles to Bernalillo, finally off I-40.

Stopped at Ute Lake State Park to shower.
Not all showers are the same.
I had to push hard on a button
every 10 seconds to keep the water running.

Back at Walmart in Bernalillo, New Mexico.

Really nice girl showed me the nail clipper I was "looking" for
instead of telling me where it would be.
I complimented her and explained my visual problems.
How hard it was to find items on a shelf
even if I knew where it was supposed to be.

Walmart was my favorite store.
Enter the zip code in the app.
And it will tell you which aisle the item would be in.

Easy to find the zip code.
Look on Google Maps.
The store address is listed.
No need to ask someone in the store for the zip code.
Interestingly, most people didn't know.
Learned afterwards to
use current location to bring up the store name.

And remember to change it at new locations.
Store aisles are not the same in every store.

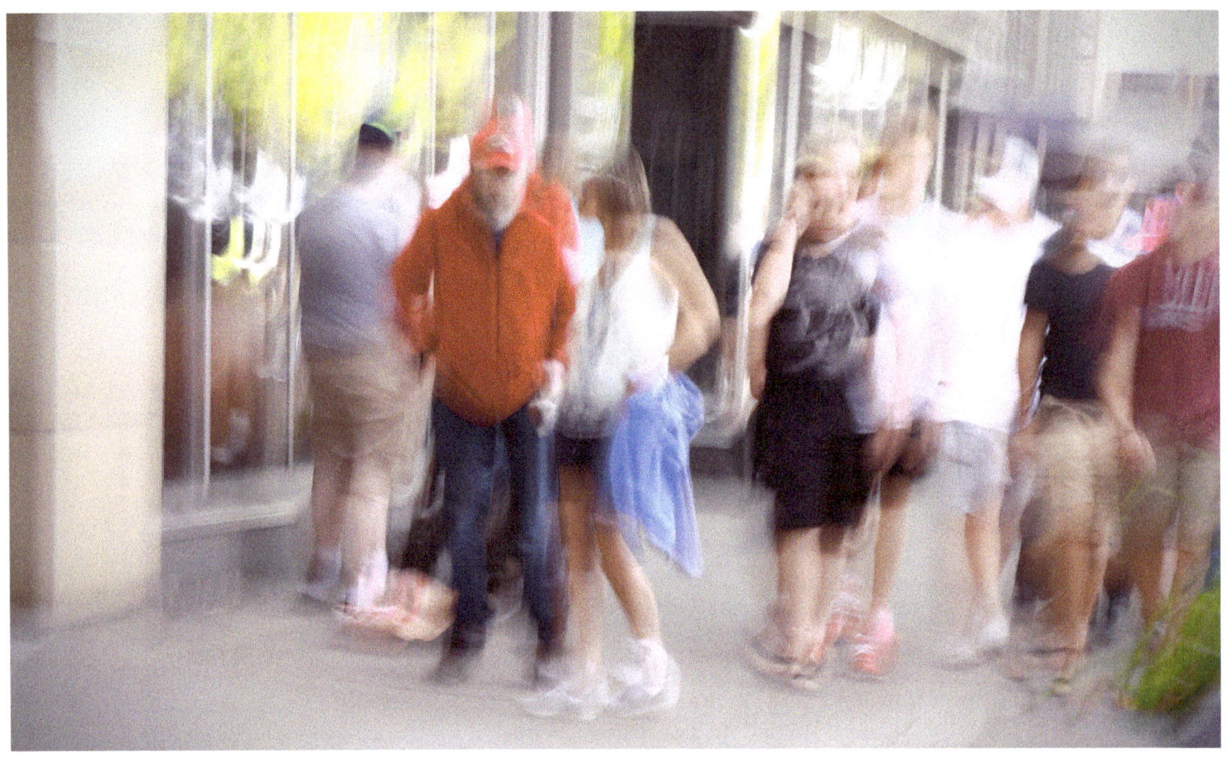

This is what it feels like in a grocery store
with people moving,
carts moving, music, noise and trying to walk straight
without knocking stuff off the shelves
when I lose my balance.

I wish my other favorite stores Albertsons and Safeway
had apps with the store layout.
It's very overwhelming when I am tired
to walk into stores
trying to find something.
Now I ask as I walk into the store instead of trying
to figure it out myself.
And the stores are all different.

It's easy to say "Read the words on the signs by the aisles."
When I look up, I lose my balance backwards.
And it takes a while to read all the words on the signs.
Reading is a SLOW process.

DAY 73 / MAY 1

I was exhausted.
Drove 1,141 miles in 4 days.

1,784 miles and 8 states since I left Corpus Christi, Texas.
Texas, Louisiana, Arkansas, Tennessee,
Arkansas again, Oklahoma, Texas and New Mexico.

Took a rest day.
A windstorm blew through.
Went to Costco to get gas.
Cleaned up the van, shopped for supplies.
I would be going back to deserted areas with limited shopping.

Had dinner at a buffet restaurant.

Talked to Daniel, just listening.
He was going through a very difficult time.
I had been divorced too.
It sucked.
I swore to never get married again.
Mark convinced me otherwise.

Daniel talked about a suicide attempt 12 years ago.
I finally let on what the real reason behind this trip was.
I didn't feel judged or hear the typical
"No, don't do it."
After the conversation he sent a message:

"Just worried about you.
I know we laugh a lot during phone calls,
but I know the pain is real."

People cross our paths in life for a reason.
A photographer became a friend,
a young man with kindness in his heart.

DAY 74 / MAY 2

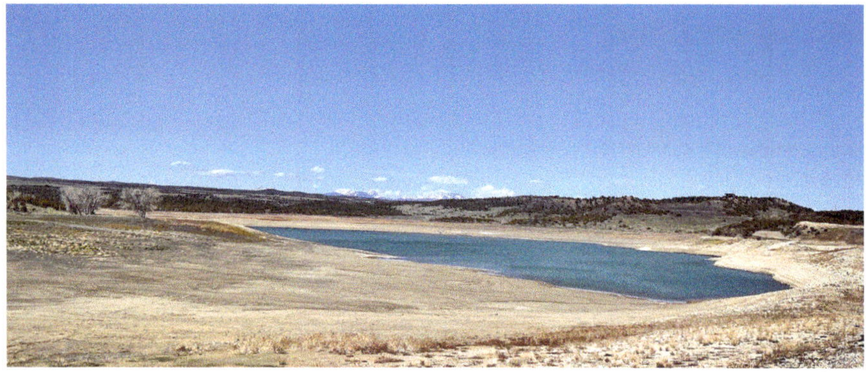

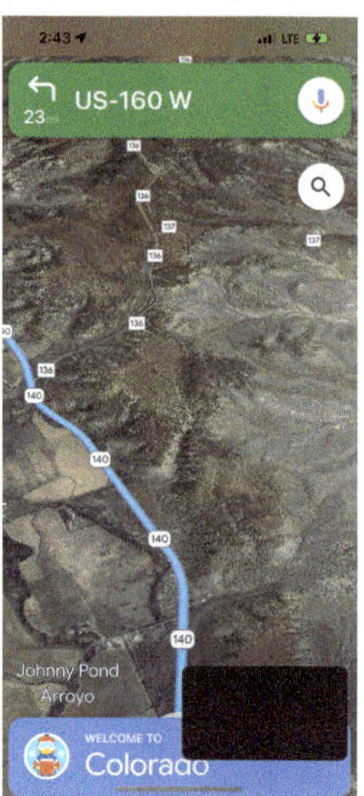

The last time I was in Colorado
was in 1998 moving from
Virginia to Idaho in a U-Haul truck.
I remembered the yellow trees and beautiful scenery.

I was very careful getting out of the van
to take pictures.
Checked if someone was approaching me.
I didn't want a repeat of the gun episode.

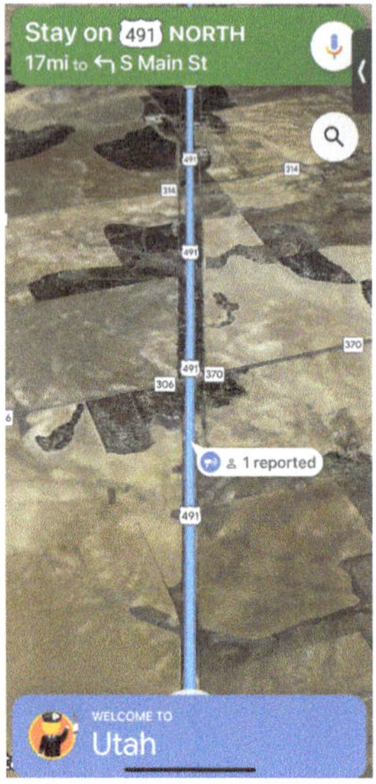

Finally, back in Utah.

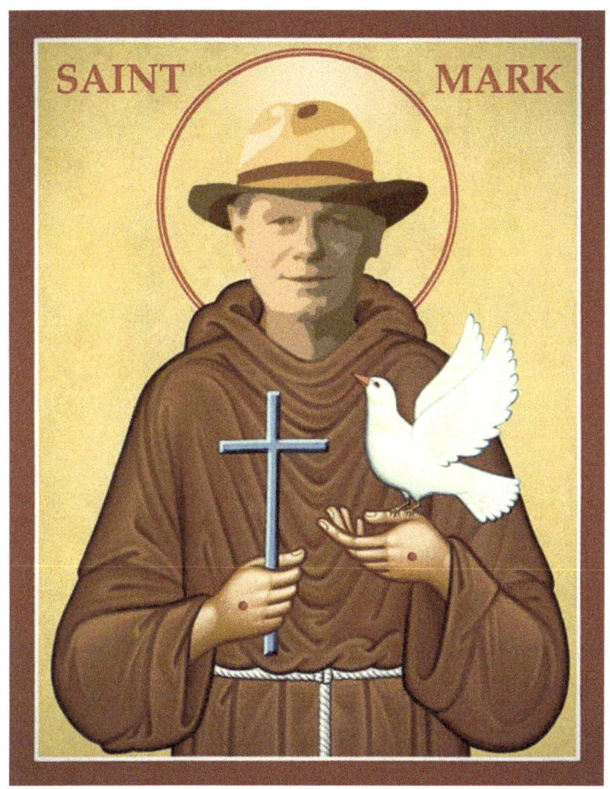

Daniel sent a picture he made of Mark.
He thought it should be "official."
My husband was a saint
for letting me go on this trip
for a long time.
And not asking when I would be home.

Daniel sent written directions for
star trails camera settings.
I had permission of two gas stations
for overnight parking
and I identified a few spots
that would work for safe parking.

I stayed at the Maverick station.
Got gas and dinner.

I was ready to go home.

DAY 75 / MAY 3

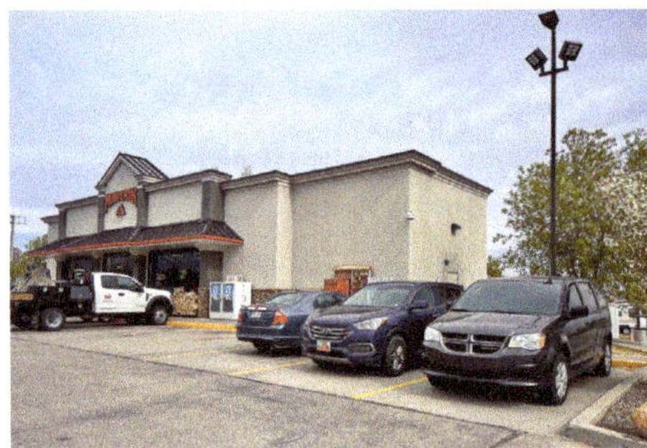

My backing-up skills were improving.
Backed into this parking spot in one move.

I called Mark to let him know of my plans.
I wouldn't have cell service for the next 24 hours.

> **Getting there** • The trailhead is on State Road 95, just east of mile marker 28, on the north side of the road. It's 2 miles southeast of the junction with State Road 276, about 19 miles northwest of the Colorado River bridge on S.R. 95, and about 28 miles southeast of the junction with State Road 24 in Hanksville. There is a short driveway to a parking lot at the trailhead.

Oh holy shit.
I screenshot these directions to a slot canyon, I think.
I didn't have a clue what it said.
And it's Times New Roman font.
Unreadable.
And I forgot which slot canyon.
Too many capital letters and numbers.
Words like north and east didn't mean anything.
I knew where Hanksville was.
Kind of.

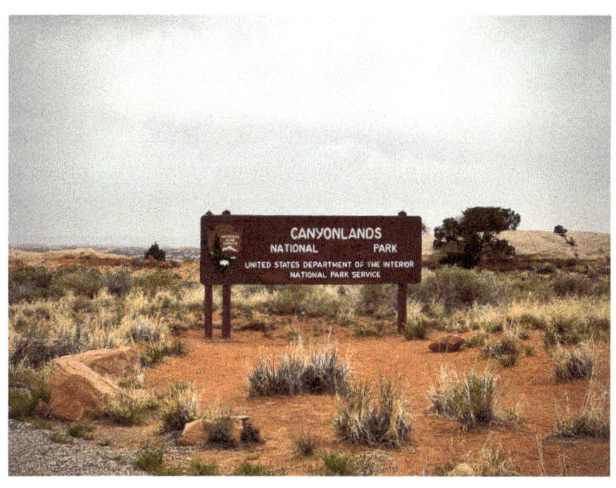

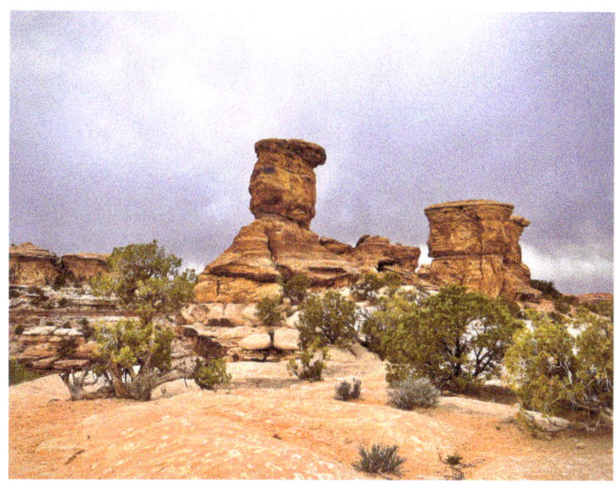

Visited the Needles part of
Canyonlands National Park.
Very deserted and isolated.
And beautiful.

Drove the two dirt roads
accessible with high clearance 2-wheel drive.
The rest of the dirt roads all required 4-wheel drive.

I was lucky to get a spot in the campground.
The disability site again.
The last one available.

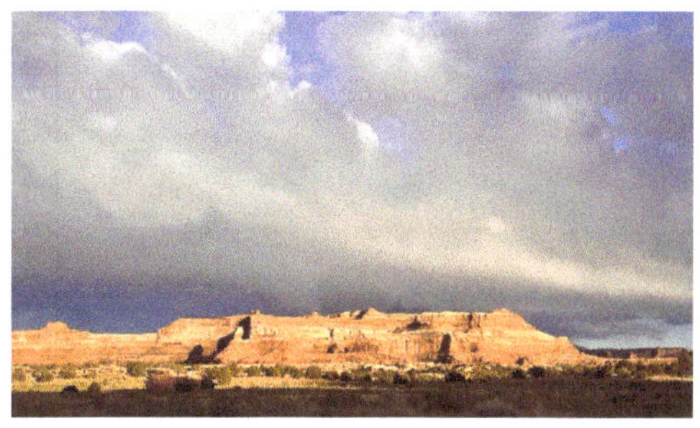

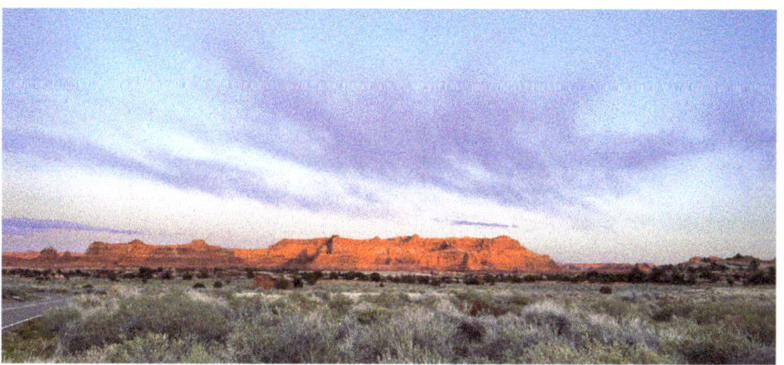

It was cloudy all day
and I didn't expect a good sunset.
I walked out of the bathroom
and the sun broke through.
Lighting the rock.
The best camera
is the one with you.
A cell phone.

DAY 76 / MAY 4 / 8,000 MILES

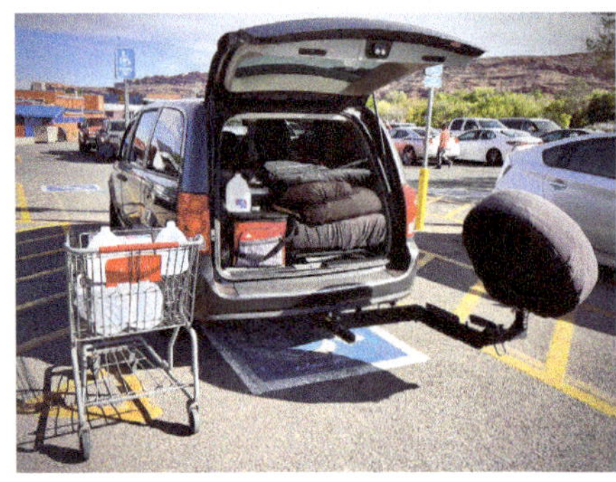

Took off for Moab.
Got gas.
Last chance to get gas for a while.
Filled up with distilled and fresh water.
8,000 miles since leaving home.

Called Mark. Not much cell service in the park.
No news is good news.

Island In the Sky part of Canyonlands National Park.

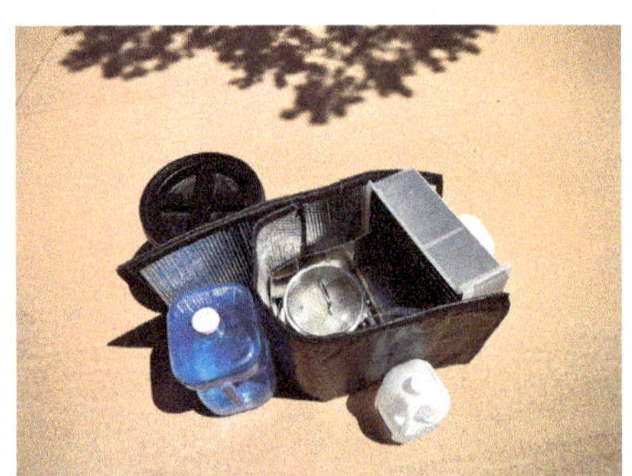

Back in my disability spot.

Paid for 4 nights.

There were other sites available,
but I should stick to the one
close to the bathroom.

Didn't want to fall in the dark.

The strategies to block the wind
while cooking evolved every day.
Made it up as I went.

Drop-dead tired.
Went to bed at 6pm.

DAY 77 / MAY 5

Well, shit.

I forgot to change the fridge
from van cigarette lighter 12-volt
to Jackery 12-volt overnight.

Drained the van battery.

Deader than dead.

11.4 volts

The electronic jump starter had no effect.

Asked the neighbor for help.
He was from New Zealand, traveling in
a rented Chevy Express van.
Good thing the jumper cables were long.

Note to self:
In future park backed in so someone
can help jump start the van.

The never-ending housekeeping tasks.
Noodles and squash for lunch.
Acorn squash reminded me of Orli.
We had it for dinner a few times in Memphis.
It's my favorite.

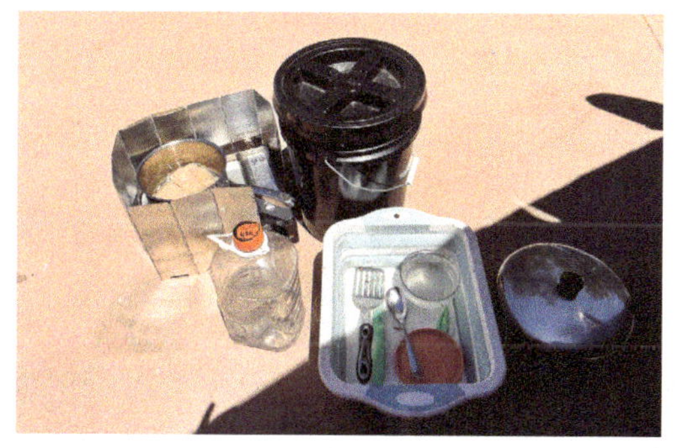

The campsite across from me was unoccupied.
A minivan with noisy people pulled up
and set up at the table.
I could tell they were not camping.
I was not in the mood for noise.
Walked over
and a man said they just wanted to have lunch
and will move on.
It's a campground, not a picnic area.

A camper pulled up looking interested in the site.
I flew out of the van
and flagged them down.
The site was available.
That's why it's not a picnic area.

Frederick, 27, and Mirte, 25, from Nederland.
Traveled in a rented RV seeing America.
I understood Dutch,
the Afrikaans background.
Understanding someone's language
is a connection point.
Great kids.
While they went for a drive someone ignored
their paid reservation stub and moved into their site.
I pointed the stub out.
When they got back,
I mentioned the incident.
They were very grateful.
They would put chairs out in the driveway
to indicate the site was taken.

I was looking for the right tree
as a foreground
for star photography.
A surprise cell signal
on the edge of the canyon.

Daniel sent reminders
for the camera settings.
And he recognized the tree
when he ate bad food
during his trip earlier
and had an unfortunate undignified "accident."
He was brave enough
to tell me about it.

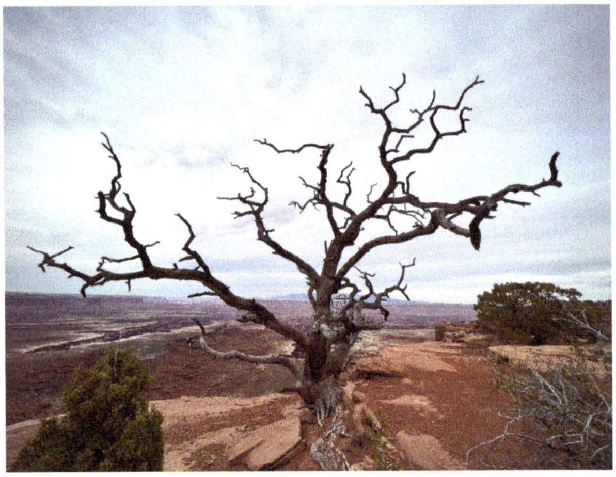

Went to bed early.
Too cloudy to hope
for a clear sky for star pictures.

I wanted to go home.

DAY 78 / MAY 6

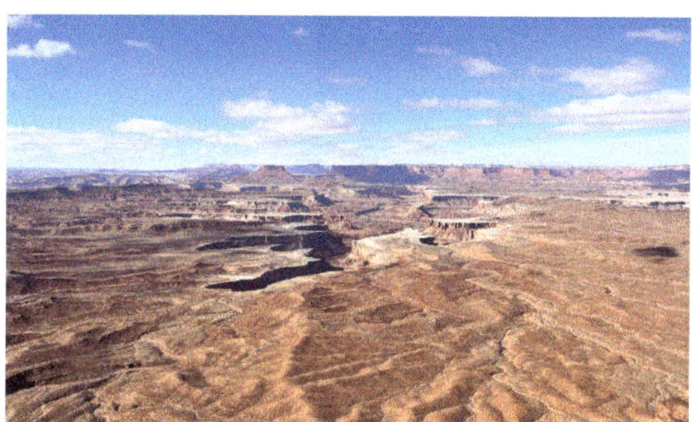

I was moving on.
The loss of $15 for the two unused nights
wouldn't bankrupt me.

Took my last walk
down to the Green River Overlook
to say goodbye to Canyonlands National Park.
Had a half-hour conversation
with a woman from Minnesota
traveling with her husband,
a retired helicopter mechanic, in their RV.
Amazing how easy it was to talk
to other travelers.

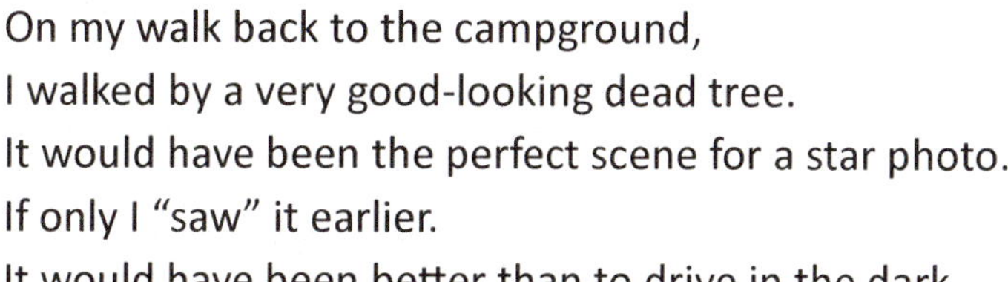

On my walk back to the campground,
I walked by a very good-looking dead tree.
It would have been the perfect scene for a star photo.
If only I "saw" it earlier.
It would have been better than to drive in the dark.

I would go to Arches National Park at 5pm.
The park required reservations to visit.
My reservation was in 3 days.
But you could go in before 6am or after 5pm
without a reservation.

Went to Moab to shower and use a good cell signal
to research the rest of the trip.

Still figuring how to get to the Bonneville Salt Flats
without driving the I-5 going through Salt Lake City.

I planned to overnight in Green River, Utah.
It was about 50 minutes' drive.
Had to leave Arches by no later than 7pm.
Didn't want to drive in the dark.

Arches National Park was breathtaking.

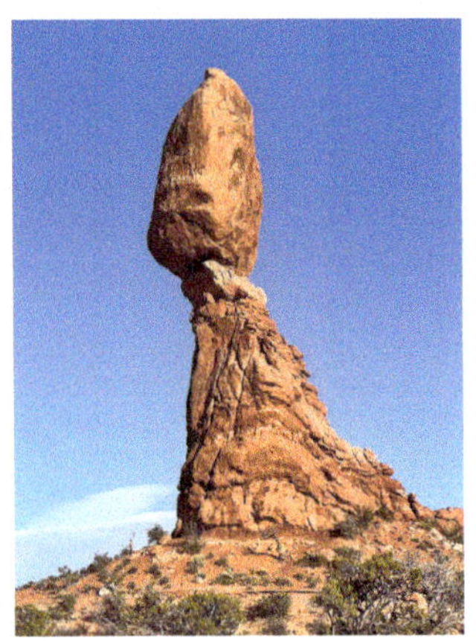

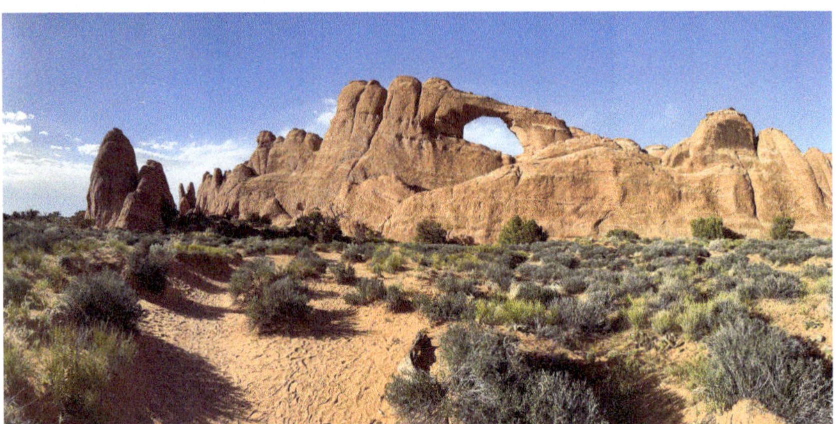

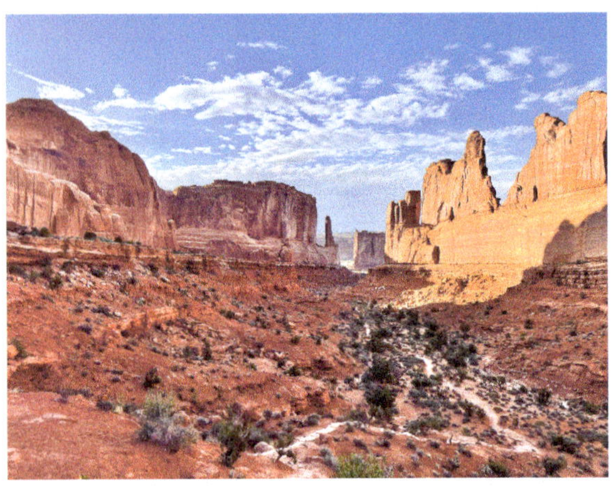

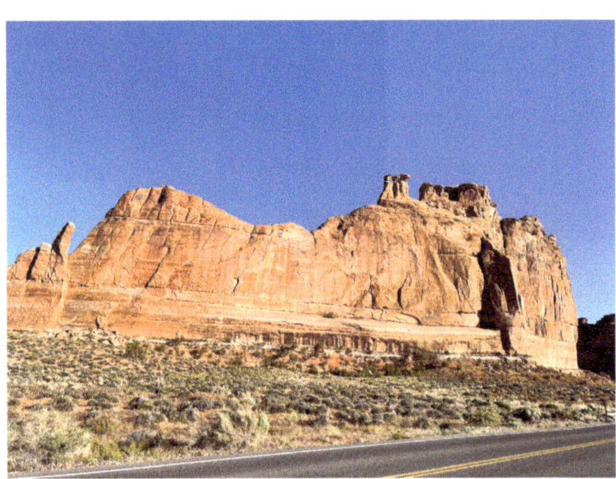

It was difficult to drive,
the sun was getting low in the sky.
Very bright and painful to look at the landscape.
I was able to get into the park
but didn't take the light into consideration.
Did a few short hikes.

The sun was setting gloriously
when I turned off the highway to Green River, Utah.
Metal donkeys on the side of the road.

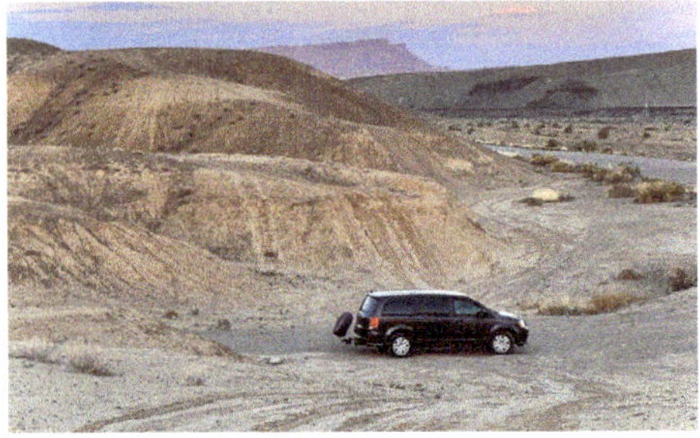

Skidded to a halt in the dirt and grabbed the phone.
Crawled in the dust for a good angle
trying not to fall off the steep embankment.
Bugs buzzed around my head.
No time to get the bug screen.
The sun was setting.

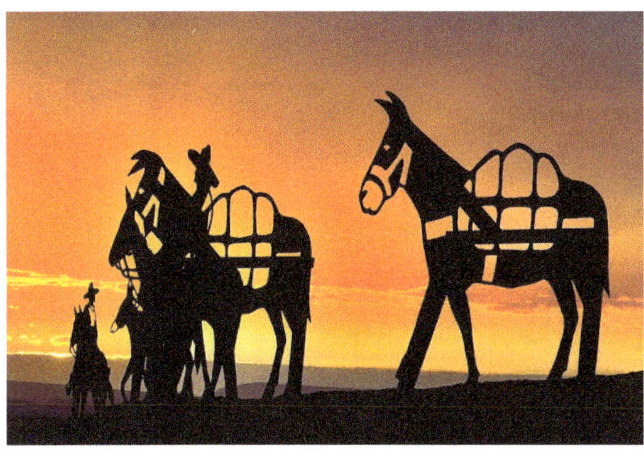

A man walked by pushing his bicycle.
Shit. Shit. Shit.
He better not be planning something.

I was ready to *"donner"*
(beat up with grievous intent)
anyone looking for shit.
Karate from 45 years ago still lingering in me.

He ignored me and kept walking.

Stayed at the Love's Truck Stop with permission.
Called Mark and sent the sunset picture.

Planned to go to Goblin Valley State Park
and Factory Butte the next day.
The ones I missed out on
during a thunderstorm.

Received a weather alert for a windstorm the next day.

Well shit.

Guessed those plans were cancelled.

DAY 79 / MAY 7

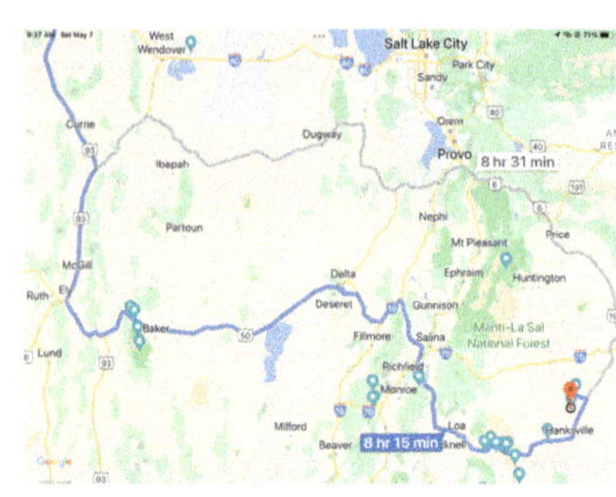

Still trying to figure how to get to
the Bonneville Salt Flats going back roads.

Windstorm warning 20-30 mph with gusts of 50 mph.

Rethought my plans: go see Goblin Valley.
Didn't have to do much outside the van,
just see if I would want to do it again in future.

While I was sitting in line at Goblin Valley State Park entrance,
an employee told me about the Little Wild Horse Slot Canyon.

Goblin Valley was spectacular.
I could see doing star photography
and it would look otherworldly.
I could also see how I would get lost in the dark.
Something I should do with a photography friend.
Someone with a sense of direction
who knew how to get back to the vehicles.

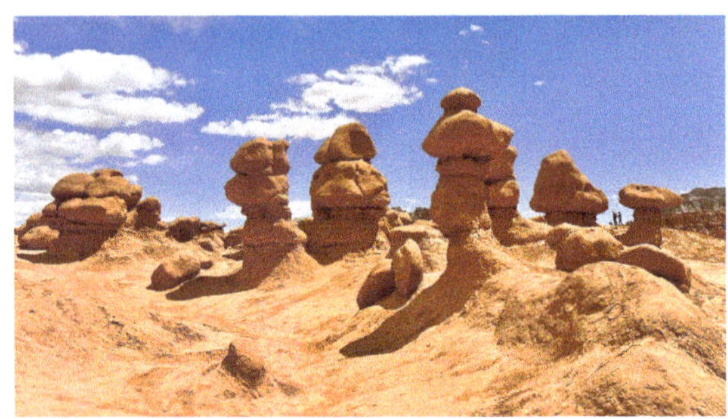

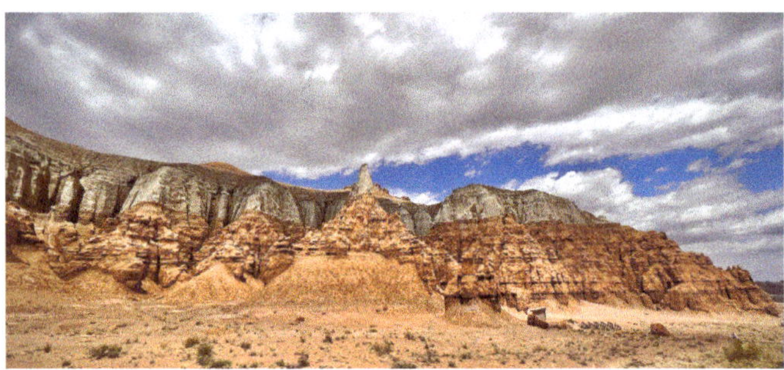

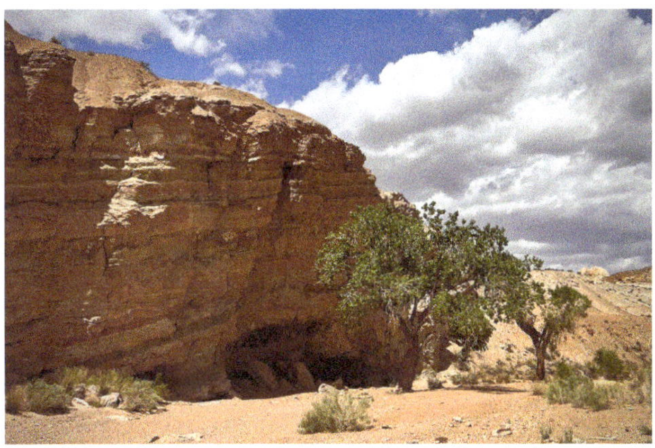

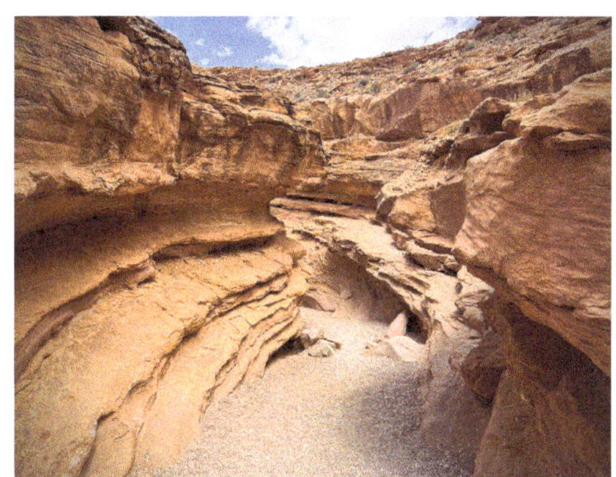

My first experience with a slot canyon
longer than 50 feet.

The colors of the rock,
the shapes,
the lines.
Wow, wow, wow.

That part of Utah was on the Colorado Plateau,
formed 200–250 million years ago.
Difficult to comprehend that much time.

I missed the sign for Little Wild Horse Canyon
and continued into Bell Canyon.

A group of people coming from
the opposite direction talked to me.
I asked about the slot canyon.
A man and woman,
who looked vaguely familiar,
acted like they have seen me before
and showed me the missed turn.
Wondering where I met them.
Canyonlands?
There was a sign, I didn't see it.

The transition was chest high,
and I made it up and down.

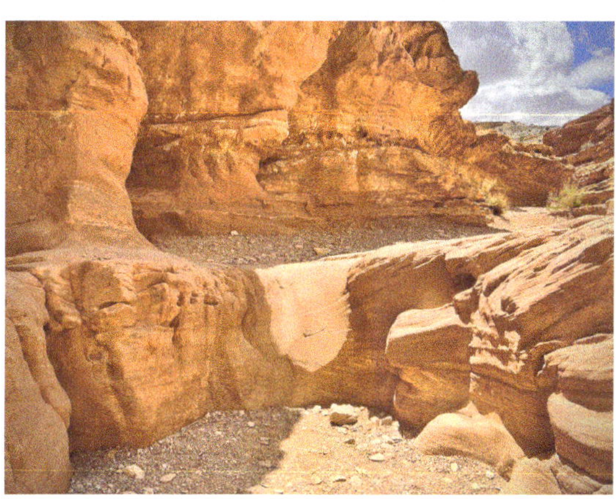

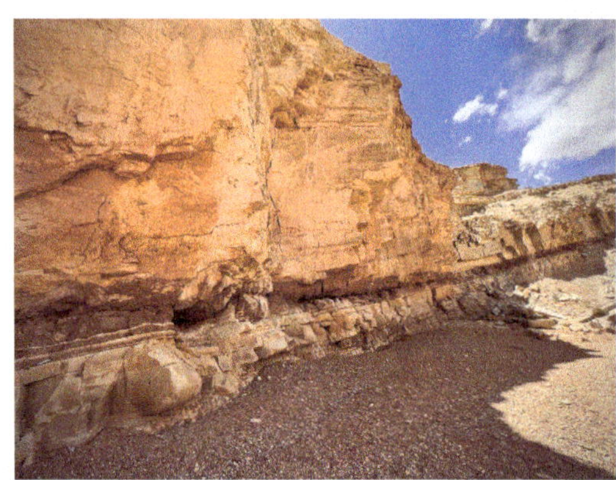

I used All Trails app to track when I hiked a trail.
It helped me get back to the van and not get lost.

I came across 2 boys on the way back
sitting in one of the big trees.
They were talkative
and it was a good time to sit on a rock,
take a break and tie my bootlaces.
They were from Hanksville
and impressed by how much I liked Utah.

I moved on to Torrey, my overnight spot.
I wanted to stop at Factory Butte,
but it was very windy
and I was tired after my 2.2-mile hike
in hot weather.

I checked on my BLM spot just outside Torrey.
It still looked good,
but I was concerned about overnight rain
and getting stuck in mud.
I asked the cashier about parking at the gas station.
I had permission to park overnight,
and the bathrooms were in great shape.
Filled up on gas and got a few treats.

Called Mark to let him know where I was.
Most of the time he could see me on the Life360 app
while I had cell service.

He was having a difficult time finding an artist
to design the front cover of his book.
I messaged Daniel who had
a design background in software interfaces.
He would talk to Mark and
point him in the right direction.

DAY 80 / MAY 8

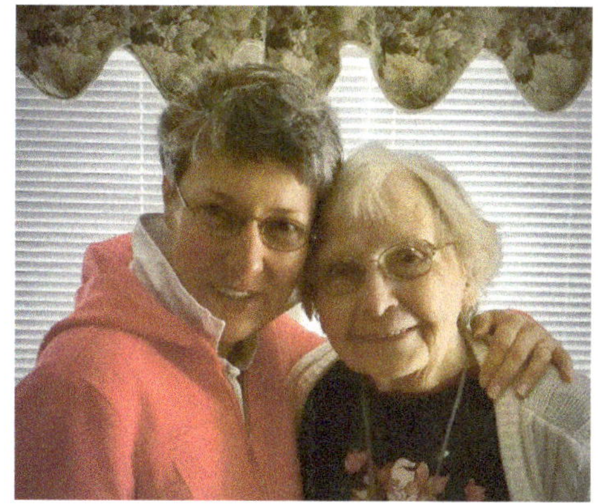

Had a very nice quiet night in my parking spot.
It was Mother's Day.
I called my mother-in-law, Loretta Ready.
I don't think anyone on this planet
has a better and nicer mother-in-law.
She was always happy to see me,
a dignified woman who invited me to visit again.
When I was still working,
it was my favorite thing to do on my break
to drop by their house and visit.
Happy Mother's Day, Mom!

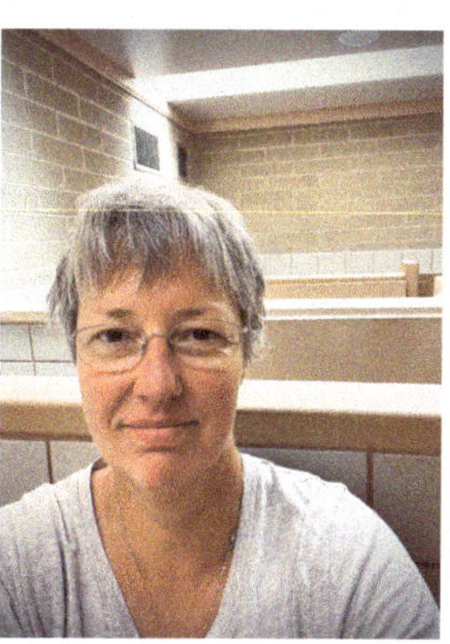

Took a break at the rest area at Annabella, Utah.
That was the one time in my life I didn't want to be tall.
I could see over the walls in the restroom
without much trouble.

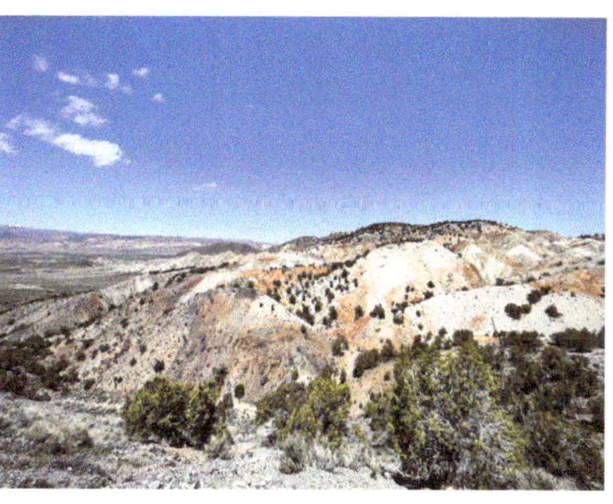

It amazed me how fast the landscape would change.
These 2 pictures were taken in the same spot,
on opposite sides of the road.

Made it to Richfield, Utah
with overnight parking at Walmart
with permission.

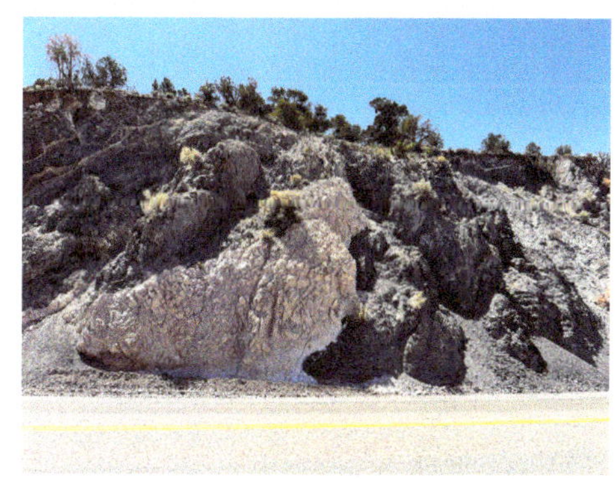

It was so windy,
it felt like the van would blow over anytime.

And I had 46 bug bites
from the other night's sunset shoot.

Mark sounded much happier
with his options of finding an artist for his book.

Messaged Daniel a thank you note.

DAY 81 / MAY 9

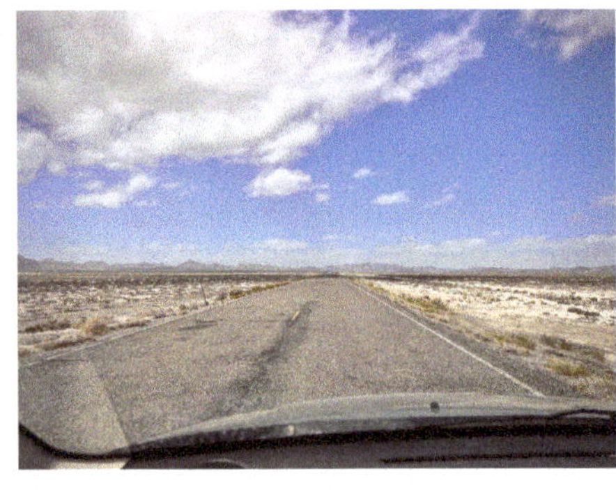

I put in Google Maps to avoid highways.
Which it did.
I was driving next to the interstate
on a dirt road.
Should have known better.
Snowed some the night before
and it was significantly colder.

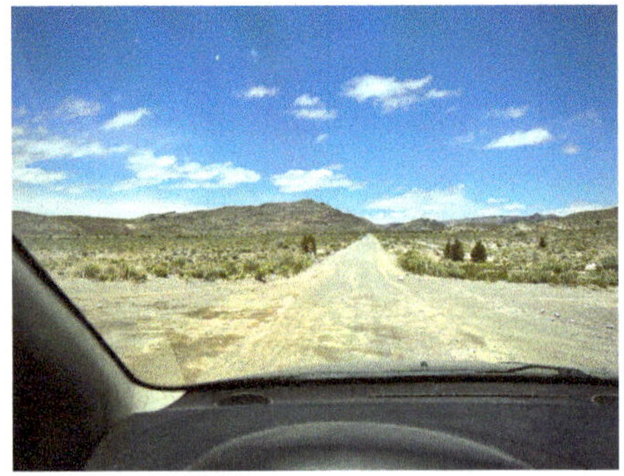

On my way to the Bonneville Salt Flats.
Hwy 174.
The road got quieter
and quieter.
Made my hair stand on end.
Very creepy feeling.
It would be the place to do 100 mph
and there would be no one
to write the speeding ticket.

Out of nowhere
the pavement stopped.
It was a dirt road.
I stopped to check the map.
All I could see on the offline map
was The Pony Express Highway.
And I didn't have a cell signal.
I couldn't call or text Mark.
Sat there, debating,
keep going, or go back to Highway 6?

That was how the people you read about on Facebook
disappeared because they followed GPS
and were found dead 2 weeks later.

A semi-truck appeared from a side road.
I jumped out of the van, tried to flag the driver down.
He gave me one look and kept driving.

The situation scared the living daylights out of me.
My legs were shaking, and my heart was beating too fast.

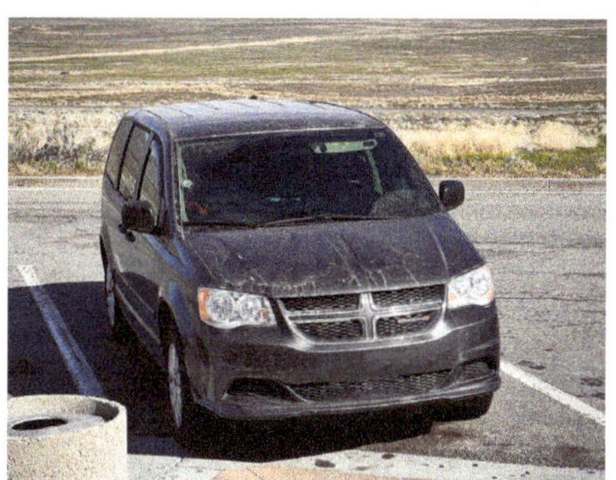

I turned around and headed back to highway 6.
It would be a 100-mile detour.

And Google Maps was redirecting me continuously
to take dirt tracks, not even roads,
to the left to get back to the Pony Express Highway.

New lesson:
Probably the most important lesson of the trip.
Don't always believe GPS.
Get a real paper map.
Also, the offline map has a lot less details
than the map you see when you have a cell signal.

I finally made it to the I-80 West.
Not the best way, but I did.
Huge learning experience.

Took a break at the Grantsville rest area.
The van needed a wash.

I stopped at the Salt Flats Rest Area Westbound on I-80.
Very impressive.
I drove to where I could access it behind the speedway.
I was too tired and stressed from the day's shenanigans
to drive onto the Salt Slats.
Did 410 miles that day.

Went to West Wendover to investigate
an overnight parking spot
while it was still daylight.
Wendover was in both Utah and Nevada.
I had permission from a few businesses.
I would decide later where I would overnight.

After a rest break and eating dinner,
I headed back to the Salt Flats.
There were other vehicles out driving and
no one seemed to have trouble driving onto the salt.

I was driving on the Bonneville Salt Flats!
And I drove 8,832 miles to get there.

I did a short run of 50 mph.
Too scared to go faster.
I was afraid I wouldn't "see" other vehicles
and get hit.

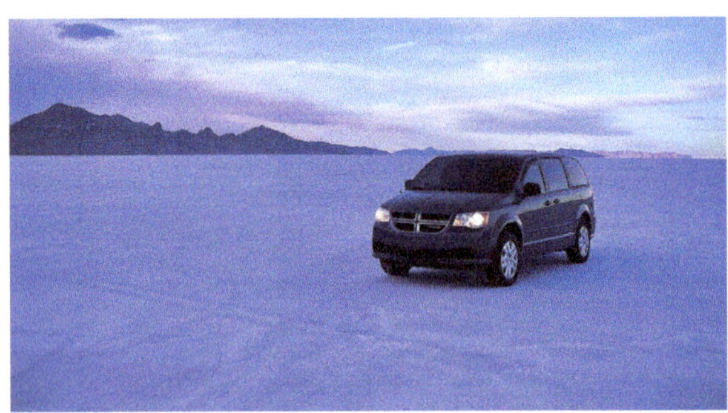

Checked off another item on my bucket list.
And overcame fear.
I was going to give up and not do it.
But I came that far, I had to do it.
Scared or not scared.

I overnight parked at a casino.
Mostly level parking lot.
Most of the businesses were on a steep slope.
It would be difficult to sleep comfortably.

Called Mark to tell him the exciting Bonneville news.

The rest of the day's news
would have to wait until I got home.
No need to stress him out.

DAY 82 / MAY 10

I felt guilty
for not cleaning the undercarriage the night before.
Went to the carwash
and the salt was welded on.
I had to put in a lot of extra effort
to get all the salt off.

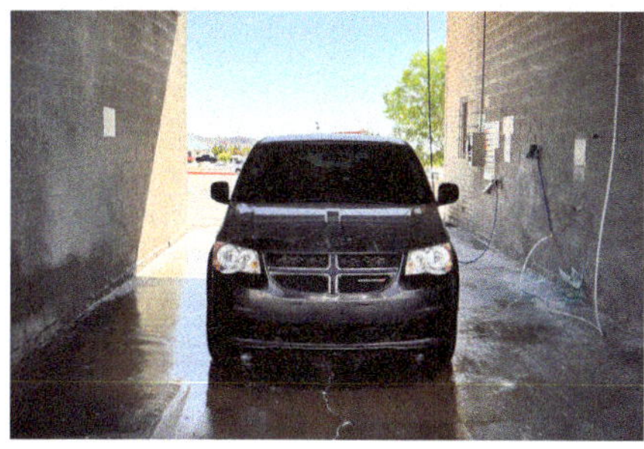

Started the journey to Twin Falls, Idaho.
Miles and miles
of
Mountains
Plains
Clouds
Snow.
All beautiful.
Stopped many times to get pictures.

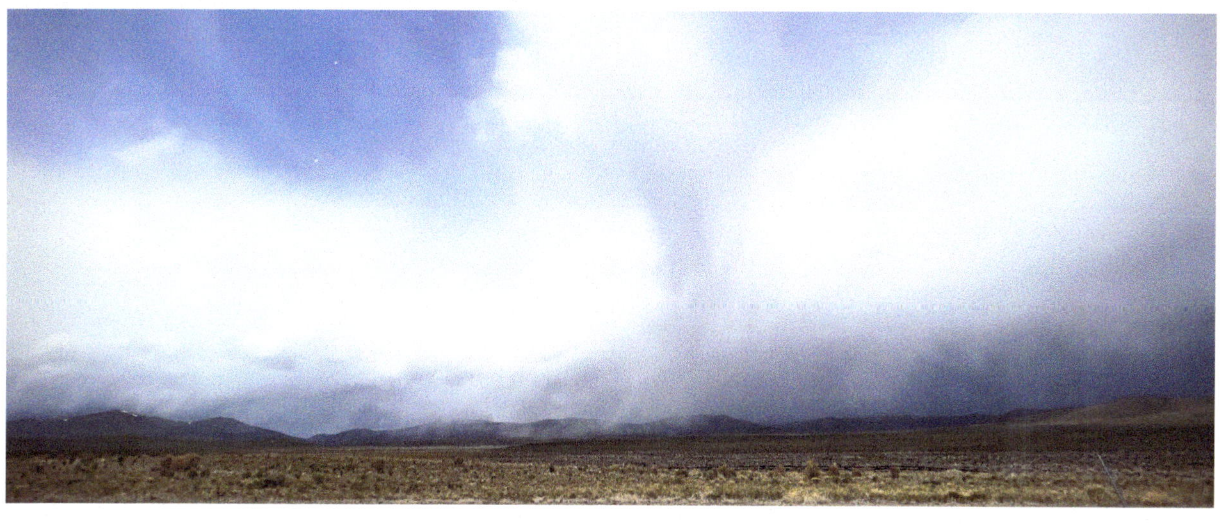

I had lived in Twin Falls from 1998 to 2001.
Hardly recognizable,
and much bigger.

The Shoshone Falls water flow
was significantly decreased.

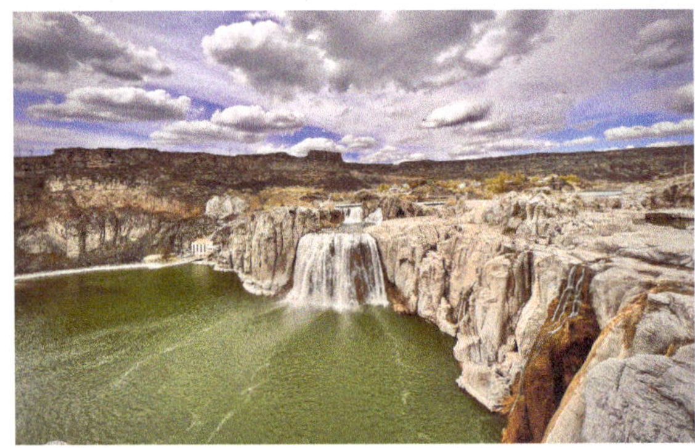

Beautiful sunset with a view
of the Perrine Bridge over the Snake River.

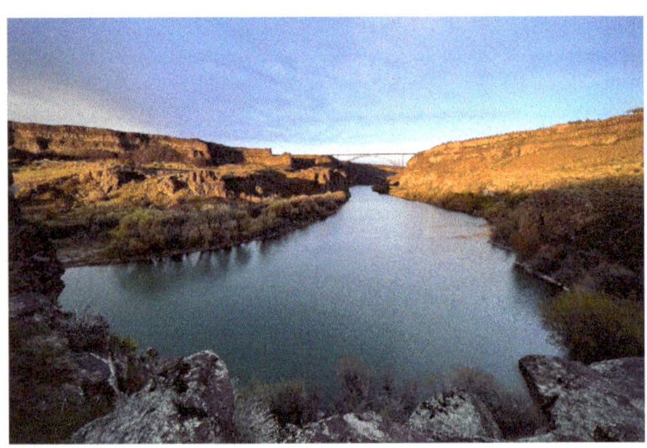

Stayed at Walmart with their permission.
A quiet evening among other travelers.

Called Mark.
I would be home the day after tomorrow.
He said he would clean up the house.

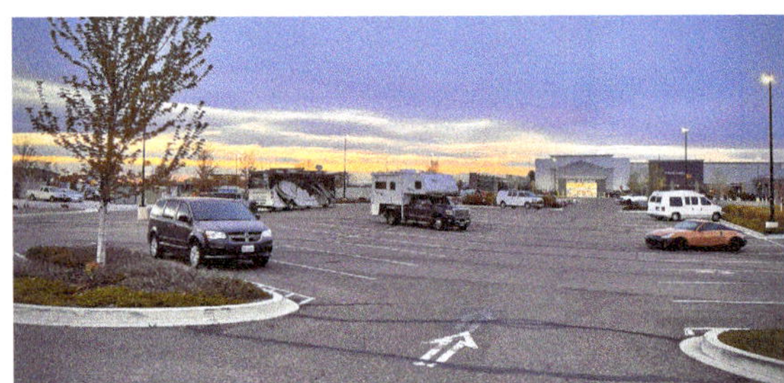

DAY 83 / MAY 11

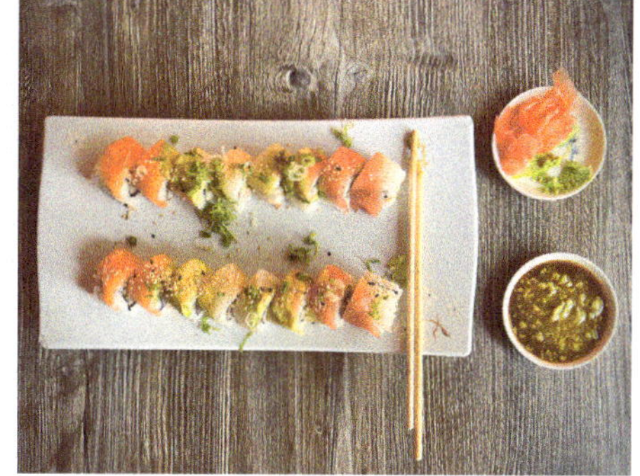

Stopped in Boise
for a buffet sushi lunch.
The waitress and her boyfriend
also traveled in a van with their two dogs.

The last night's overnight parking
would be at the same rest area
as the first night 83 days ago.
As I pulled in,
I tried to think of some eye-opening conclusions.
I had a difficult time
coming up with anything.

A Dodge Promaster van with solar panels
parked at the end of the rest area.
I saw a man only
as I walked to the bathroom.
I wouldn't approach a man on his own.
Unless he was old,
and I could outrun him.
I saw a woman with him
coming out of the bathroom.

Approached them with questions
about their experience with solar panels.
John and Janice, a photographer,
from California.
Great conversation about solar,
traveling and photography.

New insight:
I had a lot of experience with photography
locations after the trip.
I parked at the end of the parking lot,
with an almost cell signal
if the wind stopped blowing.

A car pulled in off the southbound highway,
so fast and so close to the van,
it about scraped the paint off the van.

Moved over to the opposite parking space,
out of reach of speeding vehicles.

Laid in the dark,
stuffed in the sleeping bag.
Thought about my life,
or lack of a life,
at home.

I would be home the next day.

Back in Shitville.

With the loneliness.
With the nothingness.

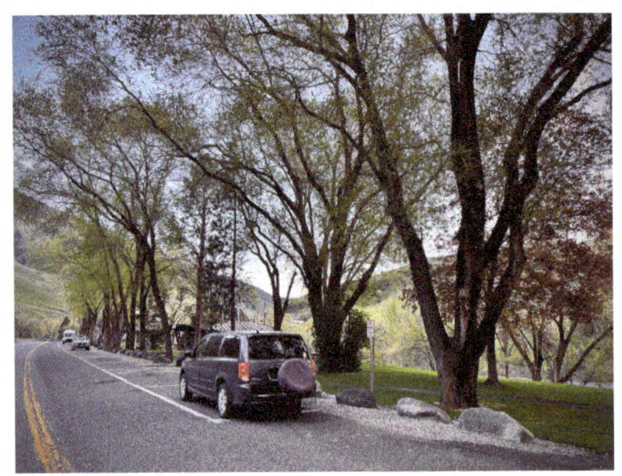

DAY 84 / MAY 12

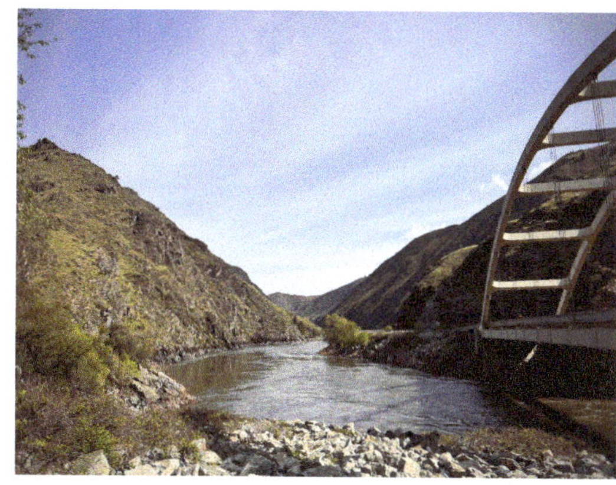

Took off around 10am.
It was just over 2 hours to get home.

Passed into the Pacific Time Zone.

I stopped in Riggins, Idaho for
my last cup of cocoa of the trip.
Called Mark to let him know
of my whereabouts.

He said he didn't have time
to clean up the house.
It sounded like he didn't do the dishes.

The view from the top
of the White Bird Grade.
Green and beautiful.
It was gray and covered
in snow 3 months ago.

Metamorphosis.

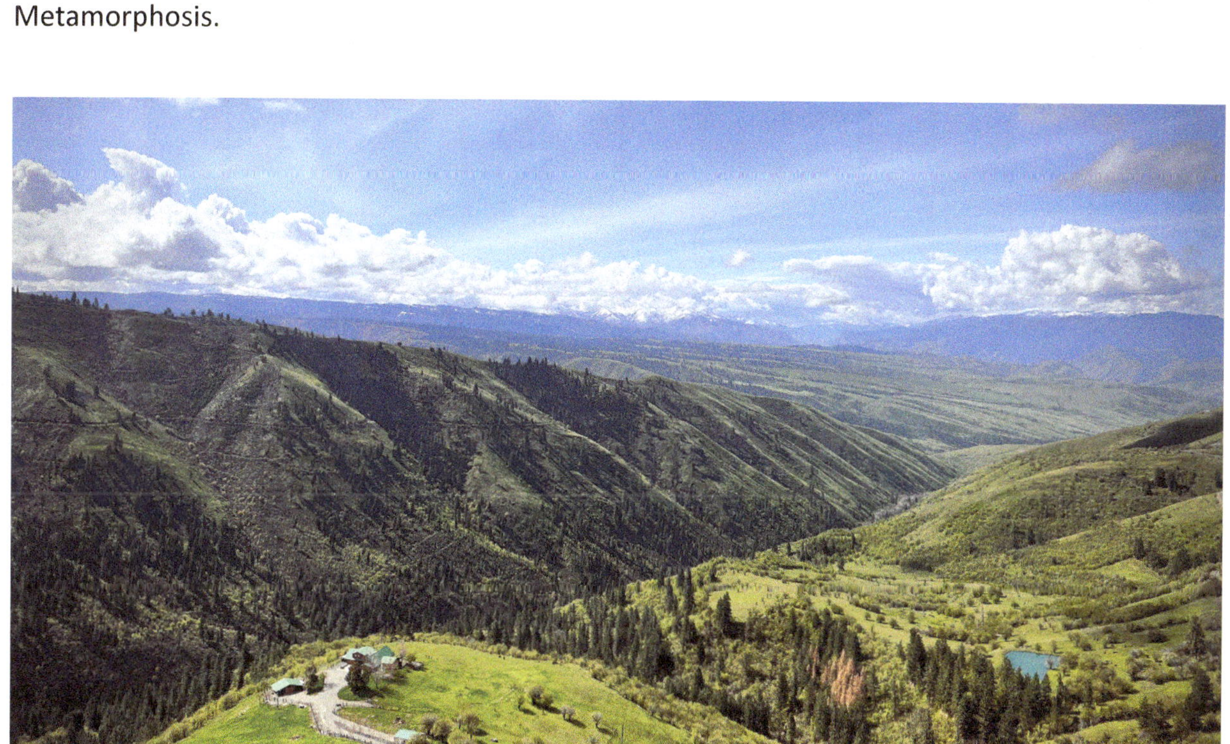

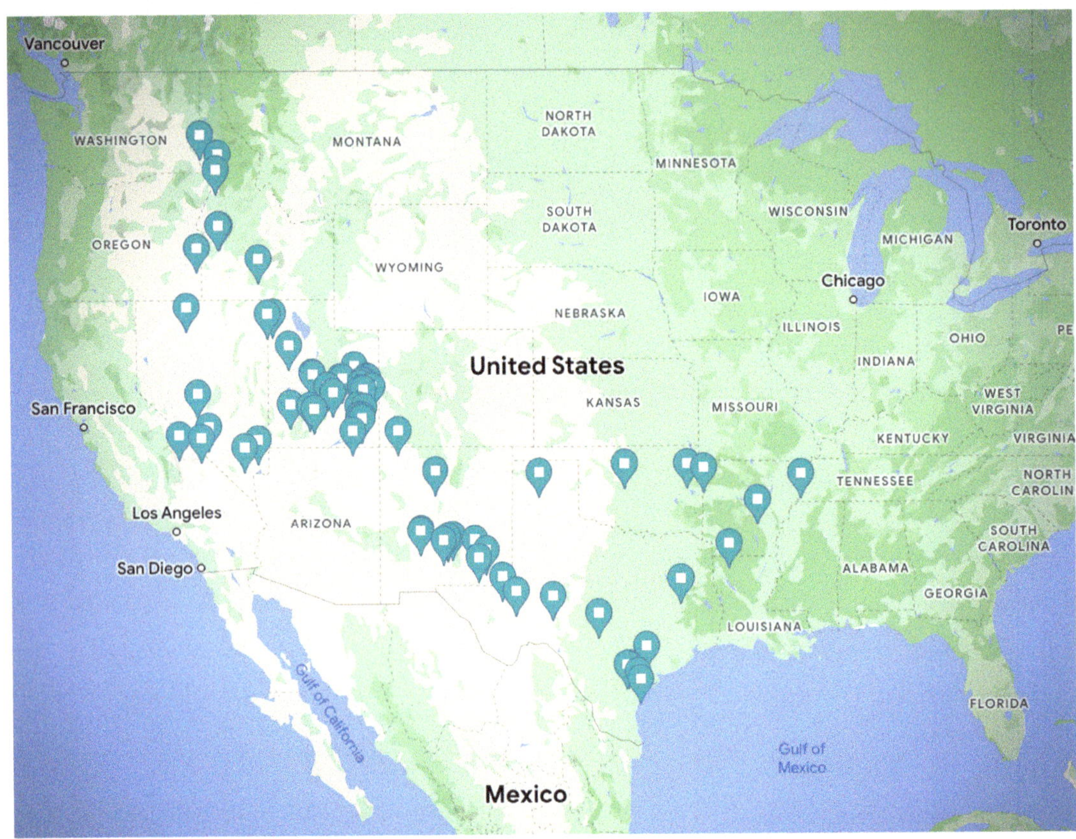

9,460.8 miles

84 days

83 nights

I made it without harming myself
or the van.
And I didn't get shot.

The dogs were barking and jumping
hysterically at the fence.
I walked into the backyard
to greet them.
The grass was super green and overgrown.
It must have rained a lot.

I unlocked the back door
and walked in.
And stopped dead in my tracks.

It looked like something exploded.
Stuff on the floor,
clothes
and laundry scattered,
papers,
dishes.
Piles of dirty dishes in the kitchen.
The counters not wiped down.
Mark's bedroom door was open.
It was chaos too.

I let the dogs into the kitchen.
Walked around slowly
staring at the disorder.
The dogs sensed my energy,
followed me quietly.

I was standing in the living room,
my phone rang.

"I'm sorry the house is such as mess."

"Are you expecting me to clean it up?"

"No."

I wasn't planning to.

I didn't really know what to do.

I kind of expected a level of disorder,
but not this bad.

Considered spending
the night at Walmart.

I forgot where the pots and pans were in the kitchen.
A black hole in my memory.
They have been in the same spot for 10 years.
Systematically opened cabinet doors until I found them.

And where was the switch for the kitchen light?

When Mark walked through the door,
the list of excuses poured out.
He didn't have time to clean house.
The dogs needed a lot of attention.
He had to do all the shopping
and cook for himself.
He tried to get a housekeeper.
And he had mowed the yard.

"Are you mad at me?"

"No. I'm disappointed."

I went upstairs
and went to bed.

That was not how I imagined coming home.

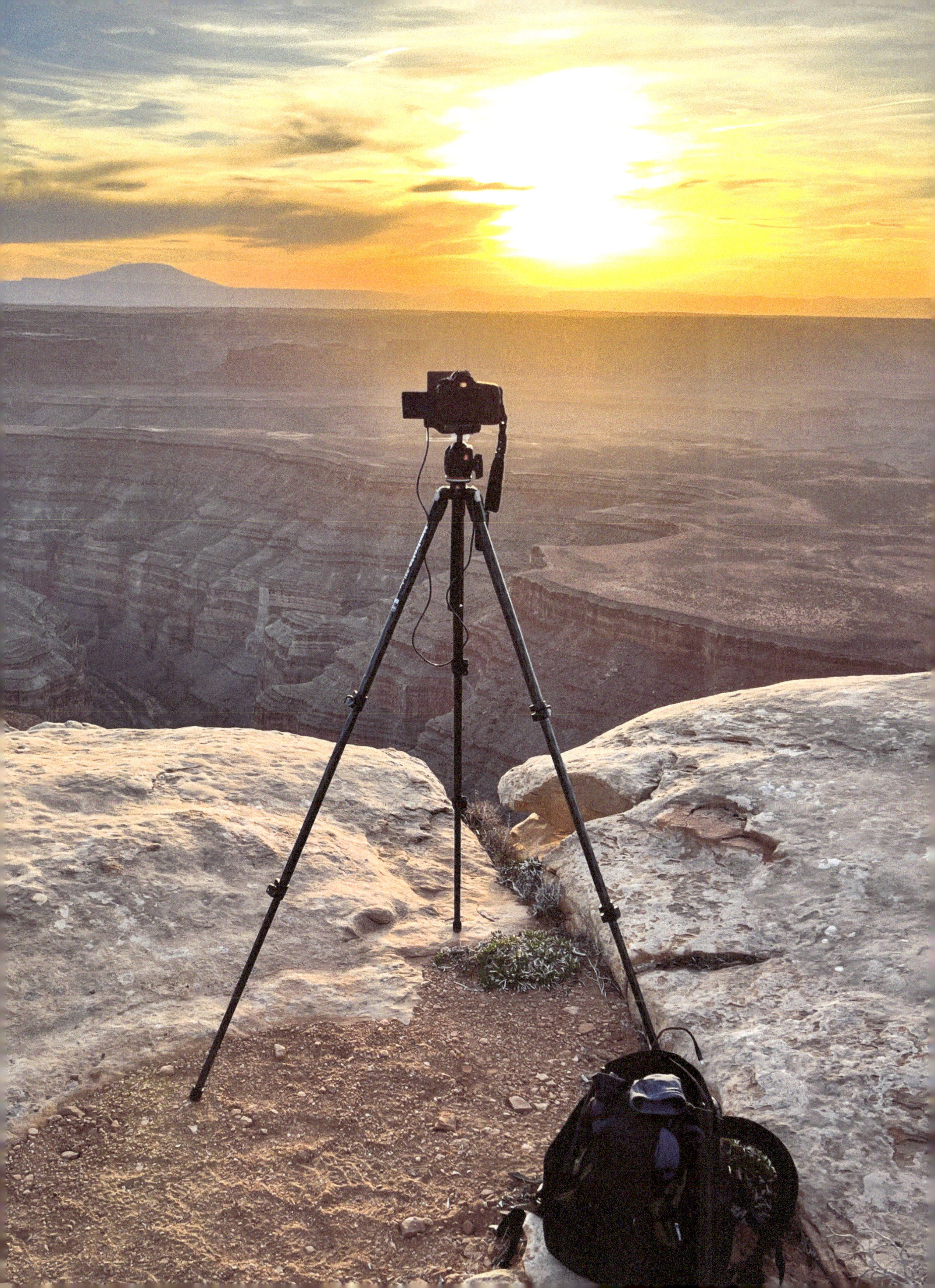

Epilogue

I had time to think about being home.

Before the brain injury, my identity was
being an occupational therapist.
31 years of comprehensive experience.
Big paycheck.
Felt accomplished.
Offered value to my patients.
Increased their independent living in the community,
their participation in meaningful activity.
I had a purpose in life.

After the brain injury,
no work,
no paycheck.
No value to others.
A disability check.
No meaning.
No purpose.
No worth.

I was Mark's wife.
I cleaned the house.
Did dishes.
Kept order in the house.
Kept track of the shopping list
and went to the store.
Bought the dog food.
Cooked dinner every night,
ready at 5pm when Mark
came home starving.
Mowed the yard.
Cleaned the driveway.
Cleaned up the workshop.

Washed the car and the van.
Took care of the garden.
And pulled weeds.
Walked the dogs.

Spent time with them.
Took them to the vet, groomer,
Home Depot and North 40.
Took them with me to the store
and they got dog treats
at the drive-thru bank and pharmacy.

I did have a job and a purpose.
I couldn't see it before I left on the trip.
I didn't value what I did every day.

It didn't meet my criteria of having purpose.

The mess I came home to,
instrumental to changing my perspective.
Mark needed me.
I knew he valued having me home.
I also knew he had new respect
for what it took to manage
the house, the dogs and the yard.

I received a small inheritance from my mother.
Enough to make a significant contribution
to paying off the house.
I heard Mark humming in the kitchen after the news.
It hit me in the chest.
I wasn't the only one living in Shitville.
He did too.
By default.
Carrying the weight of floating the boat
while I'm on disability.

I have the van.
I could go anywhere I wanted.
Any time I wanted.
Independence on wheels.

I could leave Shitville any time.
The gate is open, no one to guard it.

I had to make peace with how my brain worked
and how my life changed.

I replaced the logo on my work jacket.
I could still see the work logo inside the jacket.
But I didn't care about it that much anymore.
The logo on the outside of the jacket was what counted.

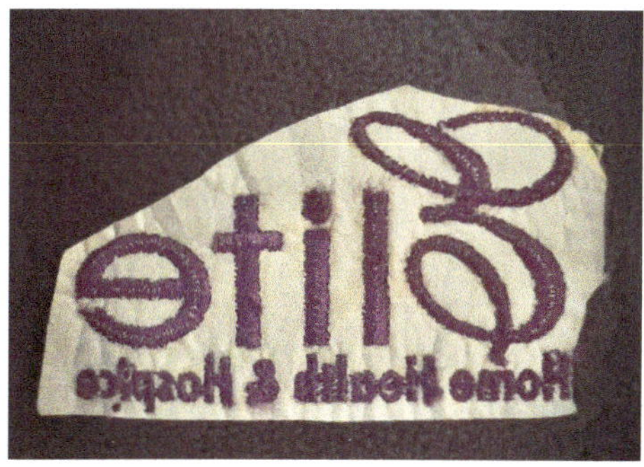

From an occupational therapist
to a traveling photographer.
I found my meaningful activity.
Which is in essence
what occupational therapy is about.
And the freedom that goes with it.

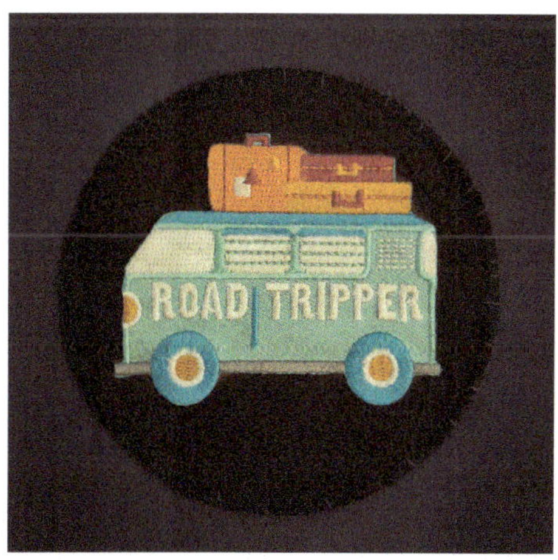

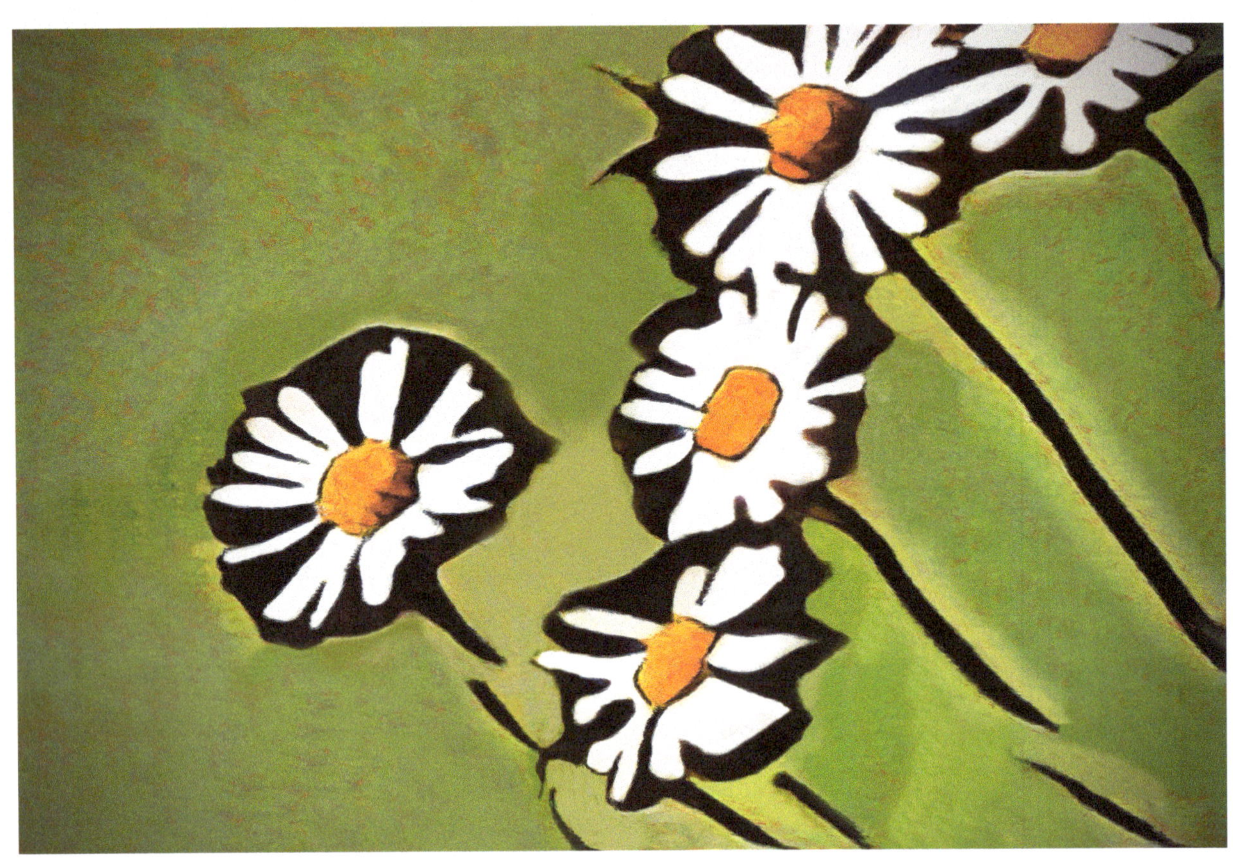

The hell I went through.
To grow through the wall
brain injury put in front of me.

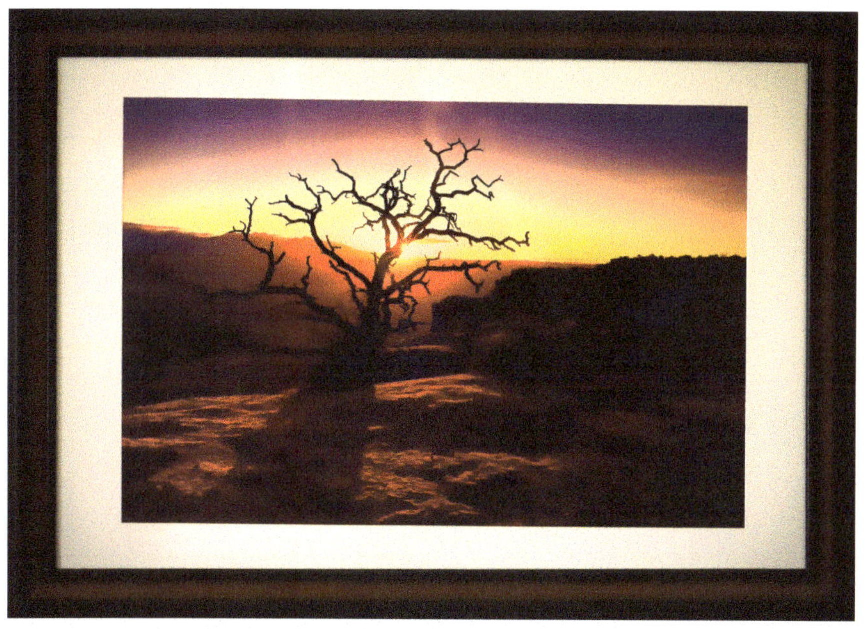

This picture is on the wall in the bedroom.
Daniel printed it on metal paper.

It looks like the light glows.

It's one of my all-time favorites.

It took a long time to realize
the answer to my question was in plain sight.

What is my purpose in life?

I am taking the best pictures ever.
I never took any time off from work to go to photography classes.
I've done several classes since the brain injury.

Here comes the sun.
The light that gives meaning to my existence.

The Light I've been looking for.

The Hope.

To not give up and call it good.

I am more than I think I am.

Mark liked to quote
"I am woman, hear me roar," a song by Helen Reddy
to encourage my independence
with everything.

I changed it to:

I am
brain
injury

Hear
Me
ROAR

On May 29, 2022, we bought a school bus.

Traveling for 2 people
and 4 dogs.

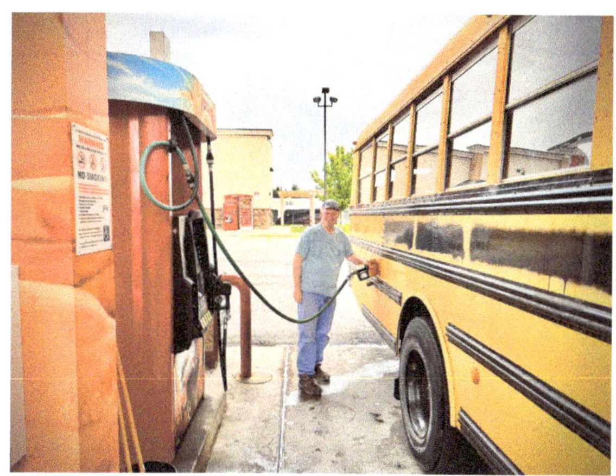

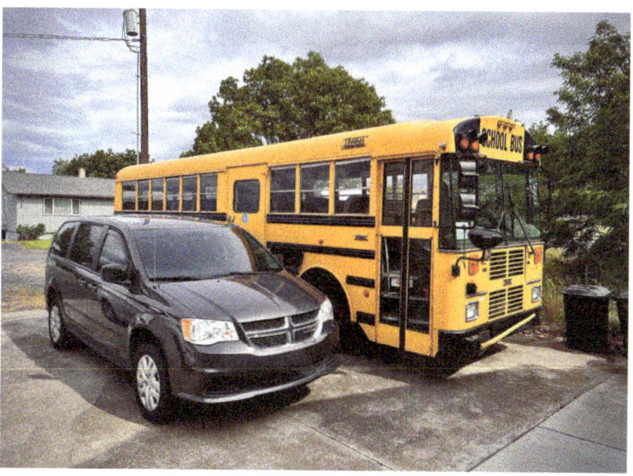

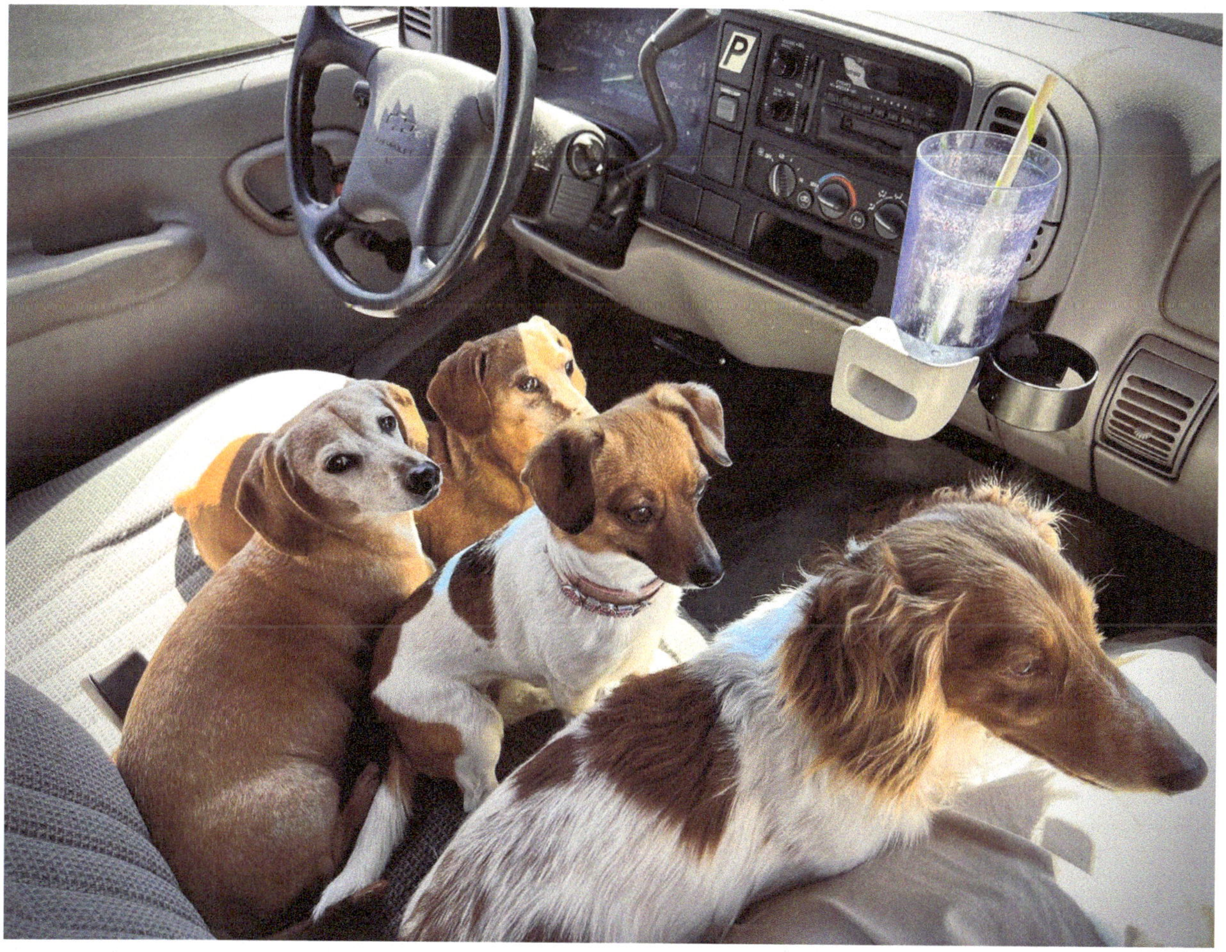

"THE VILLAGE" ACKNOWLEDGMENTS

Daniel Fairweather, "His Holy Keyboardness"
Walked the grueling book publishing road with me
as a friend, tech support, and book cover designer.
Who fixed everything I screwed up on my laptop.
"Call me so I can fix it while it's still fixable."
A fellow photographer, roadtripper and invisible disability.
And more patience than anyone I know.

Erik Jacobson, Longfeather Book Design
Took on the monumental task of
designing the book with 400 photographs.
Followed my vision for making the book easy to read.
He speaks "brain injury"
and sent me emails I could read and understand.
Got me out of "heart attack and swearing mode"
to get the book published.
Couldn't have wished for a better book designer.

SPECIAL THANK YOU TO:

Lauren Woods
Orli Weisser-Pike
Anne Rameley
Anne McLaughlin
Idaho Writers League
Patti Rae
Khaliela Wright
Lori Ready-Gorley
Neeltje Smit
Dirna Vogt
April Cox with Self-publishing Made Simple
Carol Hill
Tami Lempert

Mark Ready for putting up with the meltdowns of book publishing.

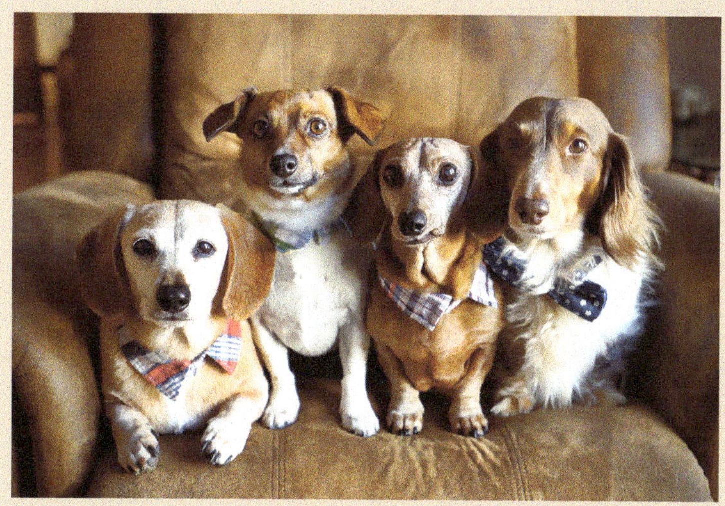

Thank you for reading
the book.
Dudley, Zoe, Daisy and Zumie

Would you please take a few minutes to leave
a review on Amazon or your favorite book retailer?

The social proof of the book
are the reviews.
Reviews help put the book in front of readers.

I appreciate your feedback.

Thank you much.

René Ready

www.ReneReady.com
Rene@ReneReady.com

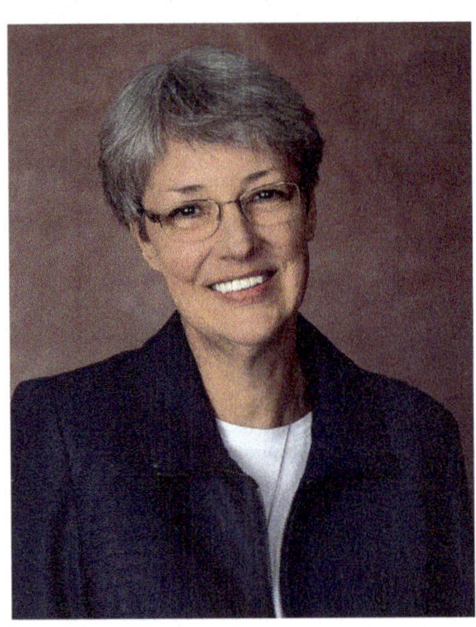

ABOUT THE AUTHOR

René Ready, an occupational therapist,
is the author of the memoir
Living in Shitville: What an Invisible Brain Injury Feels Like.

She graduated from the University of Stellenbosch, South Africa
in 1987 with a bachelor's degree in occupational therapy.
Her clinical background provides a unique perspective
of the struggles of living with an invisible brain injury.

Retired after a brain injury in 2018 during a dentist visit,
she now travels in a converted minivan
exploring and photographing the western USA.

René lives in Washington state with her husband
and 4 wiener dogs. She grows tomatoes in summer,
plans road trips and learns to drive the school bus.